# Recent Results in Cancer Research 60

Fortschritte der Krebsforschung
Progrès dans les recherches sur le cancer

# Tumors of the Male Genital System

Edited by

E. Grundmann and W. Vahlensieck

With 123 Figures

Springer-Verlag
Berlin Heidelberg New York 1977

VIIth International Symposium of the "Gesellschaft zur Bekämpfung der Krebskrankheiten Nordrhein-Westfalen e. V." Düsseldorf, October 24/25, 1975

Prof. Dr. EKKEHARD GRUNDMANN, Pathologisches Institut, Westring 17, D-4400 Münster

Prof. Dr. WINFRIED VAHLENSIECK, Urologische Univ.-Klinik, D-5300 Bonn-Venusberg

*Sponsored by the Swiss League against Cancer*

ISBN-13:978-3-642-81097-8 e-ISBN-13:978-3-642-81095-4
DOI: 10.1007/978-3-642-81095-4

**Library of Congress Cataloging in Publication Data.**
Tumors of the male genital system. (Recent results in cancer research ; 60)
"VIIth international symposium of the Gesellschaft zur Bekämpfung der Krebskrankheiten Nordrhein-Westfalen e.V., Düsseldorf, October 24/25, 1975 . . . sponsored by the Swiss League against Cancer." Includes index.
1. Generative organs, Male--Cancer--Congresses. I. Grundmann, Ekkehard. II. Vahlensieck, Winfried. III. Gesellschaft zur Bekämpfung der Krebskrankheiten Nordrhein-Westfalen. IV. Schweizerische Nationalliga für Krebsbekämpfung und Krebsforschung. V. Series. [DNLM: 1. Penile neoplasms--Congresses. 2. Prostatic neoplasms--Congresses. 3. Testicular neoplasms--Congresses. 4. Seminal vesicles--Congresses. 5. Epididymis--Congresses. 6. Neoplasms--Congresses. Wl RE106P v. 60 / WJ700 T925] RC261.R35 vol. 60 [RC280.G52] 616.9'94'008s [616.9'94'63] 76-30627



2125/3140-543210

Dedicated to the Memory of

JACQUES BOREAU (1913—1975)

Docteur en Médecine, Interne des Hôpitaux de Paris
Aide d'Anatomie à la Faculté de Paris
Chef de Clinique à la Faculté de Paris
Lauréat de l'Académie de Médecine en 1975

# Contents

# List of Participants

L. ANDERSSON, Karolinska Sjukhuset, S-10401 Stockholm.

J. BOREAU, 2, rue de Saint-Simon, F-75077 Paris.

P. BRÜHL, Urologische Universitätsklinik, D-5300 Bonn-Venusberg.

A. C. BUCK, Surgeon Lieut. Commander, Royal Naval Hospital, Mtarfa/Malta G.C., BFPO 51, Malta U.K.

P. COUDERC, Centre Hospitalier Régional de Grenoble, Laboratoire d'Anatomie Pathologique, F-38700 La Tronche.

ZOFIA DAŃCZAK-GINALSKA, Instytut Onkologii im M. Sklodowskiej Curie, P-00-973 Warszawa, ul. Wawelska 15.

G. DHOM, Pathologisches Institut der Universität des Saarlandes, D-6650 Homburg/Saar.

E. ELSÄSSER, Krankenhaus der Barmherzigen Brüder, Romanstr. 93, D-8000 Munich 19.

E. GRUNDMANN, Pathologisches Institut der Universität, Westring 17, D-4400 Münster.

P. HERMANEK, Abteilung für klinische Pathologie, Chirurgische Klinik der Universität Erlangen-Nürnberg, Maximiliansplatz, D-8520 Erlangen.

M. HIGUCHI, Dept. of Urology, Kurume University Medical School, Kurume, Japan.

H. F. HOPE-STONE, The London Hospital, Dept. of Radiotherapy, Whitechapel, GB-London E 1.

T. ICHIKAWA, National Medical Center Hospital, 1 Toyamacho, Shinjuku-ku, Tokyo 162.

D. E. JOHNSON, University of Texas System Cancer Center, M. D. Anderson Hospital and Tumor Institute, Houston, Tex. 77030.

H. KLOSTERHALFEN, Urologische Universitätsklinik, Martinistr. 52, D-2000 Hamburg 20.

F. KÖRNER, Bundeswehrkrankenhaus, Urologische Abteilung, Lesserstr. 180, D-2000 Hamburg 70.

P. LICHTENAUER, Chirurgische Abteilung der Medizinischen Hochschule, Ratzeburger Allee 160, D-2400 Lübeck.

G. T. MELLINGER, Veterans Administration, Cooperative Urological Research Group, Wichita, Kan. 67218.

F. K. MOSTOFI, Armed Forces Institute of Pathology, Washington, DC 20306.

H. NIENHAUS, Pathologisches Institut der Universität, Westring 17, D-4400 Münster.

L. PERSKY, University Hospitals, Dept. Urology, 2065 Adelbert Road, Cleveland, Ohio 44106.

B. PIERQUIN, Centre Hospitalier Universitaire Henri Mondor, Service Carcinologie Radiothérapique, 51, Avenue du Maréchal de Lattre de Tassigny, F-9400 Créteil.

E. SCHNEPPER, Radiologische Universitätsklinik, Jungeblodtplatz 1, D-4400 Münster.

G. SESIA, Divisione di Urologia, Ospedale Maggiore, di S. Giovanni Battista, I-10134 Torino/Italy.

A. SIGEL, Urologische Universitätsklinik, Maximiliansplatz, Postf. 35 60, D-8520 Erlangen.

W. J. STAUBITZ, State University of New York, E. J. Meyer Memorial Hospital, 462 Grider Street, Buffalo, N. Y. 14215.

H. TULINIUS, Icelandic Cancer Society, P.O. Box 523, Reykjavik/Iceland.

W. VAHLENSIECK, Urologische Universitätsklinik, 5300 Bonn-Venusberg.

P. C. WALSH, Johns Hopkins University, Dept. of Urology, Brady Urological Institute, Johns Hopkins Hospital. Baltimore, Md. 21205.

L. WEISBACH, Urologische Universitätsklinik, D-5300 Bonn-Venusberg.

W. F. WHITMORE, jr., Memorial Sloan-Kettering Cancer Center, Urologic Service, 1275 York Avenue, New York, N. Y. 10021.

# Introduction

E. GRUNDMANN, and W. VAHLENSIECK

In recent years tumors of the male genital system have acquired a new scientific importance in many respects: First, epidemiologic studies have revealed a striking increase of prostate carcinoma in northwestern Europe and in the USA; it is now counted among the most frequent malignant tumors in males. Geographic and ethnic distributions suggest that this tumor, too, may be triggered by exogenous factors of a still unknown nature. Histologic classification of malignant tumors of the prostate and testes has attained a certain finality, and the clinical relevance of the stages is recognized. Diagnosis by histology is now supplemented by aspiration biopsy cytology which offers a ready and reliable diagnostic potential. Its safety even surpasses that of punch biopsy histology and supports the qualification of cytology as a screening method.

In the Federal Republic of Germany prostate carcinoma was recently included in the cancer prophylaxis program of the social insurance system: Every man over 45 is entitled to one prophylactic free examination per year. Although the number of patients profiting from this opportunity is still rather small, the number of patients is steadily growing who, as a result of this prophylactic examination, received medical treatment at an early stage of the disease and with a relatively better prognosis[1]. Topical problems of social medicine are discussed in this context, as well as plans and developments of the social health service and of the supporting organizations, the federal societies for cancer campaign.

The importance of prophylaxis is enhanced by newly developed therapies, especially for prostate carcinoma and testes carcinoma. New and differentiated methods of surgery and radiology are described, and also some new aspects in chemotherapy. In general, the therapy of prostate and testis tumors has come to occupy a whole division in cancer research where success will entirely depend on the co-operation of the various disciplines. Growing interest is focused on new developments in endocrinology which may open new possibilities of medication.

Carcinoma of the penis occupies a separate position where new epidemiologic investigations have demonstrated its causes in exogenous factors, including circumcision, faulty hygiene, various infections, etc. Here, too, good progress is reported in surgical, radiologic, and chemotherapeutic methods.

---

[1] In 1975, one-third of all new cases of prostate cancer were detected in prophylactic examinations.

A review of the present status of epidemiology, diagnostics, and therapy in tumors of the male genital system has to include the tumors of the seminal vesicles and epididymis, of which more recent and comprehensive presentations are not frequent. We see a tragic event in the decease of Jacques BOREAU, one of the very few eminent experts in this field who died a few weeks after his participation in our symposium. He has presented an impressive review of his vast experience in radiology, in his paper on diagnostics and therapy of carcinomas of the seminal vesicles. His latest important and comprehensive monograph Images of the Seminal Tracts, Radiological and Clinical Comparisons had been published in 1974. During the discussion of the symposium, his contributions revealed him to be a scientist of unusual competence and personal integrity. This volume is dedicated to his memory among his colleagues.

# I. Prostate Carcinoma

## Epidemiology of Prostate Carcinoma

H. TULINIUS

Thorough and comprehensive reviews exist on the epidemiology of carcinoma of the prostate (7, 16, 19, 31). In reviewing descriptive epidemiology of the disease, this chapter will give mortality and incidence rates for carcinoma of the prostate in Iceland. It will also mention some suggestions as to etiology.

### DESCRIPTIVE EPIDEMIOLOGY

Descriptive epidemiology tries to characterize a disease in terms of its frequency of occurrence in incidence and mortality information for various groups: These may be geographically and racially defined, or in terms of other groupings such as by occupation, marital status, etc. For many diseases, including many malignant neoplasms, the age distribution is characteristic (8, 9). So it is for carcinoma of the prostate.

The mortality information, that is, how many die of a disease, is universally available, but the incidence information is often more detailed and more accurate. These data are not strictly comparable because incidence counts how often a condition - in this case malignant tumors of the prostate - is diagnosed, whereas mortality counts those who die from the condition. For some cancers, such as skin cancer, there is a great difference between the two, because relatively few people die from skin cancer. In the case of carcinoma of the prostate, this is not a problem except perhaps for the so-called latent carcinomas of the prostate (see below).

There is a great geographical variation in the frequency of the carcinoma of the prostate. It is a frequent carcinoma in northwestern Europe and in North America and extremely uncommon in the populations of the Near East and in some African, Central and South American populations. It is less frequent in eastern Europe than in western Europe. The rarity of carcinoma of the prostate in the Japanese was noted and published by STEINER (25) as early as 1954. In the last decade it has become increasingly well known that the black population of the United States has a higher frequency of the disease, both in mortality and in incidence, than the white population (18).

### MORTALITY

Table 1 shows, in order of rank, the mortality rate for carcinoma of the prostate for 1971 standardized to the so-called world population (26).

Table 1. Rank order of mortality from carcinoma of the prostate, standardized to "world" population 1971[a]

| | | | |
|---|---|---|---|
| Barbados | 22.1 | Luxemburg | 11.6 |
| Sweden | 18.4 | U.K., England & Wales | 11.2 |
| Switzerland | 18.3 | U.K., Scotland | 10.9 |
| Norway | 18.3 | Italy | 10.4 |
| Uruguay | 16.2 | Czechoslovakia | 9.7 |
| Iceland | 14.9 | Venezuela | 8.9 |
| New Zealand | 14.7 | Costa Rica | 8.5 |
| Cuba | 14.7 | Poland | 8.5 |
| Hungary | 14.5 | Israel, Jews | 7.9 |
| Australia | 14.4 | Romania | 7.9 |
| Canada | 14.2 | Malta | 7.8 |
| Netherlands | 14.2 | Panama | 7.2 |
| Portugal | 14.2 | Yugoslavia | 6.7 |
| Finland | 14.0 | Bulgaria | 6.4 |
| France | 13.9 | Greece | 6.0 |
| Germany, Federal Republic | 13.9 | Paraguay | 5.9 |
| Denmark | 13.5 | Mexico | 5.6 |
| Austria | 13.1 | Dominican Republic | 5.1 |
| Ireland | 13.1 | Mauritius | 4.3 |
| Spain | 12.3 | Hong Kong | 2.2 |
| U.K., Ireland | 12.0 | Japan | 1.9 |
| Puerto Rico | 12.0 | Egypt | 1.4 |
| | | El Salvador | 1.3 |

[a] Obtained from the World Health Organization, Geneva.

This information was obtained from the Division of Vital Health Statistics of the World Health Organization in Geneva and has been compiled from causes of death reports from the respective governments. The rates are given per 100,000. The range is between 22 and less than 2. There are a number of populations, mainly European and North American, that have rates between 20 and 10, which is fairly high for a cancer. At the lower end is El Salvador in Central America, Egypt in the Near East and Japan and Hong Kong with their Japanese and Chinese populations. Then come four populations from Central America. In the next group we find southeastern European countries, Greece, Bulgaria, Yugoslavia, Malta, Rumania, and Israel. The highest figure is from Barbados but Barbados has a relatively small population - 240,000 - interestingly enough 90% Negroes. As seen in Table 2 and Figure 1 in the preceding year, 1970, the standardized rate for Barbados was only 10.9; in 1969 it was 15.4, and in 1968 it was 17.1. These rates are not stable, presumably due to a small population. The next country however, Sweden, has a rate of 18.4 and as seen in Figure 1 these rates have been constantly 16 and above since 1958. An upward trend is seen in the figures from all these countries. The same figure shows the mortality rate from Japan, with an upward trend, from 1 to 2 over the 16-year period 1956-1971.

In those countries with a relatively high rate of prostate carcinoma this malignancy occupies one of the three top places among causes of death of malignant diseases, usually competing with lung carcinoma and stomach carcinoma.

Table 3 and Figure 2 show the age-specific and standardized mortality and incidence rates for Iceland. The mortality is obtained from the annual reports of the Director General of Health in Iceland.

Table 2. Mortality from carcinoma of the prostate for individual years from 1956 to 1971 standardized to "world" population for selected countries[a]

| | Standardized mortality rates for individual years | | | | | | | | | | | | | | | |
|---|---|---|---|---|---|---|---|---|---|---|---|---|---|---|---|---|
| | 1956 | 57 | 58 | 59 | 60 | 61 | 62 | 63 | 64 | 65 | 66 | 67 | 68 | 69 | 70 | 71 |
| Barbados | | | | | | | | | | | 17.5 | 20.0 | 17.1 | 15.4 | 10.9 | 22.1 |
| Sweden | 13.5 | 14.4 | 16.0 | 16.2 | 16.6 | 16.7 | 17.5 | 18.6 | 18.1 | 16.5 | 16.3 | 16.8 | 16.9 | 18.0 | 17.1 | 18.4 |
| West Germany | 11.7 | 11.6 | 11.2 | 11.7 | 11.4 | 11.5 | 11.9 | 12.0 | 12.2 | 12.5 | 12.9 | 12.9 | 13.0 | 13.5 | 13.6 | 13.9 |
| Czechoslovakia | 8.3 | 8.2 | 8.5 | 8.4 | 7.5 | 7.9 | 9.1 | 8.8 | 9.1 | 9.0 | 8.9 | 8.8 | 9.6 | 9.3 | 9.5 | 9.7 |
| Poland | | | | 2.9 | 3.7 | 3.7 | 4.5 | 6.3 | 7.2 | 7.4 | 7.5 | 8.1 | 8.2 | 8.0 | 8.3 | 8.5 |
| Japan | 1.0 | 1.2 | 1.4 | 1.4 | 1.4 | 1.4 | 1.6 | 1.6 | 1.9 | 1.7 | 1.8 | 1.8 | 1.9 | 2.1 | 1.9 | 1.9 |

[a] Obtained from the World Health Organization, Geneva.

Table 3. Carcinoma of the prostate in Iceland. Mortality for the ten year period 1965-1974 and incidence for the two ten year period 1955-1964 and 1965-1974, and for the twenty year period 1955-1974

| | Age Specific Rates | | | | | | | | | | |
|---|---|---|---|---|---|---|---|---|---|---|---|
| | 45-49 | 50-54 | 55-59 | 60-64 | 65-69 | 70-74 | 75-79 | 80-84 | 85- | Crude | World |
| Mortality 1965-74 | 1,9 | 4,3 | 9,9 | 31,1 | 58,2 | 125,3 | 181,9 | 386,4 | 334,5 | 13,78 | 11,69 |
| Incidence 1955-64 | 2,3 | 5,0 | 17,0 | 39,4 | 96,6 | 182,8 | 278,3 | 552,0 | 445,1 | 17,5 | 16,96 |
| Incidence 1965-74 | 3,8 | 13,0 | 24,7 | 76,3 | 160,9 | 323,9 | 382,0 | 676,3 | 907,9 | 31,5 | 27,96 |
| Incidence 1955-74 | 2,1 | 9,3 | 21,1 | 59,2 | 131,2 | 262,0 | 341,4 | 616,6 | 703,9 | 25,9 | 23,0 |

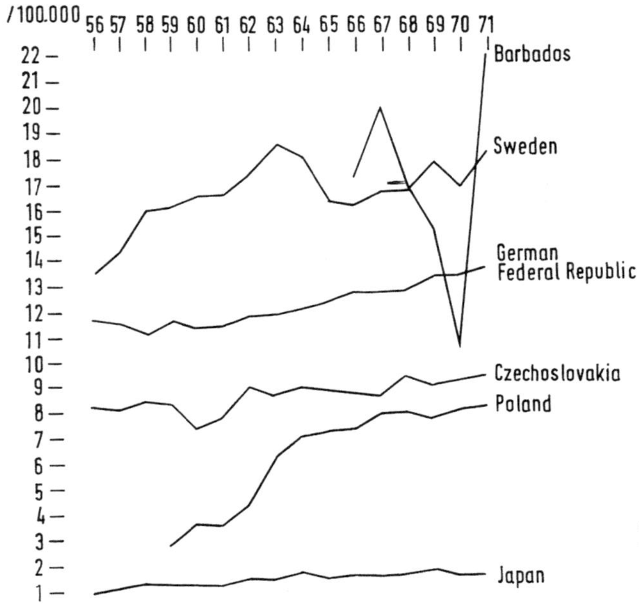


*Fig. 1. Time trends of mortality from carcinoma of the prostate for the countries listed in Table 2*

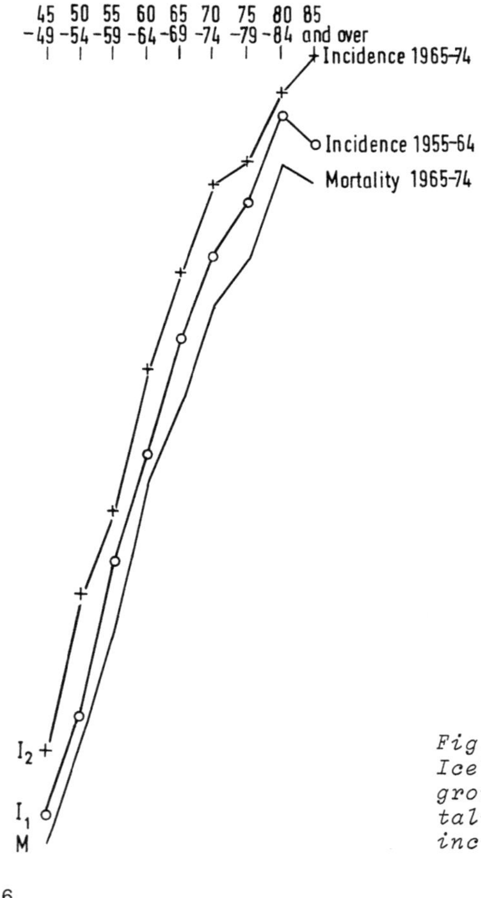


*Fig. 2. Carcinoma of the prostate in Iceland. Graph shows for 5-year age groups, logarithm of age-specific mortality for 1965-1974 and of age-specific incidence for 1955-1964 and 1965-1974*

## INCIDENCE

Apart from the data from Iceland shown in Table 3, which is from the Icelandic Cancer Registry (3-5), the incidence information is taken for the most part from Cancer Incidence in Five Continents Vol. II, which was published in 1970 (27) (see Table 4).

Here the American Negro, that is, the Negro in the Alameda County Registry in California, USA, has the highest incidence rate 65.3. Many populations have incidence rates ranging from 15 to 45/100,000. But the lowest incidence rate is for the "non-Jews" in Israel, 3.1, and in Japan, 3.2 for Miyagi prefecture and 4.3 for Okayama prefecture. In the first volume of Cancer Incidence in Five Continents the lowest figure was for the Chinese in Singapore, 0.9 (26).

There are sharp differences, both between geographical areas and between races. Migrant studies have shown that when people move from low incidence areas to high incidence areas, their risk increases. This has been shown for Polish (23) and Japanese (13) migrants to the USA. Mortality rates are, however, increasing rapidly in those countries. Table 2 and Figure 1 show a twofold increase in Japan and about a threefold increase in Poland.

All reported Chinese and Japanese populations have very low rates. The USA Negroe has the highest known rate, but the situation with Central American and African Negroes is not yet clear.

Urban areas have higher incidence rates than rural areas as seen in Norway for 1964-1966 where the respective rates are 34.1 compared with 27.3/100,000 (see Table 4).

## AGE DISTRIBUTION

Table 3 and Figure 2 show the age distribution of carcinoma of the prostate for Iceland. The peculiarity of the age distribution curve for carcinoma of the prostate, as pointed out by DOLL (8), is how late in life the rise starts and how steep the curve is. In other words, prostate cancer is relatively rare in adults and any significant frequency starts around age 60. It then rises very steeply up to the highest age groups.

Figure 3 compares the age distribution of carcinoma of the prostate in Iceland in 1957-1966 to that of stomach and colon cancer for males, and breast cancer for females (5).

## TIME TRENDS

As seen in Table 2 and Figure 1 mortality rates, at least in some populations, show a tendency to increase over time. The same can be said for incidence rates in Iceland (see Table 3 and Figure 2). This increase in standardized rates means that regardless of the age structure of the population in question, the rates for individual age groups are rising. Figure 4 shows the increase in age-specific rates for the 20-year period 1955-1974 in Iceland.

Table 4. Rank order of incidence of carcinoma of the prostate, standardized to the "world" population[a]

| | | | | | |
|---|---|---|---|---|---|
| 1. | U.S.A., California, Alameda: Negro | 65.3 | 31. | U.K., England and Wales, Liverpool | 18.2 |
| 2. | U.S.A., Hawaii: Caucasian | 43.4 | 32. | U.S.A., Texas, El Paso: Latin | 17.7 |
| 3. | New Zealand: Maori | 40.3 | 33. | U.S.A., Hawaii, Filipino | 17.6 |
| 4. | New Zealand: European | 40.0 | 34. | Finland | 17.4 |
| 5. | Canada, Saskatchewan | 39.0 | 35. | Puerto Rico | 17.2 |
| 6. | U.S.A., California, Alameda: White | 38.0 | 36. | U.S.A., Texas, El Paso: Non-Latin | 17.1 |
| 7. | Norway, Urban | 34.1 | 37. | Canada, Newfoundland | 17.0 |
| 8. | Sweden | 33.5 | 38. | U.K., England, Sheffield Region | 15.4 |
| 9. | U.S.A., Connecticut | 33.0 | 39. | U.K., Scotland | 14.1 |
| 10. | Canada, Manitoba | 31.1 | 40. | U.S.A., Hawaii: Japanese | 13.9 |
| 11. | U.S.A., Hawaii: Hawaiian | 30.0 | 41. | Israel; Jews Born Europe or America | 13.2 |
| 12. | Norway | 29.8 | 42. | Yugoslavia, Slovenia | 13.1 |
| 13. | Rhodesia, Bulawayo: African | 29.1 | 43-44. | Poland, Warsaw City | 12.8 |
| 14. | Jamaica, Kingston and St. Andrew | 28.8 | 43-44. | Romania, Banat Region | 12.8 |
| 15. | Norway, Rural | 27.3 | 45. | German Democratic Republic (DDR) | 12.6 |
| 16. | U.S.A., Nevada | 26.7 | 46. | Israel: All Jews | 12.5 |
| 17. | Canada, New Brunswick | 24.6 | 47. | Israel: Jews Born in Africa or Asia | 11.4 |
| 18. | Canada, Alberta | 23.5 | 48. | Israel: Jews Born in Israel | 10.8 |
| 19-20-21. | South Africa, Cape Prov.: White | 23.2 | 49. | Hungary, Miskolc | 10.3 |
| 19-20-21. | South Africa, Natal: Africa | 23.2 | 50. | U.S.A., Hawaii: Chinese | 9.8 |
| 19-20-21. | Colombia, Cali | 23.2 | 51. | Nigeria, Ibadan | 9.7 |
| 22. | U.K., England, Southwestern Region | 21.7 | 52. | South Africa, Natal: Indian | 9.4 |
| 23. | Canada, Quebec | 21.1 | 53. | Poland, Four Rural Areas | 9.0 |
| 24. | South Africa, Cape Prov.: Coloured | 20.4 | 54. | India, Bombay | 6.5 |
| 25-26. | Denmark | 19.5 | 55. | Hungary, County Szabolcs-Szatmar | 5.0 |
| 25-26. | Hungary, County Vas | 19.5 | 56. | Poland, Cracow City and District | 4.9 |
| 27-28. | South Africa, Cape Prov.: Bantu | 19.2 | 57. | Poland, Katowice District | 4.6 |
| 27-28. | U.K., England, Oxford Region | 19.2 | 58. | Japan, Okayama Prefecture | 4.3 |
| 29. | U.K., England, Birmingham Region | 18.4 | 59. | Japan, Miyagi Prefecture | 3.2 |
| 30. | German Federal Republic, Hamburg | 18.3 | 60. | Israel: Non-Jews | 3.1 |

[a] From Cancer Incidence in Five Continents, Vol. II (27).

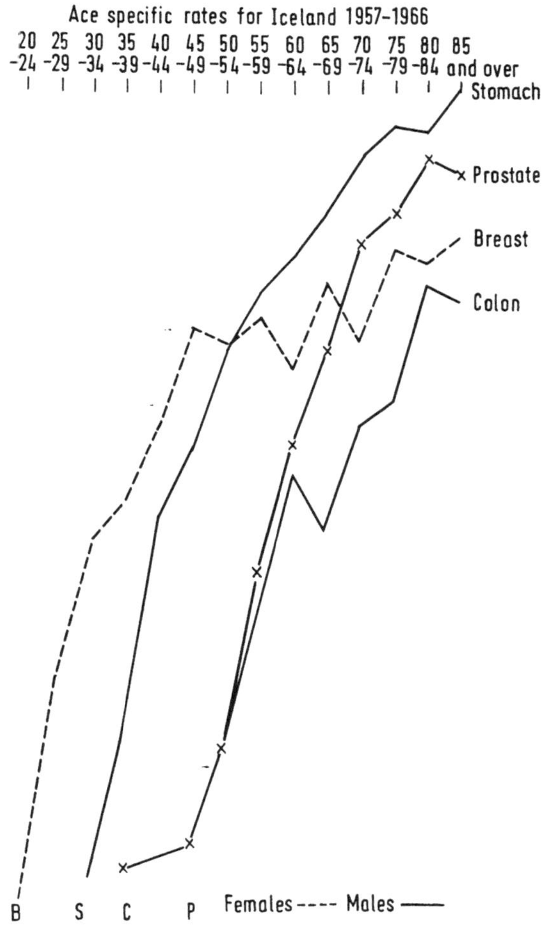


*Fig. 3. Carcinoma of stomach, colon, and prostate in males and of breast in females for the period 1957-1966 in Iceland. Logarithm of rate against 5-year age groups (5)*

It is interesting to note that in Sweden the mortality rate is rising, even though it was very high to begin with. Japan with very low rates initially, has doubled in 16 years, that is, gone from 1 to 2. This aspect of prostate carcinoma takes on a greater importance in individual countries because the age distribution of the population, is changing toward a greater proportion of old people. The age distribution of prostate cancer shows that the age groups over 60 contribute almost all the cases. These two facts will add to the number of individuals who will die from this disease unless we can prevent it, find out the causative factors, and eliminate them. Therapy may counteract this increase in mortality, but only if our present therapeutic modalities are considerably improved.

## LATENT CARCINOMA

Latent carcinomas probably exist in many organs. They have been better studied in the prostate than in other organs, but are probably also common in thyroid and lung. Adenomatous polyps of the colon are considered by many to be latent carcinomas.

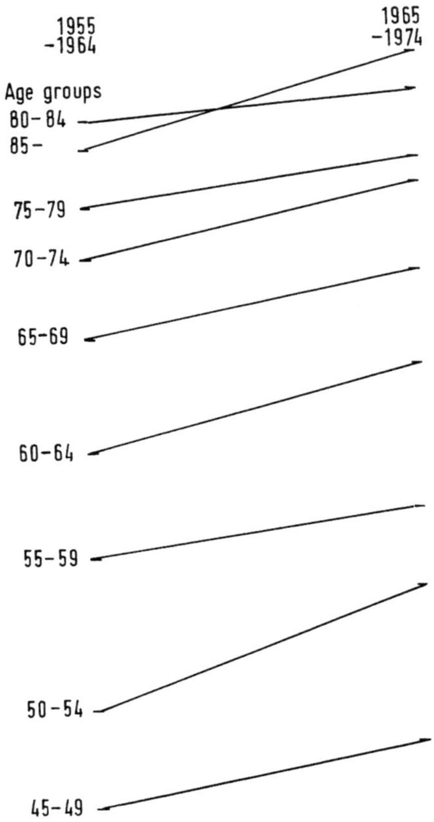


*Fig. 4. Age specific rates for carcinoma of the prostate in Iceland compared for two 10-year periods, 1955-1964 and 1965-1974 (Icelandic Cancer Registry, unpublished data)*

The fact that carcinomas are found in a fairly high percentage when prostates from autopsies and surgery are studied has been recognized since about 1935. The first observation to this effect was made by ALBARRAN in 1898 (1). Numerous studies from various parts of the world have shown that the likelihood of finding a microscopic carcinoma in the prostate of a man 45 years old and older is on the order of 1/5 (17). Translated to the terms we use for mortality or incidence, this would be 20,000/100,000. This phenomenon is closely linked to age; in other words the older the person the higher the likelihood. The average for all men 45 and older is 20%. Studies exist on men in the highest decades of life, and there the likelihood goes well over 50% (50,000/100,000).

Studies that have been published and some ongoing studies indicate that the frequency of latent carcinoma correlates fairly well in age distribution with clinical carcinoma. The published reports are conflicting about correlation between latent and clinical carcinoma of the prostate in geographical and racial comparisons.

ETIOLOGY

It is hardly an overstatement to say that almost nothing is known about the risk factors important for carcinoma of prostate. The correlation with age is unusually strong. The advanced age to which individuals attain before any appreciable number of cases begins to appear may be used to support either, or both, of the following conclusions: that this cancer has an unusually long latent period, or that the important risk factors start to operate relatively late in life. The former may receive additional support from ongoing work on latent carcinoma.

The frequency of this disease is increasing with time, at least over the last decades, suggesting that some significant risk factors are becoming more important in the "modern way of life" and it has been suggested that composition of diet (31) or air pollution (29) may be important. Much more research is needed on the nutritional aspects of cancer etiology. In support of the air pollution as a risk factor is the observation that the disease is more frequent in urban than in rural areas (7, 27).

Hormones control the prostate, and hormones can be used to affect the disease in the patient. It is therefore likely that hormones play some role in the pathogenesis of this disease. It is conceivable that differences in endocrinologic mechanisms may ultimately explain the marked racial differences.

Benign prostatic hyperplasia is also probably under hormonal control. Results are contradictory on whether there is an interrelationship between that condition and cancer of the prostate (2, 10, 12, 28). On the other hand HARBITZ and HAUGEN (14) have shown that there is no excess risk of latent carcinoma of the prostate in prostates with benign prostatic hyperplasia.

In patients with cirrhosis steroid hormone balance is altered. It has been reported (11) that the finding of cancer of the prostate at autopsy is less common in cirrhotics than in men dying from other causes.

Genetics cannot be ignored while the substantial racial differences have not been adequately explained. Studies of relatives of prostate cancer patients, both in Italy (22) and in the USA (30) have shown an excess risk in family members of cases. A frequency of bloodgroup A higher than expected in patients with carcinoma of the prostate has been reported in one study (6) but confirmation of this finding is lacking.

## SEXUAL FACTORS

Rates are higher for married men than for men who never married (7, 21) which has been taken to indicate that sexual activity increases the risk for cancer of the prostate. In a case-control study (24) it was found that hospital patients with cancer of the prostate admitted more often to sexual promiscuity than age-matched controls with nonmalignant diseases. If confirmed, two explanations have been offered. The first implicates an infectious agent or therapy for venereal diseases (15) as the etiologic agent.

The other relates to the chemical composition of semen which contains a substantial amount of zinc. Zinc is necessary as a coenzyme in several important biochemical reactions. Cadmium is an antagonist of zinc, and has been under consideration as a carcinogen. The observation has been made albeit only on a very few cases, that in a battery factory, which produced cadmium batteries, the frequency of the workers dying from prostate carcinoma was 8 times that which should have been expected (20). This observation was made some 10 years ago, and on only four cases where only half a case was expected, and has not been repeated. It, however, refers back to what was said before about air pollution since cadmium exists in particulate air pollutants (29).

## CONCLUSIONS

1. Carcinoma of the prostate is numerically one of the most important malignant causes of death in males in northwestern Europe and North America.
2. Rates are increasing, and thus its importance is increasing steadily.
3. Geographical and racial distribution shows great variability in frequency.
4. The characteristic age distribution is that of a cancer with onset later in life than most cancers.
5. Studies are needed to compare the "way of life" in populations with contrasting frequency, so that etiologic clues can be obtained.
6. Studies are needed comparing endocrinologic mechanisms among races of different frequency.
7. No concrete etiologic hypotheses seem very promising at this time.

## REFERENCES


1. Alberran, J., Hallé, N.: Hypertrophie et néoplasies épithéliales de la prostate. Ann. Mal. Org. gén. urin. 17, 797-801 (1898)
2. Armenian, H.K., Lilienfeld, A.M., Diamond, E.L., Bross, I.D.S.: Relationship between benign prostatic hyperplasia and cancer of the prostate: A prospective and retrospective study. Lancet II, 155 (1974)
3. Bjarnason, O.: Iceland. In: Cancer Incidence in Five Continents. Doll, R., Payne, P. & Waterhouse, J. (eds). Berlin-Heidelberg-New York: Springer-Verlag, 1966, Vol. I, pp. 168-178
4. Bjarnason, O.: Cancer incidence in Iceland. In: Racial and Geographical Factors in Tumour Incidence. Shives, A.A. (ed.). Pfizer Medical Monographs 2. Edinburgh: University Press, 1967, pp. 117-131
5. Bjarnason, O.: In: Cancer incidence in Finland, Iceland, Norway and Sweden. Ringertz, N. (ed.). Acta path. microbiol. scand. Sect. A Suppl. 224 (1971)
6. Bourke, J.B., Griffin, J.P.: Blood groups in benign and malignant prostatic hypertrophy. Lancet II, 1279-1280 (1962)
7. Clemmensen, J.: Statistical studies in the aetiology of neoplasms. Acta path. microbiol. scand. Suppl. 175 (1965)
8. Doll, R.: The age distribution of cancer in man. In: Cancer and ageing. Engel, A., Larson, T. (eds.). Stockholm: Nordiska Bokhandelns Förlag, 1968
9. Doll, R.: The age distribution of cancer: Implications for models of carcinogenesis. J. roy. stat. Soc. 33, 133-155 (1971)
10. Franks, L.M.: Benign prostatic hyperplasia. Lancet II, 293 (1974)
11. Glantz, G.M.: Cirrhosis and carcinoma of the prostate gland. J. Urol. (Baltimore) 93, 287-295 (1964)
12. Greenwald, P., Kirmss, V., Polan, A.K., Dick, V.S.: Cancer of the prostate among men with benign prostatic hyperplasia. J. nat. Cancer Inst. 53, 335-340 (1974)

13. Haenzel, W., Kurihara, M.: Studies of Japanese migrants. I. Mortality from cancer and other diseases among Japanese in the United States. J. nat. Cancer Inst. 40, 43-68 (1968)
14. Harbitz, T.B., Hauger, O.A.: Histology of the prostate in elderly men. Acta path. microbiol. scand. Sect. A 80, 756-768 (1972)
15. Heshmat, M.Y., Herson, J., Kovi, J., Niles, R.: An epidemiologic study of gonorrhea and cancer of the prostate gland. Med. Ann. D.C. 42, 378-383 (1973).
16. Higgins, I.T.T.: The epidemiology of cancer of the prostate. J. chron. Dis. 28, 343-348 (1975)
17. Hobach, M., Dhom, G.: Aktuelle Probleme des Prostatakarzinoms. Münch. med. W.schr. 114, 45-54 (1972)
18. Jackson, M.A., Ahluwalia, B.S., Attah, E.B., Connolly, C.A., Herson, J., Heshmat, M.Y., Jackson, A.G., Jones, G.W., Kapoor, S.K., Kennedy, J., Kovi, J., Lucas, A.O., Nkposong, E.O., Olisa, E., Williams, A.O.: Characterization of prostatic carcinoma among blacks: A preliminary report. Cancer Chemother. Rep. 59, 3-15 (1975)
19. King, H., Diamond, E., Lilienfeld, A.M.: Some epidemiological aspects of cancer of the prostate. J. chron. Dis. 16, 117-153 (1963)
20. Kipling, M.D., Waterhouse, J.A.H.: Cadmium and prostatic cancer. Lancet I, 730-731 (1967)
21. Lancaster, H.O.: The mortality in Autralia from cancers peculiar to the male. Med. J. Aust. 2, 41-44 (1952)
22. Morganti, O., Gianferrari, L., Cresseri, A., Arrigoni, G., Lovati, G.: Recherches clinico-statistiques et gênetiques sur les nêoplasies de la prostate. Acta genet. (Basel) 6, 304 (1956)
23. Staszewski, J., Haenzel, W.: Cancer mortality among the Polish born in the United States. J. nat. Cancer Inst. 35, 291-297 (1965)
24. Steel, R., Lees, R.E.M., Kraus, A.S., Rao, C.: Sexual factors in the epidemiology of cancer of the prostate. J. chron. Dis. 24, 29-37 (1971)
25. Steiner, P.E. (1954): Cited in Clemmensen (1965)
26. U.I.C.C.: Cancer Incidence in Five Continents. Doll, R., Payne, P., Waterhouse, J. (eds.). Berlin-Heidelberg-New York: Springer-Verlag, 1966
27. U.I.C.C.: Cancer Incidence in Five Continents. Doll, R., Payne, P., Waterhouse, J. (eds.). Berlin-Heidelberg-New York: Springer-Verlag, 1970, Vol. II
28. Williams, R.D., Blackard, C.E.: Benign prostatic hyperplasia and cancer of the prostate. Lancet II, 1265 (1974)
29. Winkelstein, W., Jr., Kantor, S.: Prostatic cancer: Relationship to suspended particulate air pollution. Amer. J. publ. Health 59, 1134-1138 (1969)
30. Woolf, C.M.,: An investigation of the familial aspects of carcinoma of the prostate. Cancer (Philad.) 13, 739-744 (1960)
31. Wynder, E.L., Mabuchi, K., Whitmore, W.F., Jr.: Epidemiology of cancer of the prostate. Cancer (Philad.) 28, 344-360 (1971)

# Classification and Grading of Prostatic Carcinoma

G. Dhom

There exists general agreement that the therapy and prognosis of prostatic cancer depend on the quantitative spread of the tumor within the organ and beyond. The clinical staging A-D or I-IV, as first proposed by WHITMORE (23), meets in the same way the demands which we may claim from such a classification as the TNM classification. In recent years German urologists have classified tumors according to the A-D stagings as presented by FLOCKS (1971) at the 1969 Berlin Symposium (Fig. 1). Deviating from the prior American classification (24) here stage A is a clinically palpable nodule in an otherwise well-demarcated gland, stage B is a tumor occupying a whole lobe, but still restricted to the organ, while in stage C the tumor extends beyong the organ capsule. In stage D there exist distant metastases, particularly within the skeleton, independent of the size of the primary tumor.

Before these four stages, which are made on the basis of a digital rectal finding, we put stage 0: this is the carcinoma found unexpectedly by the pathologist in tissues from TURs and adenectomies Mostofi's incidental carcinoma. We speak of latent carcinoma only when we find a prostatic carcinoma at autopsy that went unrecognized during life.

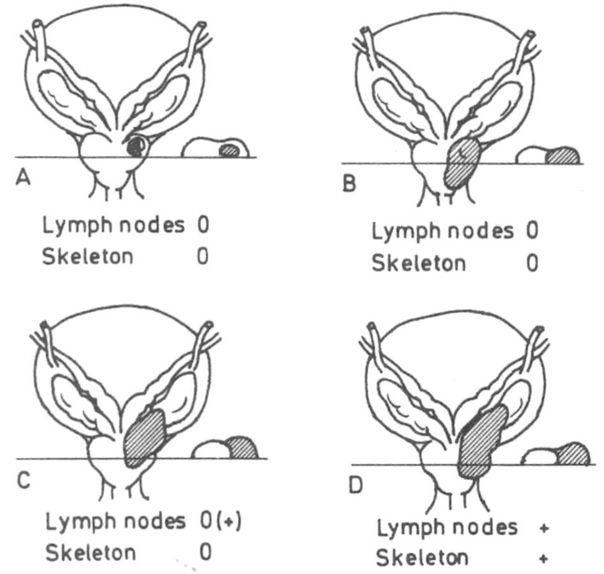


*Fig. 1. Clinical staging according to FLOCKS (11)*

At the first examination the majority of patients already show the advanced stages of categories C and D, as can be demonstrated in our material of more than 2400 cases (Table 1). In the 3 years of our register no significant changes in this distribution have taken place. It basically corresponds to the experiences of the Veterans' Administration Group (12). The value of such a clinical staging is limited in two respects:

1. The palpatory finding often does not show the true extent of a tumor. We here ignore the fact that many suspicious palpatory findings yield no carcinoma on biopsy. In about 25-50% (13) of patients with a clinical stage B, morphology shows the carcinoma to extend beyond the borders of the organ thus corresponding to a stage C tumor, BYAR and MOSTOFI (3) have shown in a comparative clinical-morphologic study how frequently a bilateral, multiple, or excessive extension of prostatic carcinoma escapes clinical diagnosis (Table 2).

Table 1. Clinical staging (at first diagnosis) Prostatic carcinoma registry, Homburg/Saar

| Stage | 1972 % | 1973 % | 1974 % |
|---|---|---|---|
| O | 7,6 | 8,8 | 9,9 |
| A | 12,6 | 14,6 | 16,3 |
| B | 38,0 | 35,6 | 30,4 |
| C | 31,6 | 30,2 | 34,9 |
| D | 10,2 | 10,8 | 8,5 |

N = 2485

Table 2. Clinical location of tumor compared to microscopic location[a]

| Unilateral vs. Bilateral | Clinical | Pathologic |
|---|---|---|
| Neither side | 52 | 0 |
| Unilateral | 111 | 34 |
| Bilateral | 45 | 167 |
| Unknown | 0 | 7 |
| **Single vs. Multiple Foci** | **Clinical** | **Pathologic** |
| No nodule | 52 | 0 |
| Single | 111 | 19 |
| Multiple or extensive | 45 | 12 |

[a] From BYAR et al. (3).

Histologically, only 34 out of 111 tumors palpated unilaterally were limited to one side. In the majority of cases prostatic carcinoma thus appears multifocal or bilateral. We were able to show recently how often palpatory findings in cases of coexisting nodular hyperplasia are subject to error when we made a histologic analysis of 141 cases of clinical stage O, i.e., incidental carcinoma (6) (Table 3). In 22 cases there were extensive carcinomas that had invaded the whole bioptic material, and in 27 cases the carcinoma had broken through the organ capsule thus corresponding to the stage C. In one of these cases a total prostatectomy was done; on histologic examination a cherry-sized carcinoma in the ventral portion of the prostate was found that had not been palpated clinically (Fig. 2).

Table 3. Expansion of the carcinoma in biopsy material, clinical stage 0[a]

| | | Cases | % |
|---|---|---|---|
| I | less than 10% | 42 | 29.8 |
| II | more than 10% | 68 | 48.2 |
| III | in the total material | 22 | 15.6 |
| | adequate assessment not possible | 9 | 6.4 |
| | Total | 141 | 100.0 |

[a] From DHOM and HAUTUMM (6).

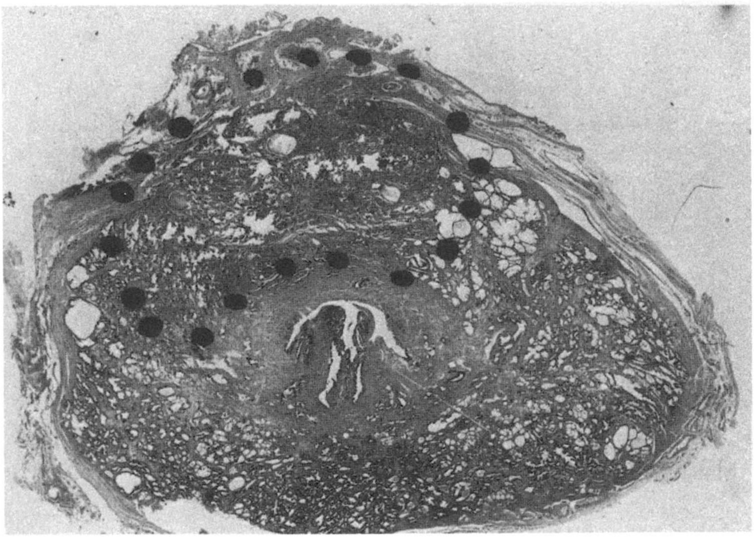

*Fig. 2. Incidental carcinoma in the ventral portion of the prostate within black dots. From DHOM and HAUTUMM (6)*

The second limitation of such a clinical staging is the result of the demonstration of metastases with special methods of examination that up to now are not in general use: some 25% of patients in stage B already have lymph node metastases within the pelvic region that can only be discovered by lymphadenectomy or lymphography (2, 4, 5, 8, 10, 14). In stage C this number is between 50 and 80% when the tumor has infiltrated the pelvic organs. Finally it has been possible to show by studying the skeleton with radioactive isotopes that bone metastases can often be demonstrated although conventional X-rays still show a normal picture (7).

Rectal examination, therefore, as a rule underestimates the true extent of a carcinoma. Nevertheless large series, especially those of the veterans' group, show that there exists a good correlation between the clinical stages based on conventional methods and the survival times of the patients (Table 4). The 5-year survival rate decreases with advancing spread (12).

Table 4. Survival by clinical stages[a]

| Stage | | No.: | Serum Prostatic Acid Phosphatase | Distant Metastases | 5 yr. survival (%) |
|---|---|---|---|---|---|
| I | | 66 | ≤ 1.0 | 0 | 69 |
| II | | 83 | ≤ 1.0 | 0 | 79 |
| III | | 504 | ≤ 1.0 | 0 | 52 |
| IV | 379 | | - | - | 25 |
| | a) | 199 | > 1.0 | 0 | 31 |
| | b) | 29 | ≤ 1.0 | + | 27 |
| | c) | 151 | > 1.0 | + | 14 |

N = 1032

[a] From GLEASON et al. (12).

Histologic classification of prostatic carcinoma is determined by the architecture of the tumor formation. A further subdivision, perhaps based on the appearance of the cytoplasm, in our opinion brings no additional gain. Each classification, however, also means schematization; this has always to be borne in mind. Necessarily there also enters a subjective factor.

We distinguish four basic types of prostatic carcinoma (Fig. 3):

1. Highly differentiated adenocarcinoma: It forms tubules with comparatively wide lumina lined by a single row of epithelium usually with a light cytoplasm. The nuclear structures can be very regular; enlarged nucleoli, however, can almost always be found. Mitotic figures are practically always absent.

2. Poorly differentiated adenocarcinoma: Here we find irregular small tubules with narrow lumina and usually with a dark cytoplasm. The nuclear pattern shows a more pronounced degree of polymorphy, enlarged nucleoli can regularly be found, and occasionally mitotic figures are seen.

3. Cribriform carcinoma: In accordance with the name large tumor masses containing no stroma but showing small openings are developed. There are formations with both light and dark cells, frequently with a pronounced nuclear polymorphy. Usually large nucleoli are developed; mitoses are found not infrequently.

4. Anaplastic solid carcinoma: The tumor cells form loose nests and cords; frequently development of large solid complexes is observed. The cytoplasm sometimes is light, vacuolized, sometimes deeply basophilic. Mitotic figures are found regularly.

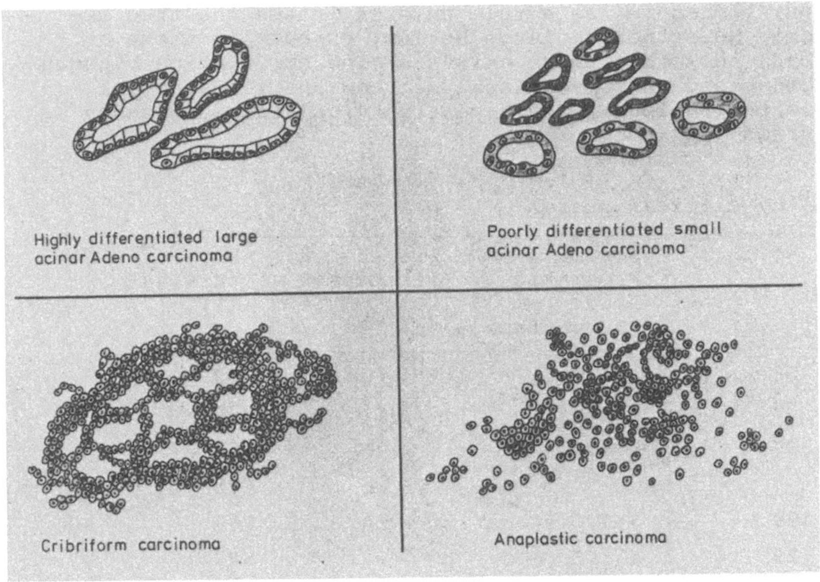


*Fig. 3. The mean histologic types of carcinoma of the prostate*

It is well known that those four basic types frequently appear combined in one single tumor. The carcinomas collected in our register therefore are subdivided into two large groups (Table 5):

1. Carcinomas of uniform architecture account for some 45% of our material. Highly and poorly differentiated adenocarcinomas are found with about equal frequency. The third and fourth place is taken by anaplastic and purely cribriform carcinomas. The rather rare urothelial and squamous cell carcinomas will be discussed below. They account for some 2% of our material.

2. About 55% of our carcinomas show a pluriform picture. Most frequently we find cribriform foci within other formations. In some of the tumors we see three or four different variants within the same slide.

The question, whether a classification is of practical value or merely l'art pour l'art, is basically answered by whether or not it is relevant regarding prognosis and therapy. There are a number of studies dealing with this question in the case of prostatic carcinoma (7, 9, 15, 20-22, 25). Two recent large studies will be compared with our own findings. One was presented by SCHROEDER et al. (19) and was based on a large number of prostatectomies (19): Among the numerous structural cytologic parameters employed for histologic grading (Table 6) the architecture of the tumor and the variability of the nuclei in regard to shape and size show the best correlation with the survival time of this group of patients who had undergone radical surgery. Figure 4 shows the different survival times of the various histologic types: patients with gland-forming carcinomas have distinctly better 10-15 year survival times than patients with solid or cribriform tumors. Based on the material in our register we are not able yet to follow the survival times of the patients, since the period of observation is still too short. We can demonstrate, however (Fig. 5), that there exists a good correlation between the clinical stage of the carcinoma and the histologic degree of malignancy. In more than 2300 cases we know the clinical stage as it was found at the time of the first examination. Of course, the findings were made by a large number of physicians whereas the histologic classification was done exclusively by myself. We find that pure gland-forming carcinomas are found less frequently in advanced tumors and more frequently in less advanced tumors. This is particularly evident in incidental carcinomas.

Table 5. Histologic classification. Prostatic carcinoma registry, Homburg/Saar

| | Carcinoma with uniform pattern | |
|---|---|---|
| | N | % |
| Highly diff. adenocarcinoma | 573 | 13.32 |
| Poorly diff. adenocarcinoma | 642 | 14.91 |
| Cribriform carcinoma | 290 | 6.74 |
| Anaplastic carcinoma | 367 | 8.52 |
| Urothel carcinoma | 72 | 1.67 |
| Squamous cell carcinoma | 10 | 0.23 |
| Mucous carcinoma | 5 | 0.12 |
| | Carcinoma with pluriform pattern | |
| Highly and poorly diff. adenocarcinoma | 282 | 6.55 |
| Cribriform and anaplastic carcinoma | 258 | 5.99 |
| Cribriform pattern in other types | 1131 | 26.27 |
| Other combinations | 675 | 15.68 |
| Total | 4305 | 100% |

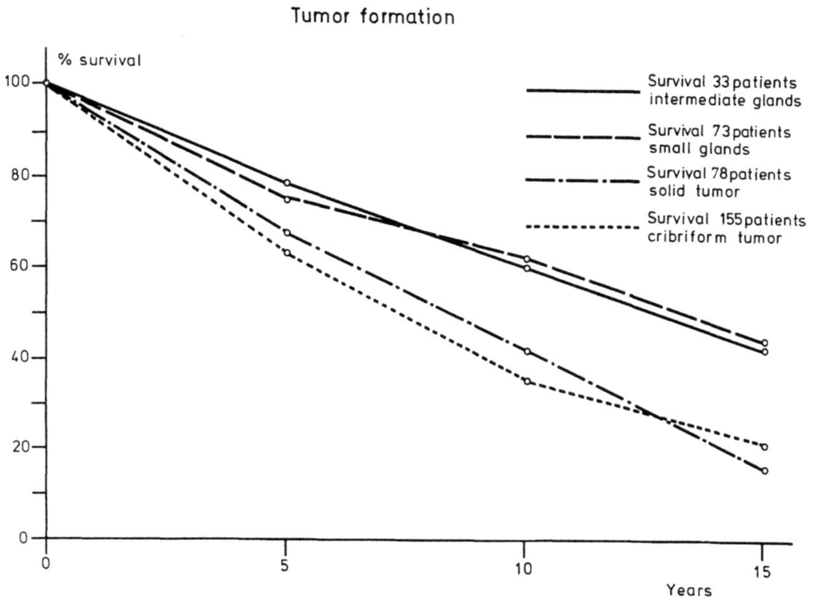


*Fig. 4. Survival and tumor formation. From SCHROEDER* <u>*et al.*</u> *(*<u>*19*</u>*)*

Table 6. Histologic grading of carcinoma of the prostate[a]

| 1. Architectural criteria | 2. Cytological criteria |
|---|---|
| Tumor formation | Cytoplasm |
| - large glands | - size |
| - intermediate glands | - clear |
| - small glands | - granular |
| - cribriform pattern | - mucin |
| - solid tumor | Nucleus |
| Amount of stroma | - size |
| Amount of tumor | - variation in size and shape |
| | - mitoses |
| | - nucleoli |
| | - vacuoles |

[a] From SCHROEDER et al. (19).

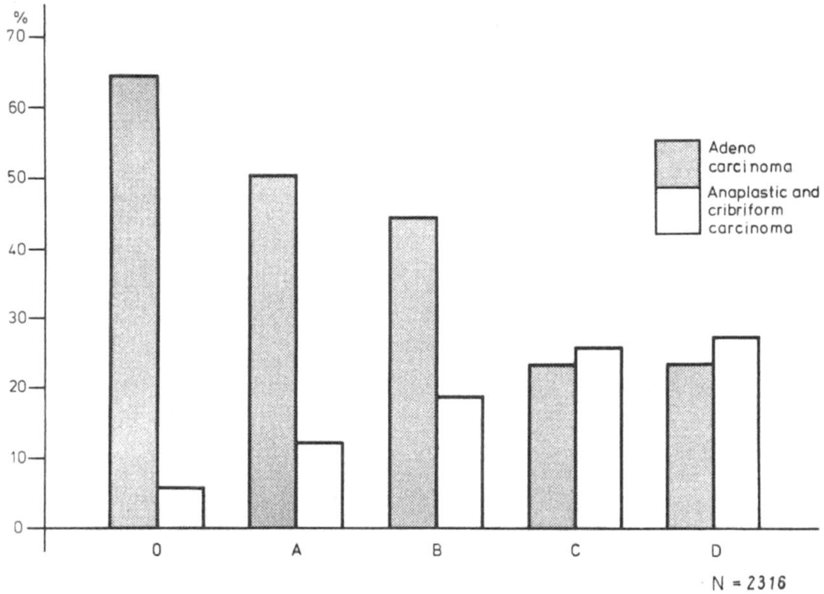


*Fig. 5. Relation between clinical stage and histologic type of prostatic carcinoma. Prostatic carcinoma registry, Homburg/Saar*

Here we find a high proportion of well-differentiated adenocarcinomas. On the other hand, in stages C and D solid and cribriform carcinomas are more frequently found than gland-forming tumors. In Figure 5 some 70% of all carcinomas are presented. The remaining 30% are represented by various mixed and combined types where often three or four variants can be found in the same tumor.

In agreement with MOSTOFI we can thus state that in addition to anaplastic solid carcinomas, purely or predominantly cribriform tumors are the ones that have a high growth potential and an unfavorable prognosis.

GLEASON, MELLINGER and the veterans' group (12) also obtained a good correlation between the degree of differentiation and survival time with their histologic grading system. For their grading they employ solely the architecture of the tumor as it appears under low power in the microscope. In order to account for the variability of the pictures each tumor is given two evaluations: one for the primary structure dominating the histologic picture and a second for the histologically less pronounced picture. Tumors with uniform structure are given two equal evaluations. The most favorable histologic evaluation, that of a well-differentiated adenocarcinoma, thus is given grade 1 plus 1 = 2, etc. To these figures the clinical stage I-IV can be added and a scale of potential malignancy is thus obtained that goes from 3 to 14 or 15. With an increase of the degree of histologic malignancy the mortality increases (Fig. 6) as calculated by the number of deaths per year of observation of the patient. This is true both for all deaths as for those that were shown to have died of prostatic cancer. It appears that the secondary picture of the tumor is of lesser significance. A similar appearance of the curve is found when clinical staging and histologic grading are combined (Fig. 7).

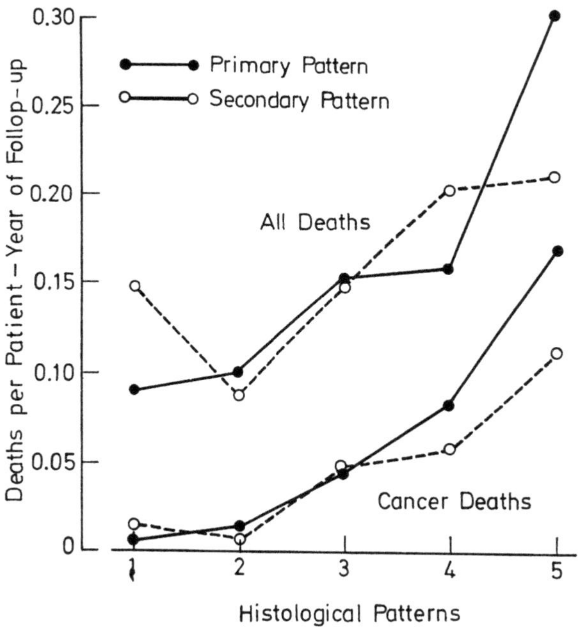


*Fig. 6. Mortality of carcinoma of the prostate and histologic grading. From GLEASON et al. (12)*

Grading and clinical staging thus can be employed for a prognostic evaluation. In regard to the question as to whether radical prostatectomy is possible or not, clinical staging with a careful search for lymph node or skeleton metastases will be of particular importance.

If, however, as is unfortunately the case in most patients, only conservative therapy is possible, the questions arise as to whether and what tumors react to withdrawal of androgens or high-voltage radiation

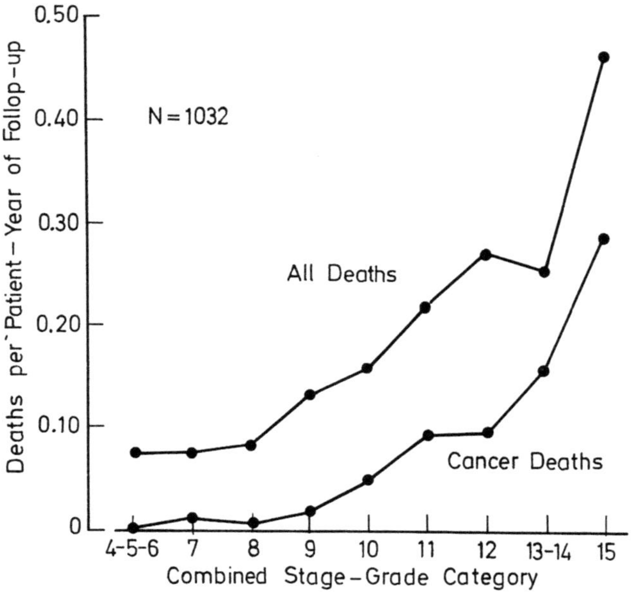


*Fig. 7. Combined stage - grading and mortality of carcinoma of the prostate. From GLEASON* et al. *(12)*

and what happens to the tumor tissue during the course of therapy. Together with our urologic clinic we have 304 patients in a long-term follow-up study. Bilateral punch biopsies were done initially at 6-month intervals and when therapy was successful, at yearly intervals. We have an average of four to five control biopsies for each patient. Having seen several hundred such biopsies we introduced a grading of regression (1). The tumor prior to treatment in the diagnostic biopsy is given 10 points. The progress of regression is indicated by a substraction of points. Here both cytologic criteria of regression such as vacuolization and shrinkage as well as the quantitative reduction in the biopsy material are taken into consideration. A tumor where only a few nests with pronounced regressive alterations are found, for example, is evaluated by us with 4 points. When we find only minute shrunken groups of cells that are hardly recognizable as carcinomas we given 2 points and when a tumor is no longer found in the biopsy material it is graded as point 0.

We thus obtained curves that can tell us something about the growth behavior of a tumor under treatment. It is, of course, necessary to adhere strictly to certain methodologic requirements. This can be demonstrated by some examples: In a tumor that responds well (Fig. 8a) the extent of the tumor and cytologic regression decrease continuously so that even in repeated control biopsies no tumor tissue can be demonstrated. In a therapy-resistant tumor the finding is essentially the same during the whole period of observation (Fig. 8b). We finally observe as a third type an initial pronounced regression, succeeded, however, in subsequent biopsies again by a massive uninfluenced tumor growth (Fig. 8c). There exists a good agreement between our morphologic findings and the rectal palpation findings. Some 20% of the tumors are resistant to hormone therapy. Of 58 irradiated prostatic carcinomas only 6 show no morphologic signs of regression. Surprising for us was the finding that the initial histologic picture allows no statement as to expectations regarding the success of hormone therapy on a certain tumor. Among the carcinomas that respond well to hormone therapy we find all types of differentiation. On the other hand there are well-differ-

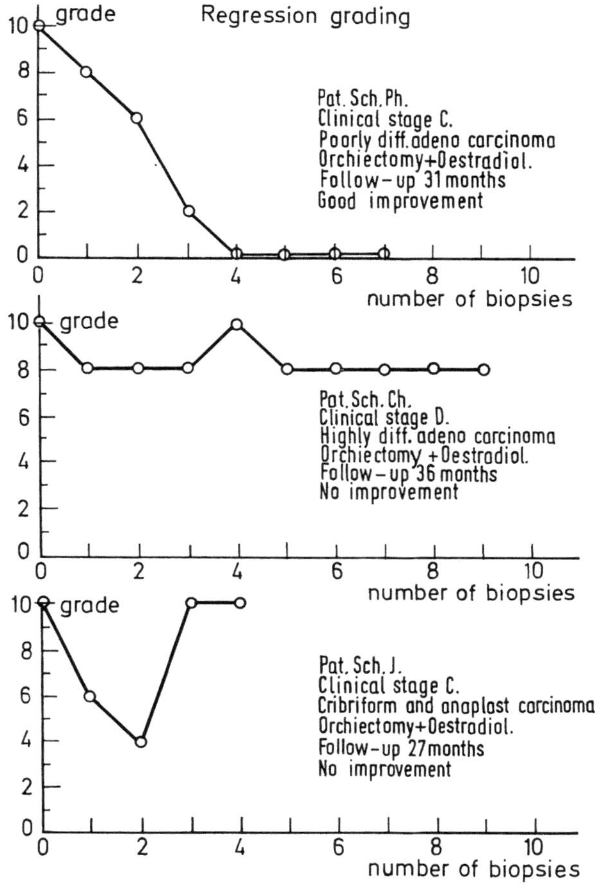


*Fig. 8. Regression grading of carcinoma of the prostate. Prostatic carcinoma registry. Homburg/Saar*

entiated carcinomas that show no regression whatsoever. So far we have - rather surprisingly - not seen any morphologically apparent complications of the repeated punch biopsies in our many hundreds of control biopsies.

Finally, some short statements regarding the urothelial or transitional cell carcinoma in the prostate. Together with the rare squamous cell carcinomas it is found in some 2% of all carcinomas. Presently we are studying and analyzing 130 cases of our own material.

Urothelial or transitional cell carcinomas appear under very different conditions within the prostate (Fig. 9):

1. In the urinary bladder without contribution of the prostate.

2. Spreading from the bladder neck to the prostate.

3. Developing primarily in the prostatic urethra and/or in the periurethral glands that are lined by urothelium.

4. Arising adjacent to or together with a typical adenocarcinoma. Here they may also arise from a transitional cell metaplasia in peripheral glands. During the course of conservative therapy there is, as a rule, a predominance of transitional cell carcinoma.

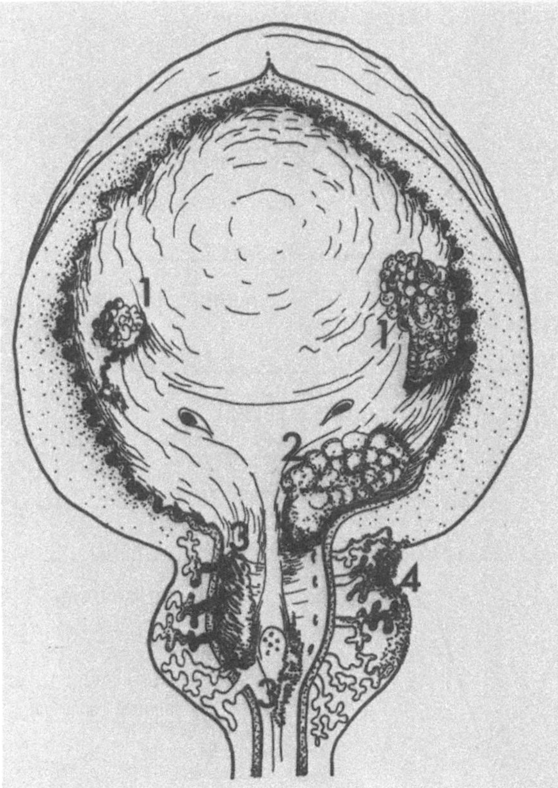


*Fig. 9. Localization of urothel carcinomas in the bladder urethra, and prostate*

The rectal-digital finding in transitional cell carcinomas of the prostate is the same as in ordinary prostatic carcinoma. The activity of acid phosphatase, however, is not elevated and skeleton metastases are rare.

They do not respond to hormone treatment or orchidectomy. The multicentric development of transitional cell tumors within the entire urinary tract has to be taken into consideration in transitional cell carcinomas of the prostate, too. A clinical search for further foci, particularly within the urinary bladder, is always necessary.

## SUMMARY

The clinical staging of prostatic carcinomas A-D or I-IV is correlated with the survival rate of the patients. The incidental carcinoma is designated as stage O. However, the rectal palpatory finding may be misleading; the morphologically proven expansion of the prostatic carcinoma frequently goes beyond the clinically recognizable stage. Already in stage B at lymphography or lymphadectomy lymph node metastases are found in 25-50% of the cases.

The histologic classification of prostatic carcinoma derives from four basic types which often appear combined within the same tumor: the highly and poorly differentiated adenocarcinomas, and the cribriform and the solid anaplastic carcinoma. Out of 4305 carcinomas in the Prostatic Carcinoma Registry of the Institute of Pathology of the Saarland about 45% are uniform and 55% of pluriform architecture. Two percent are urothelial or transitional cell carcinomas.

There exists a correlation between the histologic structure and the survival time on the one hand and the clinical stage on the other. Pure adenocarcinomas have a more favorable prognosis than cribriform or solid tumors. The morphologically proven regression of the carcinoma, induced by hormone or radiation therapy, can be followed up by needle biopsies at intervals of 6 months or a year. For this purpose a morphologic grading of regression is used. The initial histologic finding does not allow any prediction about the therapeutic responsiveness of the tumor.

The urothelial or transitional cell carcinoma in the prostate primarily may have its origin in the prostatic urethra and/or the periurethral glands. Frequently it is found combined with an adenocarcinoma, in which case it finally predominates in the course of hormone therapy, to which it does not respond.

## REFERENCES


1. Alken, C.E., Dhom, G., Straube, W., Braun, I.S., Kopper, B., Rehker, H.: Therapie des Prostatacarcinomas und Verlaufskontrolle. Urologe A 14, 112-116 (1975)
2. Arduino, L.J., Glucksmann, M.A.: Lymph node metastases in early carcinoma of the prostate. J. Urol. (Baltimore) 88, 91 (1962)
3. Byar, D.P., Mostofi, F.K., Veterans Administration Cooperative Urological Research Group: Carcinoma of the prostate: Prognostic evaluation of certain pathologic features in 208 radical prostatectomies. Cancer (Philad.) 30, 5-13 (1972)
4. Cerny, J.C., Fahra, R., Rian, R., Weckstein, M.L.: An evaluation of lymphography in staging carcinoma of the prostate. J. Urol. (Baltimore) 113, 367-370 (1975)
5. Dahl, D.S., Wilson, C.S., Middleton, R.G., Bourne, H.H.: Pelvic lymphadenectomy for staging localized prostatic cancer. J. Urol. (Baltimore) 112, 245-246 (1974)
6. Dhom, G., Hautumm, B.: Die Morphologie des klinischen Stadiums O des Prostatacarcinoms (incidental carcinoma). Urol. A 14, 105-111 (1975)
7. Emmett, J.L., Greene, L.F., Papantoniou, A.: Endocrine therapy in carcinoma of the prostate gland: 10 year survival studies. J. Urol. (Baltimore) 83, 471 (1960)
8. Erbe, W., Burchardt, P.: Lymphogene Metastasierung des Prostatacarcinoms. Urologe A 13, 127-130 (1974)
9. Evans, N., Barnes, R.W., Brown, A.F.: Carcinoma of prostate, correlation between the histologic observations and clinical course. Arch. Path. (Chicago) 34, 473 (1942)
10. Flocks, R.H., Culp, D., Porto, R.: Lymphatic spread from prostatic cancer. J. Urol. (Baltimore) 81, 194-196 (1959)
11. Flocks, R.H.: In: Life Sciences, Monograph 1. Raspe, G., Brosig, W. (eds.). Oxford: Pergamon Press; Braunschweig: Vieweg, 1971, p. 125
12. Gleason, D.F., Mellinger, G.T., Veterans Administration Cooperative Urological Research Group: Prediction of prognosis for prostatic adenocarcinoma by combined histological grading and clinical staging. J. Urol. (Baltimore) 111, 58-64 (1974)

13. Jewett, H.J.: The present status of radical prostatectomy for stages A and B. Prostatic Cancer Symposium on the prostate. Urol. Clin. North America 2, 105-124 (1975)
14. Mccullough, D.L., Prout, G.R., Daly, J.J.: Carcinoma of the prostate and lymphatic metastases. J. Urol. (Baltimore) 111, 65-71 (1974)
15. Moebius, G., Schneider, H.J., Konrath, M.: Zur biologischen Wertigkeit des Prostatacarcinoms. Urol. int. (Basel) 15, 1-21 (1963)
16. Nagel, R.: Gedanken zur Diagnostik und Behandlung des Prostatacarcinoms. Urologe B 12, 122-127 (1972)
17. Prout, G.R.: Diagnosis and staging of prostatic carcinoma. Cancer (Philad.) 32, 1096-1103 (1973)
18. Rubin, P.H.: Cancer of the urogenital tract; prostatic cancer. J. Amer. med. Ass. 209, 1695-1696 (1969)
19. Schroeder, F.H., Mostofi, F.K., Belt, E.: Carcinoma of the prostate: Grading and prognosis in 350 patients treated by total perineal prostatectomy. In press (1975)
20. Shelley, H.S., Auerbach, S.H., Classen, K.L., Marks, C.H., Wiederanders, R.E.: Carcinoma of the prostate. A new system of classification. Arch. Surg. (Chicago) 77, 751 (1958)
21. Utz, D.C., Farrow, G.M.: Pathologic differentiation and prognosis of prostatic carcinoma. J. Amer. med. Ass. 209, 1701-1703 (1969)
22. Vickery, A.L., Kerr, W.S.: Carcinoma of the prostate treated by radical prostatectomy. A clinico-pathological survey of 187 cases followed for 5 years and 148 cases followed for 10 years. Cancer (Philad.) 16, 1598 (1963)
23. Whitmore, W.F.: Hormone therapy in prostatic cancer. Amer. J. Med. 21, 697-713 (1956)
24. Whitmore, W.F.: The natural history of prostatic cancer. Cancer (Philad.) 32, 1104-1112 (1973)
25. Wiederanders, R.E., Stubber, R.V., Mota, C., Oconnel, D., Haslarn, G.J.: Prognostic value of grading prostatic carcinoma. J. Urol. (Baltimore) 89, 881 (1963)

# On the Significance of Sex Hormones in Producing Experimental Prostate Tumor in the Rat

M. HIGUCHI

If any exact method to produce carcinoma in a certain target organ is established, detailed investigation of possible tumor morphogenesis will be facilitated. Its establishment has added significance because the study of the developmental progress of experimental tumors will provide a clinico-pathologic basis for the production of human tumors. Furthermore, establishment of a model of an experimental tumor not only clarifies pathomorphologic development of tumors but contributes analogously to a pathophysiologic explanation of human cancers. With its experimental support, rapid progress will be made possible in the field of early diagnosis and therapy of human cancers.

Next is the important problem of how to establish a method to make an exactly transplanted carcinoma by using the primary tumor focus in the experimental animal.

The place of transplanted carcinomas in experimental tumor study may be compared to the role of successive pure cultivated strains of microorganisms in the field of bacteriology. Hence, the transplanted carcinoma is a tumor with wide application. In fact, the majority of cancer investigators use transplanted carcinomas as their material.

There have been many reports of experimental tumor formation in the prostate since the first experiment of MOORE and MELCHIONA (18) in 1937 who produced squamous cell carcinoma in the prostate by injecting 1:2 benzpyrene, one of the hydrocarbon compounds, directly into the rat prostate.

Other carcinogenic substances used to produce experimental prostate tumors are benzpyrene, methylcholanthrene, 4-nitroquinoline-N-oxide, etc., administered in various ways. MIRAND (17) and WOJEWSKI (33) inserted crystals of carcinogenic substances into the prostate. MOORE (18), HORNING (10), KÄLLÉN (15), TAKENAKA (29) and HIGUCHI (9) injected solutions of carcinogenic substances. DUNNING (5) and NAKANISHI (21) implanted pellets containing carcinogenic substances, and HORNING (10) adopted a special method in which a crystal of 20-methylcholanthrene wrapped in mouse prostate epithelium was lodged in the subcutaneous region of another mouse of the same strain.

Pathohistologically, experimentally produced prostate tumors are frequently squamous cell carcinomas. However, the human prostate tumors that urologists encounter are usually adenocarcinomas. For this reason it is extremely dangerous to draw conclusions applicable to human cancer from these experimental carcinogenic processes. The first task for tumor investigators is to produce experimental adenocarcinoma similar to human prostate adenocarcinoma.

On the other hand, there is an experimental view that androgen acts to inhibit the proliferation of tumors while estrogen exerts a stimulative action on it.

HUGGINS and HUDGES (14) clarified that prostate carcinoma is an unusual excess proliferation on the mature prostate epithelium, the proliferation still having features of the epithelium which was the originating matrix tissue. They further observed experimentally that the abnormal epithelial proliferation tended to regress or atrophy following castration or administration of estrogen. This is today a principal basis of the therapy of prostate cancer. The effects of sex hormones on the carcinogenic mechanism of prostate cancer, which has been considered to be androgen-dependent, remain to be elucidated.

## I. THE EFFECTS OF SEX HORMONES ON EXPERIMENTAL PROSTATE TUMOR FORMATION

### Materials and Methods

Animals used were 5-week-old male and female Donryu rats weighing about 70 g. Each rat was fed in its metal cage in a room maintained at 24°C. Animals were fed with CE.2 (a solid feed for rats), and water was given ad lib.

Carcinogenic substances used in this experiment were 20-methylcholanthrene (20-MC) and 4-nitroquinoloine-N-oxide (4-NQO), both manufactured by Wako Pure Chemical Ltd. These chemicals were administered in the form of crystal or 1% olive oil solution.

Sex hormones used were hexestrol (4,4'-dihydroxy-$\alpha$,$\beta$-diethylbibenzyl disodium phosphate) from Chugai Pharmaceutical Co. and testosterone propionate (17$\beta$-hydroxyandrost-4-ene-3-one propionate) from Teikoku Zoki Co. Ltd.

In the direct injection group, 0.1 ml of 1% 20-Mc or 4-NQO olive oil solution was injected into the ventral lobe of the prostate of male Donryu rats after median scrotal skin section under ether anesthesia.

In the group receiving 20-MC or 4-NQO crystal, the following procedure was done: 5-week-old Donryu rats were administered testosterone propionate s.c. in a daily dose of 2.5 mg per rat for 4 consecutive days (total dosage: 10 mg). They were then sacrificed by bleeding, the ventral lobe of the prostate was aseptically extirpated and its capsule was removed. The prostate parenchymal tissue was cut to a size of about 2 $mm^3$, spread on gauze immersed in warm Puck's solution, and 0.1 mg of crystal of 20-MC or 4-NQO was wrapped in this tissue, inserted into the subcutaneous region of male and female Donryu rats of the same strain and age.

In the group combined with sex hormone application, 0.5 mg of hexestrol per rat or 2.5 mg of testosterone propionate per rat was injected s.c. every day.

The duration of the experiments was 6 months, and all surviving rats were killed up to the 200th day after birth. Otherwise, at suitable times during this period, one or two rats were sacrificed by bleeding in order to observe the state of tumor formation together with weighing, and palpation of the tumor. In all animals, the angioarchitecture of both the prostate which was directly injected with carcinogenic substances and the subcutaneous tissue at the site of transplantation was observed, and macroscopic examination and the weight of the tumor mass and various organs, plus a check for tumor metastases were made.

The extirpated tumor mass was further transplanted subcutaneously to male and female rats of the same strain and age after sectioning in as aseptic a manner as possible. Some of these sections were for pathologic studies.

## Results

1. Occurrence of Experimental Tumor. When the rats which were given 20-MC or 4-NQO as carcinogenic substance were sacrificed or died during the experimental period, the rate of occurrence of experimental tumor could be summarized as follows. In the direct injection group, the rate was 50% (20 of 40 rats) in rats administered 20-MC and 51.3% (20 of 39 rats) in those given 4-NQO. In the group receiving transplantation of wrapped carcinogenic substances, the rate was 27.8% (15 of 54 rats) for 20-MC and 19.6% (10 of 51 rats) for 4-NQO.

The difference in rate of occurrence of tumor by carcinogenic substance was significant between the cases given 20-MC and those given 4-NQO. As to the carcinogenic rate according to administration procedure, the rate of tumor formation after direct injection of carcinogenic substance was evidently higher than that after carcinogenic crystal wrapped in transplanted tissue.

The rate of tumor formation in the group with direct injection of carcinogenic substances into the prostate was 44.4% (4 of 9 rats) after 20-MC injection and 40% (4 of 10 rats) after 4-NQO injection. When testosterone propionate was injected after 20-MC or 4-NQO application, the rate of tumor formation was 33.3% (4 of 12 rats) with the former and 36.3% (4 of 11 rats) with the latter, the rate being definitely higher in the direct injection group.

When the carcinogenic substance was directly injected into the prostate immediately after castration, tumor formation was observed in 60% (6 of 10 rats) after 20-MC and in 66.6% (6 of 9 rats) after 4-NQO administration. However, when direct injection of carcinogenic substance immediately after castration was combined with continuous administration of hexestrol, the tumor formation rate was 66.6% (6 of 9 rats) with 20-MC and 66.6% (6 of 9 rats) with 4-NQO. There was no significant difference between the cases with only castration and the cases with estrogen application after castration. In summary, the rate of experimental tumor occurrence was clearly higher in the rat group with castration or with estrogen administration after castration, in addition to carcinogenic substance, than in the rat group given only carcinogenic substance.

Androgen administration resulted in a decrease in the rate of tumor formation (Table 1a and b).

When carcinogenic substances wrapped with transplanted prostate tissue pieces were subcutaneously inserted into rats, the tumor formation rate was 27.2% (3 of 11 rats) with 20-MC and 11.2% (1 of 9 rats) with 4-NQO. When testosterone propionate was injected into rats with subcutaneous tranplantation, the tumor formation rate was 25% (2 of 8 rats) with 20-MC and 9.1% (1 of 11 rats) with 4-NQO. Androgen administration had no significant effect on the tumor formation rate.

The tumor formation rate was increased in the rats with tranplantation after castration: the rate was 33.3% (3 of 9 rats) with 20-MC and 37.5% (3 of 8 rats) with 4-NQO. In the rat group A injected with hexestrol after castration, there was a significant difference in the tumor formation rate between 20-MC (50%, 6 of 12 rats) and 4-NQO (33.3%, 4 of 12 rats).

Table 1a. Occurrence of experimental tumor: 20-methylcholanthrene directly injected into the prostate

| Group A | Experimental method | Rats No. | No. of tumors | Occurrence of tumor (%) | Tumors | | | | Remarks |
|---|---|---|---|---|---|---|---|---|---|
| | | | | | Adeno-carcinoma | Adenoma | Squamous cell carcinoma | Sarcoma | |
| Group I | 20-methylcholanthrene | 9 | 4 | 44.4 | | | 1 | 3 | Pneumonia 1 |
| Group II | 20-MC and testo-sterone propionate | 12 | 4 | 33.3 | | 1 | 1 | 2 | Bladder stone 1<br>Pneumonia 2 |
| Group III | 20-MC and castration | 10 | 6 | 60.0 | | 1 | 2 | 3 | Bladder stone 1<br>Hydronephrosis 1 |
| Group IV | 20-MC, castration and hexestrol | 9 | 6 | 66.6 | | 1 | 3 | 2 | Hydronephrosis 2 |

Table 1b. Occurrence of experimental tumor: 4-nitroquinoline-N-oxide was directly injected into the prostate

| Group A | Experimental method | Rats No. | No. of tumors | Occurrence of tumor (%) | Tumors | | | | Remarks |
|---|---|---|---|---|---|---|---|---|---|
| | | | | | Adeno-carcinoma | Adenoma | Squamous cell carcinoma | Sarcoma | |
| Group V | 4-nitroquinoline-N-oxide | 10 | 4 | 40.0 | | | 1 | 3 | Metastasis to bladder 1<br>Hematuria 1 |
| Group VI | 4-NQO and testo-sterone propionate | 11 | 4 | 36.3 | | 1 | 2 | 1 | Bladder stone 1<br>Hydronephrosis 1 |
| Group VII | 4-NQO and castration | 9 | 6 | 66.6 | | 1 | 2 | 3 | Bladder stone 2<br>Hematuria 1 |
| Group VIII | 4-NQO, castration and hexestrol | 9 | 6 | 66.6 | | 1 | 3 | 2 | Metastasis to lymph node 1<br>Pneumonia 1 |

When carcinogenic substance wrapped with transplanted prostate tissue pieces was further transplanted subcutaneously into the female rats, tumor occurred in 7.1% (1 of 14 rats) with 20-MC and in 9.1% (1 of 11 rats) with 4-NQO.

Following transplantation of carcinogenic substances wrapped with prostate tissue pieces, androgen caused no significant change in the rate of tumor formation, whereas castration or estrogen application with castration significantly increased the rate. However, the tumor formation rate was lower in female rats with transplantation than in male rats undergoing the same procedure (Table 2a and b).

2. Pathologic Findings. First, the vasculature was examined. In the rats injected with carcinogenic substances into the ventral lobe of the prostate, an early change was new vascularization in the prostate capsule, which was considered to be a living reaction to foreign substance. In these cases, the extent of new vascularization became marked in parallel to the advance of the tumor formation. Its detailed pattern could not be investigated because of adhesion to nearby organs. In an early stage of the experiments of tumor formation by transplantation, transplanted tissue pieces capable of passing through the carcinogenic substances did not show new building of blood vessels but were frequently changing to necrotic masses. New or further vascularization became marked with increasing size of the tumor mass.

Macroscopic examination of the rats directly injected with carcinogenic substances indicated that formation of tumors of various sizes was recognized at sites corresponding to the sites of injection. In some cases the tumor grew as large as an infant's fist, and thus occupied the whole abdominal cavity (Fig. 1).

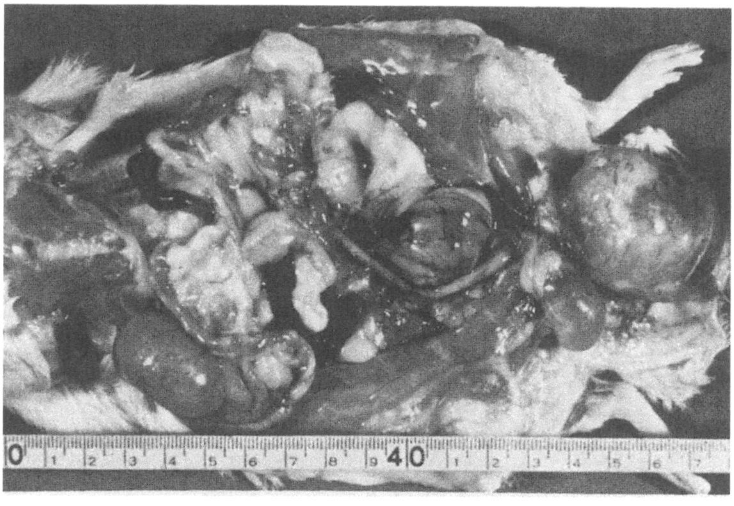

*Fig. 1. Rat injected directly with carcinogenic substance showing formation of tumors of various sizes*

When tumor was produced by transplanting wrapped carcinogenic substances , the site of the tumor was identical to the site of transplantation. Also, the size of the tumor thus formed was varied and irregular, as in the tumors of the rat group directly injected. The transplanted tumors were characterized by strong adhesion to the subcutaneous or muscular layer of the abdominal wall (Fig. 2).

Table 2a. Occurrence of experimental tumor: 20-methylcholanthrene wrapped with tranplanted prostate tissue pieces subcutaneously inserted into rats

| Group B | Experimental method | Rats No. | No. of tumors | Occurrence of tumor (%) | Tumors | | | | Remarks |
|---|---|---|---|---|---|---|---|---|---|
| | | | | | Adeno-carcinoma | Adenoma | Squamous cell carcinoma | Sarcoma | |
| Group I | 20-methylcholanthrene | 11 | 3 | 27.2 | | 1 | 1 | 1 | |
| Group II | 20-MC and testosterone propionate | 8 | 2 | 25.0 | | | 2 | | Pneumonia 1 |
| Group III | 20-MC and castration | 9 | 3 | 33.3 | | 1 | 1 | 1 | |
| Group IV | 20-MC, castration and hexestrol | 12 | 6 | 50.0 | | 3 | 2 | 1 | |
| Group V | 20-MC and female rat | 14 | 1 | 7.1 | | | | 1 | |

Table 2b. Occurrence of experimental tumor: 4-nitroquinoline-N-oxide wrapped with transplanted prostate tissues pieces subcutaneously inserted into rats

| Group B | Experimental method | Rats No. | No. of tumors | Occurrence of tumor (%) | Tumors | | | | Remarks |
|---|---|---|---|---|---|---|---|---|---|
| | | | | | Adeno-carcinoma | Adenoma | Squamous cell carcinoma | Sarcoma | |
| Group VI | 4-nitroquinoline-N-oxide | 9 | 1 | 11.2 | | | 1 | | |
| Group VII | 4-NQO and testosterone propionate | 11 | 1 | 9.1 | | | | 1 | |
| Group VIII | 4-NQO and castration | 8 | 3 | 37.5 | | 1 | 1 | 1 | |
| Group IX | 4-NQO, castration and hexestrol | 12 | 4 | 33.3 | | 1 | 1 | 2 | |
| Group X | 4-NQO and female rat | 11 | 1 | 9.1 | | 1 | | | |

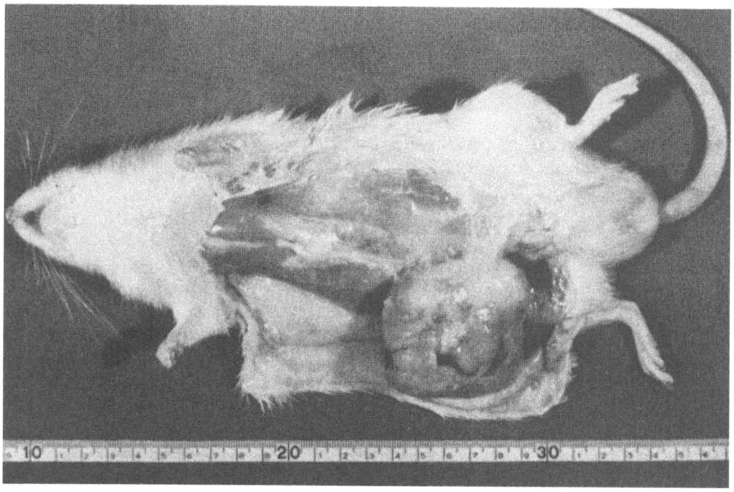

*Fig. 2. Tumor produced by transplanting wrapped carcinogenic substances. Site of tumor was identical to site of transplantation*

Histologically, these tumor masses were multiform. Among 40 rats in which tumors were induced by direct injection of carcinogenic substances, adenoma was observed in 6 rats (15%), squamous cell carcinoma in 15 rats (37.5%), and sarcoma in 19 rats (47.5%). In 25 rats with tumor formation following transplantation, adenoma was seen in 8 (32%), squamous cell carcinoma in 9 (36%), and sarcoma in 8 (32%).

Weights of the tumors ranged from 0.324 to 12.31 g (mean ± SD 4.547 ± 1.238 g) in the rat group with direct injection of carcinogenic substance into the prostate, and from 0.238 to 3.872 g (mean ± SD 0.934 ± 0.279 g) in the rat group with transplantation of carcinogenic substances wrapped with the prostate epithelial tissue.

When the change in endocrine milieu was combined with the experimental conditions, tumor weight ranged from 0.379 to 8.271 g (4.327 ± 0.719 g) in the rat group receiving direct injection of carcinogenic substances, from 0.324 to 8.777 g (4.446 ± 0.811 g) in the rat group administered androgens, from 0.783 to 12.31 g (5.891 ± 1.121 g) in the rat group given estrogens, and from 0.831 to 9.7 2 g (4.001 ± 1.212 g) in the castrated group. In the rats direct injected with carcinogenic substances, tumor weights ranged from 0.342 to 1.244 g (0.721 ± 0.031 g) in the group receiving only carcinogenic substances, from 0.238 to 1.231 g (0.741 ± 0.120 g) in the castrated group, from 0.742 to 3.872 g (2.093 ± 0.271 g) in the group given estrogens, and from 0.241 to 0.274 g in the group with transplantation into female rats. Tumor weights were evidently increased by estrogen application.

3. Complications and Metastasis. In the group receiving direct injection of carcinogenic substances into the prostate, the most frequently observed complication was flow disturbance in the urinary tract following an increase in tumor size. Less frequent or rare complications were hydronephrosis, ureter hydrops, retentive bladder and consequent bladder stone formation, and hematuria due to tumor. In the early stage of the experiments, pneumonia was sometimes observed.

Metastasis to various organs took place. Metastasis to the pelvic lymph nodes and metastatic infiltrates in the vesical wall were seen in all the rats injected with 4-NQO. No remote metastases were recognized.

In the rat group receiving transplantation of wrapped carcinogenic substances, only one rat died of pneumonia in the early stage of the experiments, and no metastases were seen.

In the group administered sex hormones, a detailed examination of the cardiovascular system was done, but no special changes were observed.

4. Histogenesis. The normal structure of the ventral lobe of the rat prostate was the glandular tissue which was covered by the single, high-columnar epithelium. When glandular secretion was poor, many papillary extrusions toward the lumen were observed. The cells located at the base of the high-columnar epithelium had relatively large nuclei and a basophilic cytoplasm. When the glandular lumen was filled with a secretion which was stained lightly with eosin, the glandular internal space looked like a simple cyst, the epithelium reduced its height or size in a flat or cuboid pattern, and the basophilic stainability of the cytoplasm tended to decrease. The glandular parenchymal portion was formed with a few lobules, and development of interstitial tissue between them was poor (Fig. 3).

The pathohistologic reaction of the prostate tissue into which carcinogenic substances were directly injected was successively followed up. First, tissue destruction at the site of injection was locally observed. A type of inflammation began to take place as a reaction to the foreign carcinogenic substances. Then, granuloma was formed involving the carcinogenic crystal. Directly near the granuloma, giant cells for foreign bodies were seen. Surrounding the granuloma, infiltration of the round cells and proliferation of fibrogranular cells were observed. Sometimes there was abcess formation. At that time, the granular portion adjacent to the site of injection was cystically expanded, frequently in association with epithelial destruction or necrotic alteration.

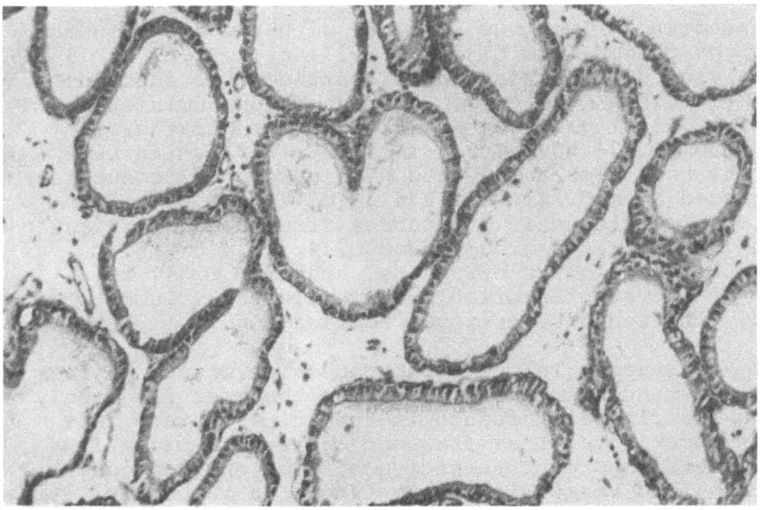

*Fig. 3. Normal structure of ventral lobe of rat prostate*

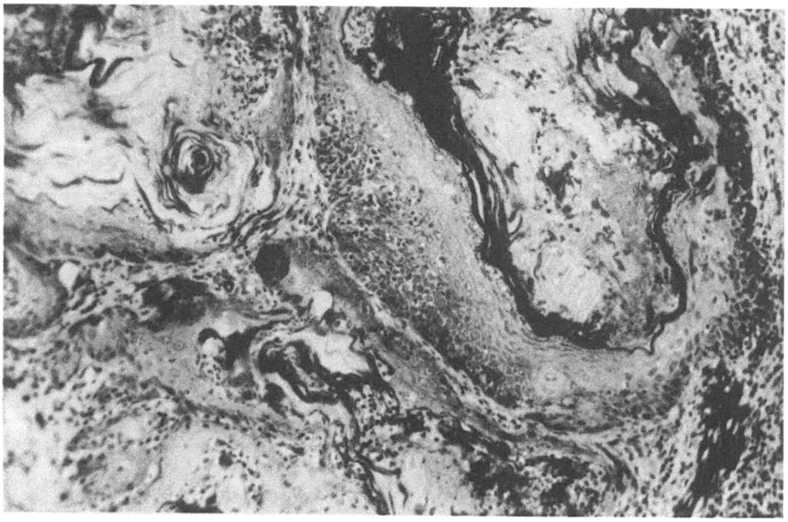

*Fig. 4. Tumor showing transition to squamous cell carcinoma, planoepithelial metaplasia of the epithelium*

The pathohistologic changes in the prostate tissue into which wrapped carcinogenic substances were transplanted, were also successively traced. The region in contact with the wrapped material showed remarkable tissue destruction, and near this region, inflammatory reactions to foreign body were observed. Next, infiltration of giant cells to the foreign body appeared in parallel with granuloma formation.

In the tumor showing transition to squamous cell carcinoma, planoepithelial metaplasia of the epithelium appeared at about the 100th day. At the time, the glandular epithelium was morphologically impressed and became flat. The greater part of the glandular internal spaces was filled with secretion showing the dark tone of eosin, and with fallen epithelial fragments. Thus, the glandular epithelium tended to become hyperplastic, changed to squamous epithelium with multilayer and marked cornification, and partly infiltrated the interstitial tissue (Fig. 4). Thus, the squamous cell cancer focus, characterized by almost complete loss of glandular structure and hyperplasia of the cornified epidermal and prickle cell layer and by its strong cornifying tendency, was definitely established.

In the cases in which the artificial tumor changed to a sarcoma, the transition took place suddenly, indicating extremely rapid proliferation of the tumor tissue. Histologically, all the sarcomas thus transformed were leiomyosarcomas. The sarcomas were composed of almost oval cells. The cellular bodies were long and slender and their cellular bundles mixed and in disarray. This leiomyosarcoma differed from leiomyoma in that the cellular component was abundant, cell size was irregular and unequal, and a necrotic pattern was found here and there. The site of mitosis was directly associated with the presence of giant cells and the mitotic cells were highly atypical (Figs. 5 and 6).

In the cases of artificial tumor that changed to adenoma, epithelial cells were found around the crystal, the structure of the acinus was not observed in the proliferated cell population, the septum composed

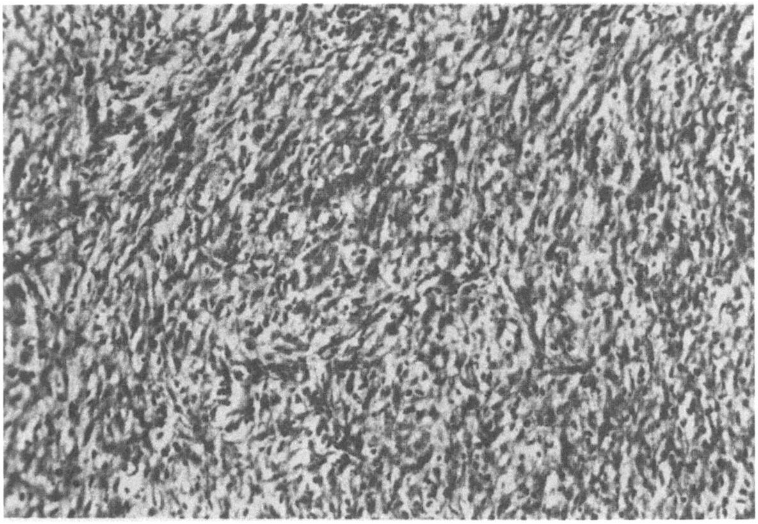

*Fig. 5. Sarcoma composed of almost oval cells of which cellular bodies were long and slender. Cellular bundles are mixed and in disarray*

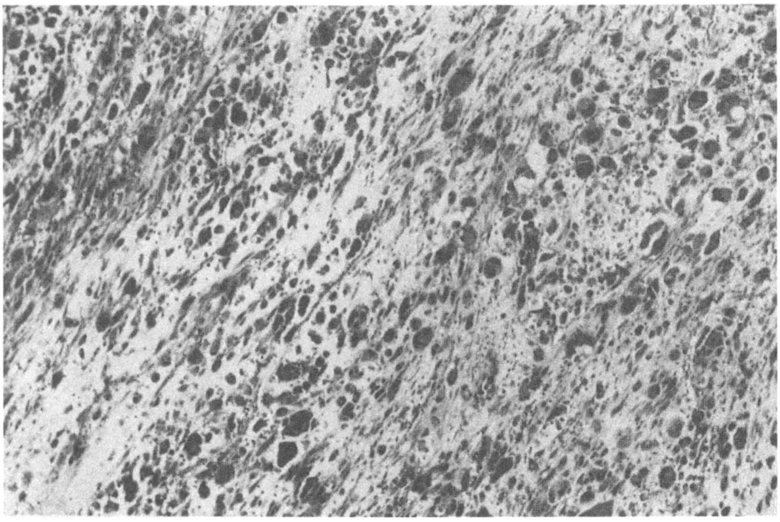

*Fig. 6. Magnification of Fig. 5*

of connective tissue disappeared, and the blood vessels and sinuses were filled with erythrocytes. In this type of adenoma, the cell arrangement was properly irregular and the cells were atypical (Figs. 7-9). Near the cells, were blood vessels expanded by filling up with erythrocytes. Acinar multiplication was marked, and in addition each acinar population was separated by fine connective tissues. One acinus was composed of five to eight cells and the nuclei of the cells located at

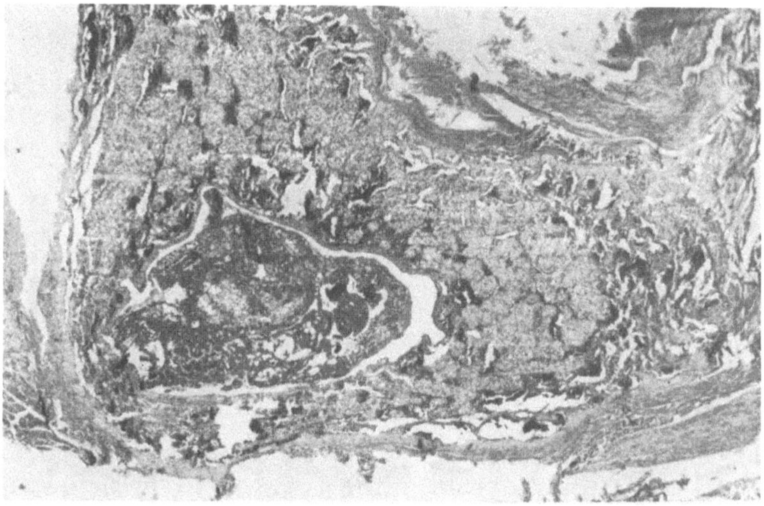

*Fig. 7. In cases of artificial tumor which changed to adenoma, epithelial cells surrounded the crystal*

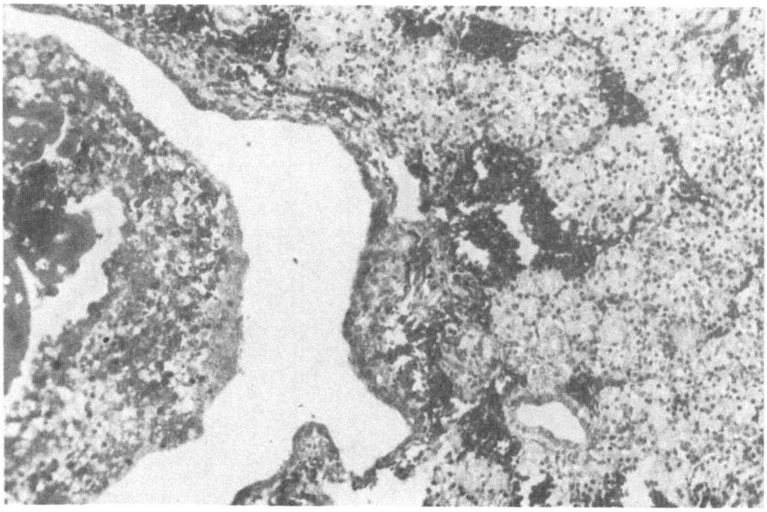

*Fig. 8. Structure of acinus was not observed in proliferated cell population, the septum composed of connective tissue disappeared, and blood vessels and sinuses were filled with erythrocytes*

the nuclear peripheral region were of equal sizes. Sometimes, vascular degeneration was observed (Fig. 10).

The change in endocrine circumstances did not result in any special histologic alteration.

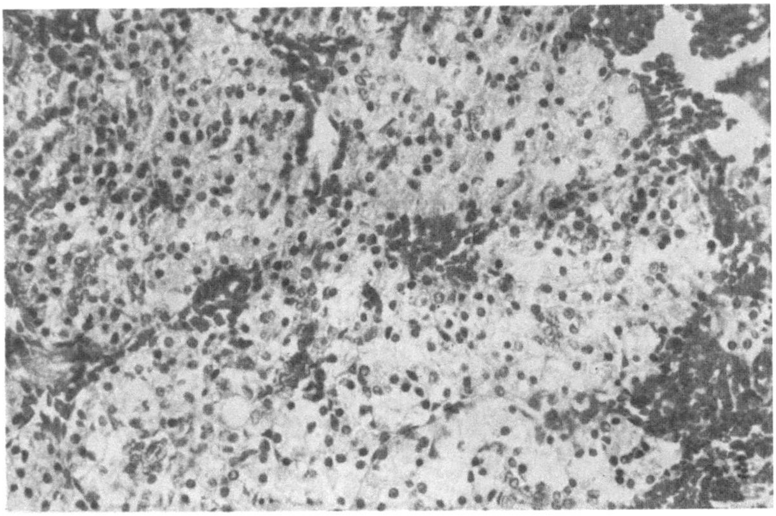

*Fig. 9. In this type of adenoma, cell arrangement was properly irregular and cells were atypical*

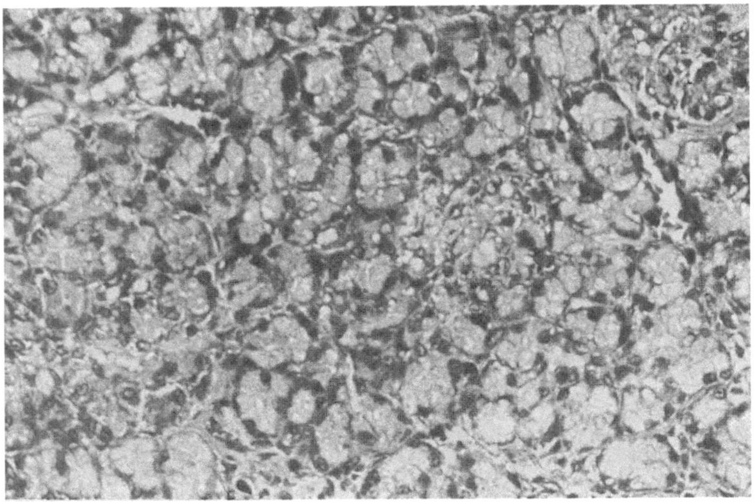

*Fig. 10. One acinus was composed of 5 to 8 cells. Nuclei of equal size were located at the periphery. Sometimes, vascular degeneration was noted*

## II. THE EFFECTS OF THE CHANGE IN ENDOCRINE MILIEU ON TRANSPLANTATION OF EXPERIMENTALLY FORMED PROSTATE ADENOMA

### Materials and Methods

The tissue for transplantation was made as follows. After injection of 20-MC or 4-NQO, the ventral lobe of the prostate was extirpated at a suitable time, and spread out. Carcinogenic substances were wrapped in it and the tissue mass was transplanted to another rat. An artificial tumor mass detected at a relatively early stage was extirpated. Carcinogenic substances, if retained, were removed on a gauze immersed in Puck's solution using a magnifying glass. Some of the tissue was histologically examined, and some of the tissue pieces which demonstrated adenoma were selected for transplantation (Figs. 11 and 12).

Some pieces of adenoma tissue thus obtained were transplanted subcutaneously to 5-week-old male and female Donryu rats. The rats were classified into five experimental groups in order to observe the effects of the change in their internal endocrine milieu. The first group consisted of untreated male rats, the second was injected with testosterone propionate 2.5 mg per rat daily, the third group was castrated, the fourth was injected with hexestrol 0.5 mg per rat daily after castration, and the fifth was the female rat group. The experimental conditions were similar to those described above.

### Results

1. Rate of Successful Transplantation. The rate of successful transplantation was 51.25% (41 of 80 rats) in the male rats.

Pathohistologic changes in transplanted tumors were as follows: adenocarcinoma 5% (4 of 80 rats), squamous cell carcinoma 5% (4 rats),

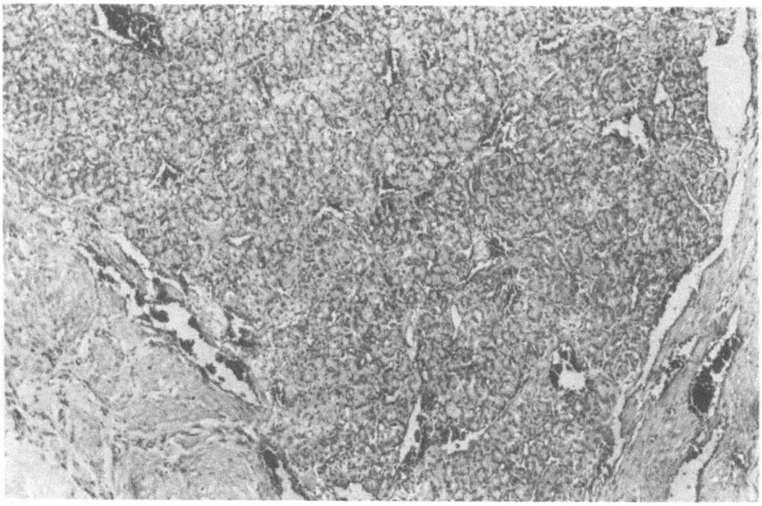

*Fig. 11. Adenoma of tissue for transplantation*

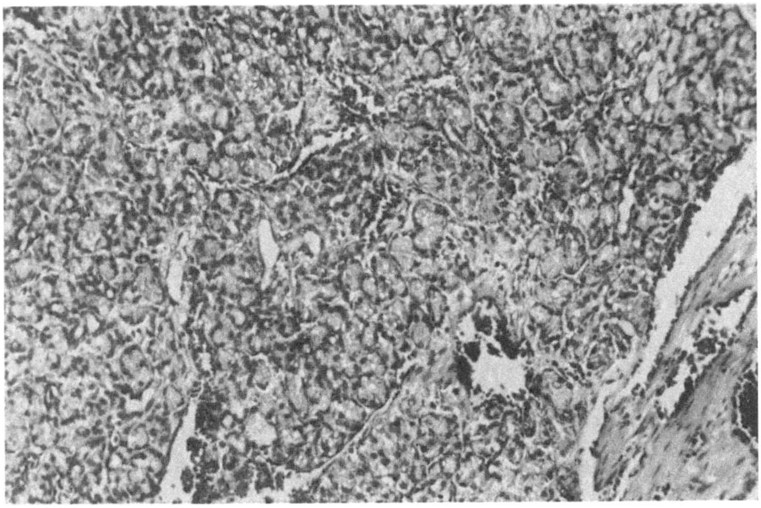

*Fig. 12. Adenoma. Magnification of Fig. 11*

sarcoma 5% (4 rats), adenoma unchanged 36.25% (29 rats), necrotic alteration 46.25% (37 rats), and death 2.5% (2 rats).

In the examination of 32 rats at the end of the 15th experimental week, the figures were: adenoma unchanged 37.5% (12 rats), necrosis 56.25% (18 rats), and death 6.25% (2 rats).

In the survey of 48 rats that survived for more than 15 weeks of the experimental period, adenocarcinoma was seen in 8.33% (4 rats), squamous cell carcinoma in 8.33% (4 rats), adenoma unchanged in 35.42% (17 rats), and necrosis in 35.58% (19 rats).

There was a significant difference between these two types of observations. The results suggested that transplanted adenoma tended to become malignant with increasing time after transplantation.

The rate of successful transplantation was 40% (10 of 25 rats) in the female rats.

Pathohistologically, the changes were as follows: adenocarcinoma 4% (1 rat), adenoma unchanged 36% (9 rats), necrotic alteration 52% (13 rats), and death 8% (2 rats). Necrotic alteration of the transplanted mass was observed in 7 rats until the 15th week and in 6 rats after the 15th week. Among these tumors, transplanted adenoma without any additional change remained for a period longer than 15 weeks.

<u>2. The Effects of the Change in Internal Endocrine Milieu on Transplantation</u>. In the 20 male rats, the rate of successful transplantation was 55% and the rate of production of adenocarcinoma from adenoma was 0%. In 20 rats injected with testosterone propionate, the rate of successful transplantation was reduced to 40%, but the adenocarcinoma rate remained 0%.

In the 20 castrated rats, the rate of successful transplanation was 45.0% and the rate of production of adenocarcinoma was 0%.

In 20 rats injected with hexestrol after castration, the rate of successful transplantation was increased to 65% and the rate of production of adenocarcinoma was increased to 20%.

On the other hand, in the 25 female rats the rate of successful transplantation was 40% and the rate of production of adenocarcinoma was 4% (Fig. 13).

The rate of adenoma which was unchanged throughout the course of the experiments will indicate the effect of the internal endocrine milieu on artificial tumors. This rate was 42.5% (17 of 40 rats) in the male rats or the rats administered testosterone propionate, 30% (12 of 40 rats) in the castrated rats or in the rats given hexestrol after castration, and 36% (9 of 25 rats) in the female rats. In summary, these results indicated that castration and hexestrol injection after castration in male rats reduced the self-maintaining ability of an adenoma with a consequent tendency to malignancy; in other words, the ability to maintain the property of an adenoma tended to decline.

3. Histogenesis. Pathohistologic changes of transplanted adenoma were successively followed up. Necrotic alteration, regardless of procedure, was seen in 46.25%. This change might result from necrotic change of the transplanted tissue itself, inflammation in response to foreign transplanted tissue, and incomplete angioarchitecture in the vicinity of the transplanted tissue.

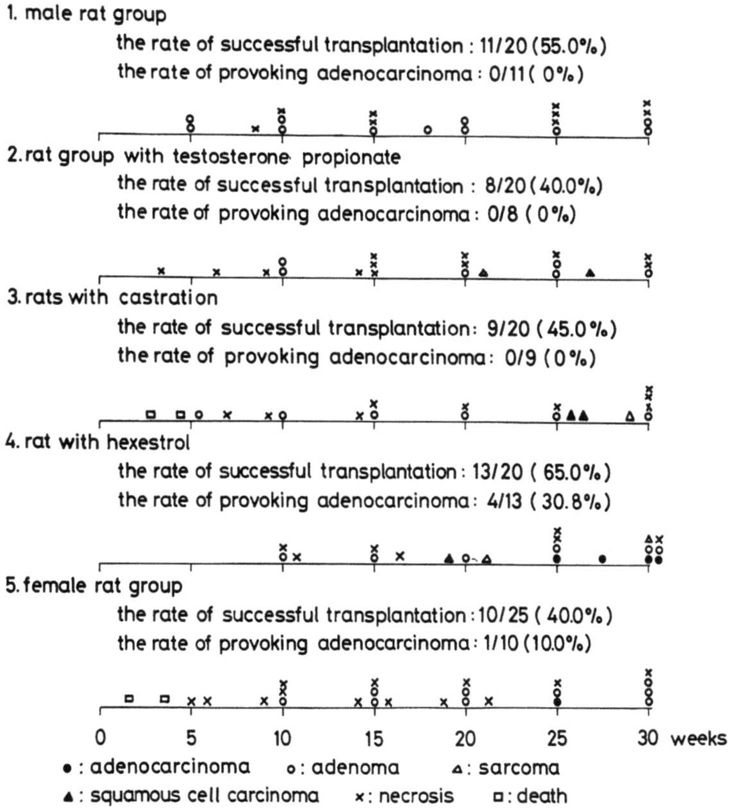


*Fig. 13. Effects of change in endocrine milieu on transplantation experimentally formed prostate adenoma*

The mechanism by which squamous cell carcinoma or sarcoma develops from transplanted adenoma may not be explained by the change in the adenoma itself caused by the endocrine environmental change, but may be the result of carcinogenic substances remaining attached in the transplanted adenoma and inducing cancer or sarcoma by stimulating the tissue in a way that remains to be elucidated (Figs. 14 and 15).

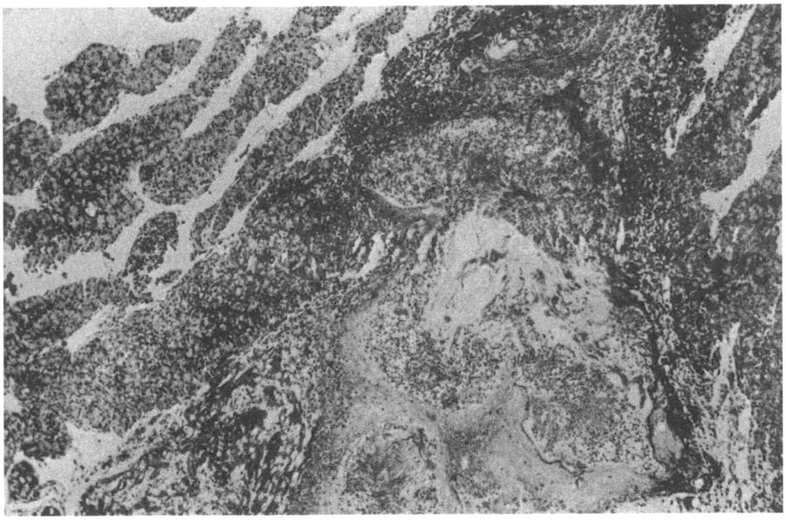

*Fig. 14. Squamous cell carcinoma from transplanted adenoma*

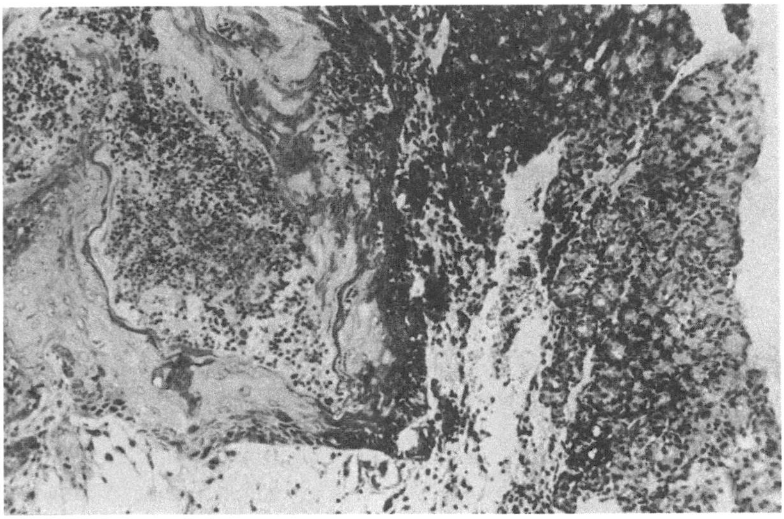

*Fig. 15. Magnification of Fig. 14*

In all rat groups, transplanted adenoma tissue which remained without specific pathological changes in fine structure was recognized.

The transitional progress from transplanted adenoma to adenocarcinoma could not be actually observed. It is my impression that when the transplanted tumor mass is extirpated and examined after suitable periods it has already turned into adenocarcinoma, especially in the cases presenting a change to adenocarcinoma.

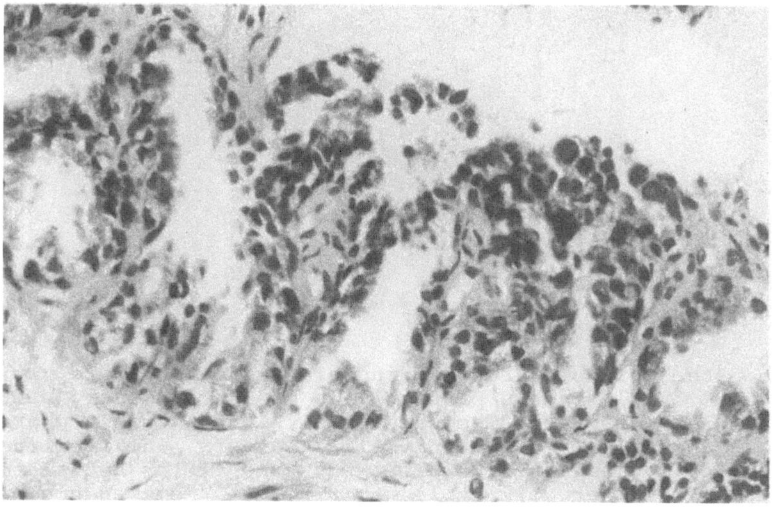

*Fig. 16. Adenocarcinoma in castrated male rat injected with hexestrol 0.5 mg daily*

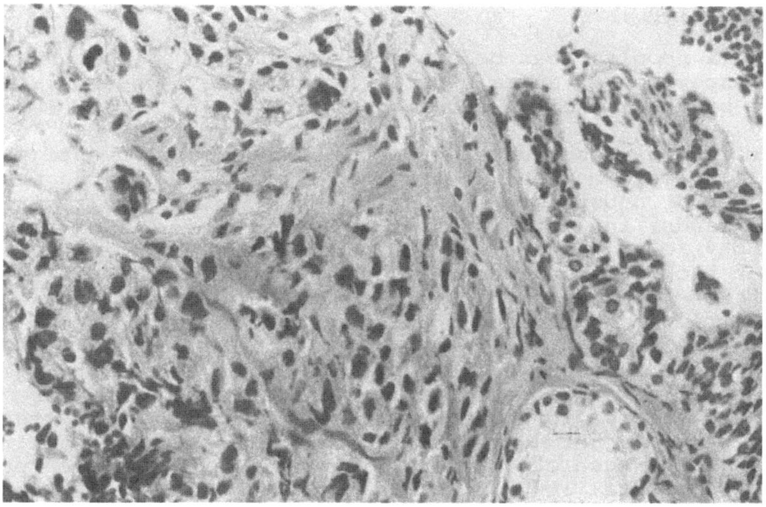

*Fig. 17. Adenocarcinoma in castrated male rat injected with hexestrol 0.5 mg daily*

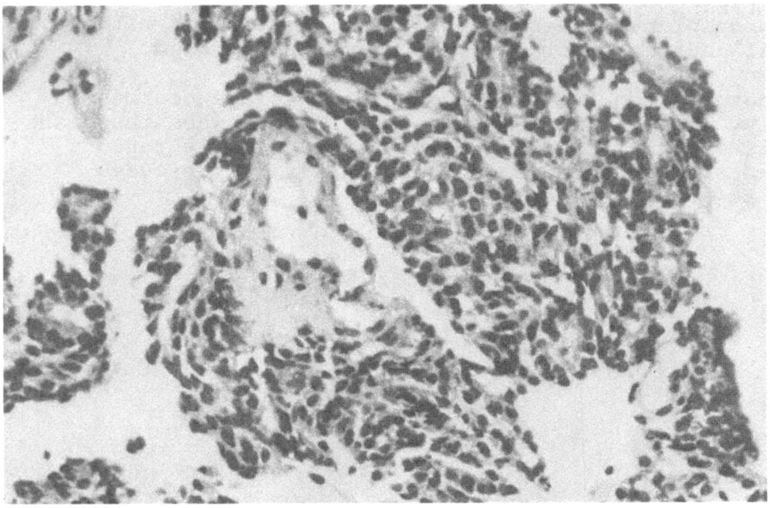

*Fig. 18. Adenocarcinoma in female rat*

The pathologic pictures of transplanted tumors were various, and in general little tumors particularly had a relatively well-differentiated glandular structure. The cancer cells were usually characterized by low columnar or a cubic epithelial pattern, and the intercellular boundary was evident. However, the tone of the cytoplasm of the cancer cells was either dark or light (Fig. 16). Some adenocarcinomas had a specific property of papillary proliferation. Another type of adenocarcinoma showed marked cancerous infiltration into interstitial tissue, so that the adenocarcinoma was in an acinar form demonstrating small lacunar spaces (Figs. 17 and 18).

## Discussion

When a neoplasm can be produced by administering certain substances to experimental animals using an adequate procedure, such substances can be designated as carcinogenic.

Carcinogenic substances have been thoroughly investigated, and their carcinogenic mechanisms analyzed chemically. At the present time, the number of substances supposed to be carcinogenic is in the hunderd thousands, including synthesized chemicals. All of them, however, are nonphysiologic and are practically nonexistent in the living organism. Even though cancer can be induced experimentally in animals or humans by these substances, it is incorrect to suppose that all naturally occurring cancers are produced by carcinogenic chemicals.

Since the frequency of cancer rises with increasing age, it is thought that administration of carcinogenic substances causes metabolic disorders similar to those observable in aging, and certain by-products unexpectedly formed through normal metabolic pathways may contribute to this carcinogenic process. This possibility has been proposed by some investigators. In 1933, COOK et al. (3) opined that abnormal metabolic process of steroids in vivo produced a carcinogenic hydrocarbon compound. In 1934, COOK et al. (3, 4) succeeded in synthesizing 20-MC from desoxycholic acid. Subsequently, many experiments were done with regard to the carcinogenic ability of 20-MC which bore a striking resemblance to dibenzanthracene or benzpyrene of hydrocarbon compound. It is interesting to note that these compounds can be synthesized from a substance similar to steroids that are normally present in the human body. For this reason, it may be that these substances cause cancer spontaneously by bringing about abnormal metabolic processes similar to subtle reactions in the living organism.

20-MC, a powerful carcinogenic chemical, has made tumor study possible in various fields, but experiments of prostate tumor formation using 20-MC are relatively few in number and rudimentary.

20-MC was artificially synthetized by OCHIAI (22) in 1943 and was shown to be carcinogenic by NAKAHARA (20) in 1957 and to be locally carcinogenic by MORI (19) in 1961. 4-NQO has been thought to have a particular carcinogenic capability by which tumors are formed in distant regions. The present author attempted to produce experimental prostate tumor by using 20-MC and 4-NQO.

In the author's experiments with injection of carcinogenic substances into the ventral lobe of the prostate, experimental prostate tumor was formed in 50% with 20-MC and in 51.3% with 4-NQO. MOORE (18) obtained a 78% tumor formation rate after application of benzpyrene to rats, MIRAND (17) 35%, DUNNING (5) 50%, and TAKENAKA (29) 53.9%.

In the author's study, the tumor formation rate was 27.8% using 20-MC and 19.6% with 4-NQO, lower than the 40% reported by HORNING (10) using the same chemical.

In carcinogenic experiments, besides the property of the carcinogenic substance, special attention should be paid to such factors as dosage, the nature of the solvent, method of administration, duration of use, strain and age of experimental animal, and feeding conditions. In particular, when tumor formation experiments are performed over a long term, the presence of new additional parameters should be considered. Pure strains such as the C3H mouse which shows a high tumor formation rate is favourable for breast cancer or liver cancer, but there are no reports as to animals for use in prostate tumor experiments.

HORNING et al. (12) gave 20-MC to two strains of mice: tumor incidence was 37.8% in the strong A strain and 47.5% in mice of the RIII strain. TAKENAKA (29) produced tumor in 53.9% of Wistar rats. The author obtained a similar rate in rats of the Donryu strain. All these values indicate that when experimental conditions are almost identical, experiments will give similar results. The results of KÄLLÉN et al. (15) are interesting in that tumor incidence was low in the rats, and young mice were able to form tumors. These facts should be taken into consideration since human prostate carcinoma is considered to be an aging phenomenon. The author has utilized young rats in his experiments because the prostate is a hormone-sensitive organ and so juvenile animals are thought to be favourable for this purpose.

Up to the present time, sufficient or excess dosage of relatively powerful carcinogenic substances has been applied for exact formation of tumors. However, ARTHUR and EASTLICK (1) have proposed a concept of carcinogenic threshold concentration above which tumor formation occurs in all cases. SEVERI et al. (27) reported that increased application of carcinogenic substances resulted in shortening of latency and elevation of the tumor formation rate. In order to explain subtle carcinogenic mechanisms, it is necessary to determine the minimum effective dose that will provoke a tissue reaction. MATAKE and IMAI (16) emphasized that, because higher concentrations of carcinogenic substances caused necrosis and sequentially reduced cancer formation rates, not only dosage but concentration might be related to carcinogenicity. In my results, the experimental cancer formation rate was much higher when the carcinogenic substance injected was dissolved in olive oil than when a technique employing direct contact with the cells was used. The former procedure facilitates permeation into the tissue and a more lasting effect on the cells.

In many carcinogenic experiments, most of the tumors formed are squamous cell carcinomas. HORNING (10) developed an ingenious procedure employing homogeneous subcutaneous transplantation of the prostate epithelial tissue. He observed that homogeneously and subcutaneously transplanted prostate epithelial tissue acted to stimulate locally the cellular vital activity which was reduced because of the resting state of the secretory phase. He also reported that transplantation caused histologic splitting of the nucleus or karyoconcentration in the low columnar cells which were located in the relatively basic portion of the acinus.

HADDOW (7) considered a decrease in cellular activity or vitality as a background field in which the carcinogenic substance acted to transform or change normal metabolic reactions in an unknown specific manner. VASILIEV and GUELSTEIN (30) observed that tumors originated from injured cells. HIEGERS et al. (8) reported that tumors arose from somatic cells by mutation. ORR (24) hypothesized that, although intermediate forms between normal and tumor cells could not be recognized, tumor cells might occur by loss of normal metabolic regulation after qualitative changes in metabolic, nutritive, and supporting tissues induced by the carcinogenic substance.

The author introduced a new method of transplanting prostate tissue homogeneously and subcutaneously adapted from HORNING 's original method. My modification consists of wrapping the carcinogenic substance with extirpated, finely cut, and spread but injured tissue. These procedures, as indicated by ORR, brought about (1) various changes in supporting or nutritive tissues at the site of subcutaneous insertion, (2) a change in vascular architecture, and (3) qualitative change in cellular metabolic processes.

HUGGINS and HODGES (14) concluded that prostate cancer represented an abnormal proliferation of the mature prostate epithelium with the original histologic properties of the prostate epithelium, and the castration or estrogen administration caused regressive atrophy of prostate cancer. The present-day hormone therapy of prostate cancer is based on this conclusion.

The cell activity of prostate cancer is dependent upon the grade of secretion of androgen, and therefore tumor cell growth stops when the androgen supply is interrupted by castration. Clinically, it is generally accepted that growth of prostate tumor is inhibited by castration or estrogen administration whereas prostate cancer is exacerbated when androgens are administered. It is believed that estrogen alleviates the pain of human prostate cancer. Sex hormones may be related to the normal growth of the prostate, and the dysharmonic state of the hormones is probably connected to prostate tumor formation.

Practically, when androgen is injected, hypertrophy and hyperfunction of the male sexual or accessory sexual organs are widely observed, but tumor formation is not noticed (33-35).

Thus, the author attempted experiments to determine the effect on tumor formation in the rat prostate in the presence of an abnormal sex hormone milieu. In the group injected with carcinogenic substance into the prostate, castration and estrogen administration caused higher rates of formation. In the group administered androgen, the tumor formation rate was reduced. In the group given carcinogenic substances wrapped in prostate tissue, estrogen application resulted in an increase in the tumor formation rate. Transplantation to female rats showed a lower tumor formation rate than that to male rats. The increase in the tumor formation rate was statistically significant in the group administered estrogen.

In general, prostate tumors androgen-dependent occur at a higher rate and become exacerbated when estrogen is additionally applied. Estrogen administration or estrogen dominance, which is to be expected in castrated and female rats, somewhat inhibits tumor formation.

In summarizing the results of other investigators, DUNNING et al. (5) reported that proliferation of transplanted prostate tumor by 20-MC was more marked in female than in male rats. HORNING (11) observed that estrogen administration facilitated carcinoma formation, and TAKENAKA (29) proposed an estrogen dominance hypothesis.

On the other hand, MOORE and MELCHIONNA (18) found that the time of occurrence of experimental tumor was hastened by castration but the incidence was reduced, while a combination of castration and androgen administration resulted in an increase in tumor formation. WOJEWSKI et al. (33) also reported that castration promoted carcinogenicity in the prostate induced by 20-MC, whereas estrogen as well as androgen had no special effect on tumor formation.

There are no definite conclusions on the carcinogenic effects of hormones. RÖHL (25), in summarizing his experiments on the effects of various hormones on tissue-cultured prostate cancer tissue, concluded that although the effects of hormones were dependent upon the grade of differentiation of cancer cells, mature prostate cancer was androgen-dependent but immature cancer was not.

There is doubtless a subtle regulatory process of hormone reception at certain sites of prostate cells or prostate carcinoma cells. The next problem will be to answer the question by what mechanism or how the sensitivity of these sites is changed after transplanting the prostate epithelial tissue.

When steroid hormone is given to animals, the hormone raises specific reactions in the cells after passing through the cell membrane of the target organ. This process is explained by the hormone-gene theory, which interprets the effects of sex hormones as follows. Estrogen exercises its physiologic action on the cells of the uterus without any metabolic alteration, whereas the androgenic action of testosterone is by combining dihydrotestosterone changed by 5α-reductase with in the nucleus. In the prostate, which is a target organ of androgen, testosterone demonstrates its specific action through the reduction of testosterone to dihydrotestosterone in the prostate. FARNSWORTH (6) and SHIDA et al. (28) consider that estrogen produces its direct therapeutic antiandrogenic effects on the prostate cell itself by inhibiting the activity of 5α-reductase.

At the time of testosterone injection in rats, testosterone may demonstrate androgenic influence after changing to dihydrotestosterone. This kind of change is difficult at the time of transplantation of the prostate epithelial tissue because the entry of testosterone is comprimised by reason of the incomplete vasculature. In addition the sequential change of testosterone to dihydrotestosterone is difficult due to the qualitative cellular changes in the prostate. Accordingly, the effects of androgen on prostate cancer cannot be interpreted by a target organ concept.

Estrogen, when it has entered into the cell, inhibits the activity of 5α-reductase and therefore the action of androgen on the prostate. In the rats injected with estrogen, there may be an estrogen advantage endocrinologically.

As discussed above, the effects of sex hormones on the development and production of tumor tissue are not clear. Female as well as male sex hormones may play a role as initiating factors but as accelerating factors. Although the mechanism has not been clarified in detail, it is reasonable to assume that sex hormones play an accessory or secondary role in carcinogenicity.

Therefore, all prostate cancers are not androgen-dependent. It is impossible to conclude or designate an initiating factor for prostate cancer, probably because the prostate becomes qualitatively different from the normal prostate, especially in its ultrastructure. As far as the author's results are concerned, endocrine dysfunctions, including sex hormone imbalance, may offer a condition favorable for carcinogenesis. Promotion of tumor formation under conditions of estrogen dominance indicates that estrogen and androgen behave through the same mechanism.

The experiments in which the endocrine medium was changed in association either with direct injection of 20-MC and 4-NQO or after wrapping them with prostate epithelium, demonstrated that the histology of the tumors had no immediate correlation to carcinogenic substances. In the group with direct injection to the prostate, adenoma was seen in 7.5%, squamous cell carcinoma in 18.98%, and sarcoma in 24.04%, and in the wrapped prostate epithelium group, adenoma was seen in 7.59%, squamous cell carcinoma 8.57%, and sarcoma in 7.61%; the formation of the clinically frequent adenocarcinoma was not seen.

Experimentally, adenocarcinoma was formed in 2 of 30 tumors by MIRAND (17), in 1 of 6 tumors by KÄLLÉN and RÖHL (15), and in 11 of 12 tumors by HORNING (10) following implantation of wrapped carcinogenic substances. The majority of carcinomas reported were squamous cell carcinomas, sarcoma ranked second.

The author paid special attention to the adenomas composed of glandular prostate tissue. The purpose was to form adenocarcinoma by transplanting the adenoma thus produced and changing the endocrine milieu. Only the adenoma of which the cellular origin could be confirmed as prostate tissue was used for transplantation. The adenomas were transplanted in rats that received wrapped carcinogenic substances. Tissue specimens were naturally small in size but the carcinogenic crystal remained in the central region of the specimen. Therefore, experiments were made as follows: A portion of adenoma distant from the central crystal was cut off, the crystal was washed as thoroughly as possible and the tissue piece was transplanted subcutaneously into rats whose internal endocrine milieu had been artificially changed. The results were the following: Most of the transplanted tissues were necrotic, some remained adenomas, and transplantable tumors were seen in 9.75% (4 of 41 rats) of male rats, and in 10% of female rats (1 of 10 rats).

Administration of androgen to male rats did not produce adenocarcinomas from adenoma, whereas adenocarcinomas were produced in female rats and male rats given estrogen after castration.

Whether the tumor used by the present author was a complete adenoma and whether the tumor was in a precancerous state or not are possible objetcions. Transformation from adenoma to adenocarcinoma was not so frequent, but the change to carcinoma occurred quite suddenly and irreversibly.

Many pathologists including WILLIS (31) have thought that the carcinogenic process is characterized by preceding graded focal changes requiring a relatively long peroid, and that the ultimate change was represented by the malignant tumor (23). This suggested the presence of a precancerous stage. ROUS (26), however, explained carcinogenesis in terms of mutation of latent cells capable of forming carcinoma.

Another concept of the carcinogenesis of prostate carcinoma is that this carcinoma is a manifestation of aging phenomena as previously proposed by THIERSCH and COHNHEIM, among others. Considering the fact that prostate carcinoma frequently originates from glandular tissue showing senile atrophy, it is likely that the cancer arises by mutation of cells in physiologic declines, and at a time when the presence of a latent cancer-promoting factor is postulated.

Although the author's experimental results do not approach the final stage of investigation of human tumor formation, they will give a clue to the problem of prostate carcinogenesis. However, if further efforts demonstrate clinically that there are cases of prostate cancer not amenable to such hormone therapy as antiandrogen treatment through castration, the significance of sex hormones in producing human prostate cancer will be certainly increased.

## Conclusion

Experimental production of prostate cancer in animals may contribute to diagnosis and therapy of human prostate cancer by providing a model for provocation, initiation, and pathophysiology of the cancer.

It is interesting and important to know in detail the effects of sex hormones on the carcinogenic mechanism of prostate cancer which has been considered to be androgen-dependent. The author investigated the influence of sex hormones upon experimental prostate tumor formation as follows:

1. In Donryu rats, which have a low rate of spontaneous tumor formation experiments in tumor formation were performed by direct injection of 1% 20-MC or 4-NQO olive oil solution to the ventral lobe of the prostate and by subcutaneous transplantation of 20-MC or 4-NQO crystals wrapped in prostate epithelial tissue. In addition, the effects of the endocrine milieu on the rate of tumor formation were investigated.

2. The rate of tumor formation was as follows: In the rat group with direct injection of carcinogenic substance to the ventral lobe of the prostate the tumor occurred in 50% using 20-MC and in 51.3% with 4-NQO; in rats receiving transplanted wrapped carcinogenic substances the tumor formation rate was 27.8% with 20-MC and 19.6% with 4-NQO.

The results of the cases associated with change in endocrine milieu could be summarized as follows. In the rat group with direct injection of carcinogenic substances, the castrated rats or rats administered estrogen after castration showed a higher rate of tumor formation than the rats who only received carcinogenic substances; androgen administration caused a reduction in tumor formation rate regardless of method. In the group receiving transplanted wrapped carcinogenic substances, although there was no significant difference in the tumor formation rate between the rats receiving carcinogenic substances only and those given androgen, castration or estrogen administration after castration obviously resulted in an increase in the tumor formation rate. However, the tumor formation rate was clearly lower in female rats with subcutaneous transplantation than in the male rats undergoing the same procedure.

3. The tumors formed experimentally were classified histologically as follows. In the direct injection group, adenoma was seen in 15%, squamous cell carcinoma in 37.5%, and sarcoma in 47.5%. In the subcutaneous transplantation group, adenoma was observed in 32%, squamous cell carcinoma in 36%, and sarcoma in 32%. Estrogen administration resulted in an evident increase in the weights of the tumors formed.

In summary, the author has failed to provoke experimentally prostate adenocarcinoma, which constitutes a majority of human prostate cancers.

Thus, special attention was paid to the adenomas that were formed. Experimentally produced adenoma originated from the glandular tissue of the prostate. This type of rat prostate adenoma could be transplanted subcutaneously to other rats of the same strain. An attempt was made to clarify the effects of a change in endocrine milieu on the transplanted adenoma, and the following results were obtained.

1. The rate of successful transplantation was 51.25% in the male rats and 40% in female rats.

2. Histologic classification of the transplanted tumors was as follows: in male rats, adenoma was seen in 5%, squamous cell carcinoma in 5%, and sarcoma in 5%. Transplanted adenoma tended to alter to a malignant one with increasing time after transplantation.

In female rats, transplanted adenoma changed to adenocarcinoma in 4%, while 36% remained unchanged.

3. When the endocrine milieu was experimentally changed, the results were as follows: In rats given hexestrol after castration, the rate of successful transplantation was 60% and the rate of adenocarcinoma was 20%. In female rats, the rate of successful transplantation was 40% and the rate of adenocarcinoma was 4%. Estrogen dominance promoted the transition from adenoma to adenocarcinoma.

4. It was difficult to determine whether the adenoma used was in a precancerous state or not. From the experimental results, carcinogenic progress from adenoma to adenocarcinoma was not confirmed. This transition may take place extraordinarily and suddenly.

## References


1. Arthur, J.W., Eastlick, H.L.: The relationship between dose and carcinogenic response obtained by injecting methylcholanthrene into the peritoneal cavity of chickens. Growth 27, 199-204 (1963)
2. Buu-Hoi, N.P.: The role of experimental chemical carcinogenesis in research on the etiology of tumors. Arzneimittel Forsch. 11, 813-819 (1961)
3. Cook, J.W., Hieger, I., Kennaway, E.L., Mayneord, W.V.: Cancer production by pure hydrocarbones. Proc. roy. Soc. 111, 455-484 (1932)
4. Cook, J.W., Kennaway, E.L., Kennaway, N.M.: Production of tumors in mice by deoxycholic acid. Nature (Lond.) 145, 627 (1940)

5. Dunning, W.F., Curtis, M.R., Segaloff, A.: Methylcholanthrene squamous cell carcinoma of the rat prostate with skeletal metastases, and failure of the rat liver to respond to the carcinogen. Cancer Res. 6, 256-262 (1946)
6. Farnsworth, W.E.: A possible mechanism of regulation of rat prostate function by testosterone. Biochim. biophys. Acta 150, 446-451 (1958)
7. Haddow, A.: Chemical carcinogens and their modes of action. Brit. med. Bull. 14, 79-92 (1958)
8. Hieger, I.: Carcinogenesis, London: 1961, Academic Press
9. Higuchi, M., Uremura, K., Eto, K., Gohara, S., Hirata, S.: Occurrence and ultrastructure of experimentally produced tumors in rat prostates. Kurume med. J. 19, 205-219 (1972)
10. Horning, E.S.: Local action of 20-methylcholanthrene and sex hormones on prostatic grafts. Brit. J. Cancer 6, 80-88 (1952)
11. Horning, E.S.: Induction of glandular carcinomas of the prostate in the mouse. Lancet II, 829-830 (1946)
12. Horning, E.S.: The effects of castration and stibestrol of prostatic tumors in mice. Brit. J. Cancer 3, 211-230 (1949)
13. Horning, E.S., Dmochowski, L.: Induction of prostate tumors in mice. Brit. J. Cancer 1, 59-63 (1947)
14. a. Huggins, C.: Endocrine factors in cancer. J. Urol. (Baltimore) 68, 875-884 (1952)
b. Huggins, C.: Biological activities of Steoids in Relation to Cancer. New York: 1960, Vol. I, Academic Press
c. Huggins, C., Hodges, C.V.: Studies on prostatic cancer I. The effect on castration, of estrogen and androgen injection on serum phosphatases in metastatic carcinoma. Cancer Res. 1, 293-297 (1941)
15. Källên, B., Röhl, L.: Tissue culture studies on a rat prostatic cancer induced with 20-methylcholanthrene. Acta path. microbiol. scan. 50, 283-290 (1960)
16. Matake, H., Imai, T.: Contribution on the development and growth of the benzpyrene skin cancer in mice. Gann. 49, 156-157 (1958)
17. Mirand, E.A.: Prostatic neoplasms in rats. Exp. Med. Surg. 14, 318-331 (1956)
18. Moore, R.A., Melchionna, R.H.: Production of tumors of prostate of white rat with 1 : 2-benzpyrene. Amer. J. Cancer 30, 731-741 (1937)
19. Mori, K.: Preliminary note on adenocarcinoma of the lung in mice induced with 4-nitroquinoline-N-oxide. Gann. 52, 265-270 (1961)
20. Nakahara, W., Fukuoka, F., Sugimura, T.: Carcinogenic action of 4-nitroquinoline-N-oxide. Gann. 48, 129-137 (1957)
21. Nakanishi, K.: Tumorogenic action of 4-nitroquinoline-N-oxide on the prostate of rats. Jap. J. Urol. 62, 838-857 (1971)
22. Ochiai, E., Ichikawa, M., Sai, Z.: Nitro-action of 4-nitroquinoline-N-oxide. J. pharm. Soc. Nippon 63, 280-282 (1943)
23. Ohota, K.: Precancer. Saishin-Igaku, 13, 2-6 (1958)
24. Orr, J.W.: The mechanism of chemical carcinogenesis, with particular reference to the time of development of irreversible changes in the epithelial cells. Brit. med. Bull. 14, 99-101 (1958)
25. Röhl, L.: Hormone dependency of prostatic cancer studies by cell-culture technique. Brit. J. Urol. 30, 450-453 (1958)
26. Rous, P., Kidd, J.G.: Conditional neoplasms and subthreshold neoplastic states: A study of the tar tumors of rabbits. J. exp. Med. 73, 365-390 (1941)
27. Severi, L., Squartini, F., Olivi, M.: Tumor induction methylcholanthrene in mice: Sites of tumor growth as related to the carcinogen dose and to endogenous hormonal stimulation. Acta Un. int. Cancr. 18, 25-29 (1962)
28. Shida, K., Shimazaki, J., Urano, E., Kurihara, H., Takahashi, H., Furuya, N., Taya, M.: Studies on mechanism of the action of androgens on the prostate; Reduction and its role on the action of testosterone to prostate. Jap. J. Urol. 63, 14-26 (1971)

29. Takenaka, I.: Experimental studies on prostatic tumors. Acta urol. Jap. 10, 745-758 (1964)
30. Vasiliev, J.M., Guelstein, V.I.: Sensitivity of normal carcinogenic substances. J. nat. Cancer Inst. 31, 1123-1151 (1963)
31. Willis, R.A.: Pathology of Tumors, 3rd ed. London: Butterworths, 1960, pp. 589-599
32. Wojewski, A.: The evaluation of methods applied in diagnosis of prostatic cancer. Urol. int. (Basel) 14, 140-159 (1962)
33. Wojewski, A., Laska, A.: Experimental cancer of the prostate. Urol. int. (Basel) 17, 223-229 (1964)
34. Zahler, H.: Die Auffrischung greisenhafter Hunde mittels Hodenwirkstoffen und ihre Auswirkung im Hoden un Prostata. Virschows Arch. path. Anat. 305, 65-107 (1939)
35. Zuckerman, S., Sandys, O.C.: Further observation on effects of sex hormones on prostate and seminal vesicles of monkeys. J. Anat. (Lond.) 73, 597-616 (1939)

# Aspiration Biopsy Cytology of Prostate Carcinoma

H. NIENHAUS

Aspiration biopsy cytology was inaugurated by FRANZÉN, ZAJICEK and ESPOSTI in 1950 from their Institute of Clinical Cytology at Karolinska Academy, Stockholm; the method attained high technical and diagnostical standards during the following years (24). Besides exfoliative cytology and histology, aspiration biopsy cytology must be accepted as an independent approach to morphologic diagnosis and as an instrument of research. In contrast to routine preparations in exfoliative cytology or in histology, the needle preparation allows detailed and parallel examination of the cell and of the histologic structure, resulting in better documented diagnosis. As in various other organs, e.g., in the thyroid or in the breast, the detection of a carcinoma in the prostate is 10% more safe by aspiration biopsy than by mere histologic biopsy. Subsequent histologic counter-checking seldom fails to confirm a positive diagnosis based upon needle preparations (5, 6, 10, 14, 15, 21).

With a fine needle of 0.6-mm maximum diameter very small tissue particles are punched suitable for squeeze preparation. Filling the needle with particles is enforced by aspiration. Eventually, the quantity of tissue extracted is much greater than in conventional histologic preparations, and the sample represents a much larger area of tissue.

The advantages of aspiration biopsy, namely high diagnostic evidence with minimal inconvenience to the patient, may be diminished or suppressed by faulty technique, as often happens in newly developed methods. We therefore want to emphasize the methodologic aspect of aspiration biopsy from the prostate, and to outline its clinical, diagnostic, and scientific values.

The instrumental equipment designed by FRANZÉN (12) consists of a 10-ml syringe (Fig. 1). A handle attached to the piston allows vigourous aspiration and secure guiding with one hand. The 0.6-mm needle No. 16, length 20 cm, fixed with a Luer's nozzle, is inserted into the prostate through a tube guided by the palpating finger.

The point of the needle has to be firmly inserted in the tumor or in the suspicious area, before aspiration can be performed. During the procedure the tumor tissue may be punctured in various depths and directions. After pressure compensation by releasing the piston, the needle is withdrawn from the tumor. Now the needle is removed and then expelled on a glass slide by means of the air-filled syringe, without lifting the point of the needle from the slide. The obtained tissue particles are gently squeezed with a coverslip and smeared in one direction. The success of the aspiration should be estimated at this moment; whenever the material appears insufficient, the puncture may be repeated immediately in the same session, even several times if necessary. In

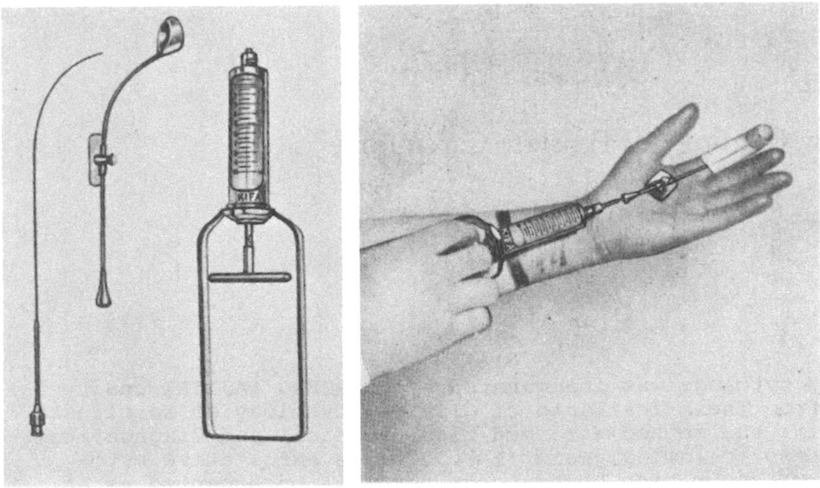

*Fig. 1. Original equipment for aspiration biopsy cytology of prostate designed by FRANZÉN (12)*

opposition to punch biopsy, essential complications or contraindications were not reported, and the procedure requires neither anesthesia nor any other preliminaries (14, 24).

Papanicolaou and May-Grünwald-Giemsa staining have proved most adequate for the diagnostic problems of the prostate. Papanicolaou staining - hematoxylin and eosin in alcoholic medium - requires wet fixation of the tissue. Smears that have dried by air contact may not be stained according to Papanicolaou but only with May-Grünwald-Giemsa. The neglect of these staining rules is often an obstacle to conclusive comparison of results between different authors (Fig. 2). Since smear preparations are liable to dry very fast, fixation must follow immediately after smearing the sample on the glass slide. By using no other technique but May-Grünwald-Giemsa staining, several steps can be saved and mistakes in fixing are avoided. After a technically perfect needle puncture the glass slide will be densely covered with epithelia, and diagnosis may proceed on histologic criteria.

Normal prostate epithelium forms coherent, monolayered complexes of uniform cells with regular intervals between nuclei and distinct cell borders (Fig. 2). As a rule, there are no intracellular secretory granules, nuclei are symmetrical and homogeneously stained, and small round nucleoli are visible in some parts. Sometimes these epithelia contain brown clodlike or granular inclusions. Besides epithelia some light eosinophilic secretion, lamellar bodies or small stromal complexes are found.

Atypical prostate epithelium shows more or less marked swelling of nuclei, clearly characterized by an increased nucleo-cytoplasmic ratio (Fig. 3). Despite considerable variations in size the contours of the nuclei remain smooth. We may also find a trabecular or alveolar disarray of cells. The histologic equivalents to these features are seen in hyperplastic cribrous and pseudopapillary clusters of epithelium inside ectatic glands. Atypical hyperplasia may occur at various stages. Their respective prognostic value is derived from the fact that severe atypias are often observed in association with carcinomatous epithelia in one

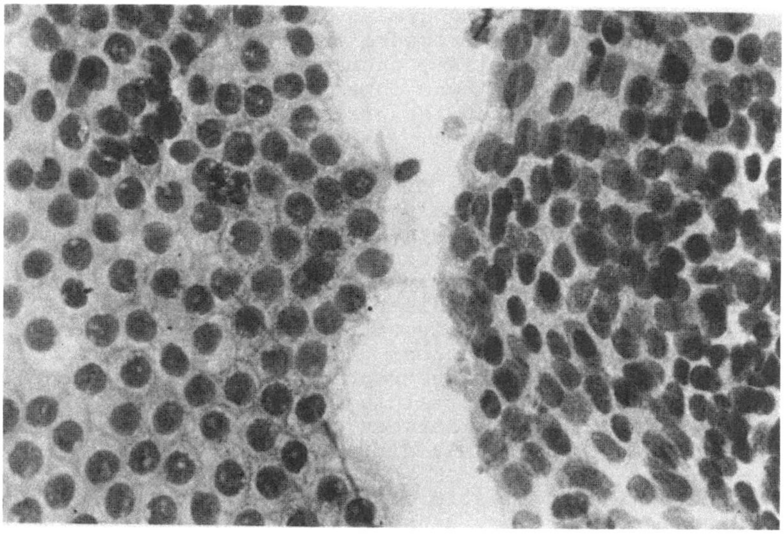

*Fig. 2. Normal prostate epithelium (left) compared to carcinomatous epithelium (right) in the same preparation. Poor staining due to technical mistakes (Aspiration biopsy, dry fixation, Papanicolaou staining). Patient aged 82.* x *440*

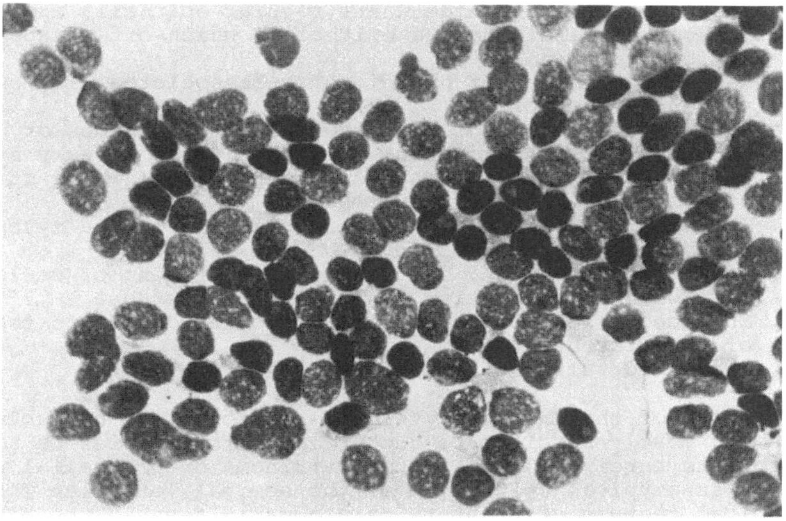

*Fig. 3. Prostate epithelium, severe dysplasia: anisokaryosis, swelling of nuclei, alveolar grouping of cells. Dark basal cells, light acinar cells (Aspiration biopsy, dry fixation, May-Grünwald-Giemsa). Patient aged 51.* x *600*

preparation (17). Here we are moving on the borderline between dysplasia and carcinoma. For the prostate this borderline is less clearly defined than for portio epithelium, stomach, and breast. As far as we know, it was only McNEAL (16) who interpreted his serial histologic examinations in terms of a stepwise grading from dysplasia to carcinoma in situ and to real carcinoma.

In prostate carcinoma the disarray of cells is the most striking feature (Fig. 4). Solid, tubular, or alveolar formations no longer show any parallel or radial orientation of nuclear axes, but rather a random arrangement of them. The loss of polar orientation in cells and in their nuclei is very clearly marked. Electron microscopy reveals corresponding apolar disorganization inside the cells (13). Since aspiration biopsy obtains chiefly vital tumor tissue, we may not expect the classical criteria of nuclear polymorphism and hyperchromasia which become apparent only in dystrophic tumor tissue. Whenever nuclear polymorphism is more or less failing, such microadenomatous changes in cell populations, and disorders of cellular polarity may serve as reliable criteria for highly differentiated adenocarcinoma (23).

With increasing anaplastic dedifferentiation the coherence of cells is abandoned. We find very dense nuclear crowding, or the tumor cells are arranged in small group or are solitary. Increased functional swelling of nuclei appears as a correlate to proliferation intensity in living tumor cells. Since anaplastic carcinomas usually have the highest proliferation rate, their heterochromatin content should be rather low, and nuclear hyperchromasia will not be found (Fig. 4) (4).

The following cytologic criteria of malignancy are deduced from these facts:

1. Irregular swelling of nuclei in distinct gradation of sizes, seen most clearly on a slide where regular epithelia appear in the neighborhood of carcinomatous epithelia, which often happens in circumscribed carcinomas
2. Marked lobulation of nuclei, often associated with an increased number of nucleoli
3. Increased translucence together with filamentous or fine granular condensation of chromatin, or with blurred streaky structures. The pattern is clearly seen in dry preparations where it resembles that of prophase
4. Split-off particles of nuclear chromatin in the cytoplasm appearing as so-called micronuclei
5. A marked distension, deformation, and fading of nucleoli, occasionally with vacualization and numerical increase
6. Enhanced basophilia of cytoplasm corresponding to the accumulation of undifferentiated RNA (22)
7. Increased vulnerability of cells and nuclei

In spite of their gross cytologic polymorphism the nuclear patterns remain mostly specific to the organ, which enables us to distinguish prostate carcinoma from rectum carcinoma or urothelial carcinoma and from an atypical epithelium of the seminal versicles (18). One very typical feature of prostate carcinoma is seen in the bigger nucleoli.

Several attempts were made to coordinate the findings of aspiration biopsy cytology with histologic classifications of prostate carcinoma (Figs. 4 and 5) (9, 11). As a rule, the correspondence appears convincing when well-differentiated intermediate and anaplastic variants are compared. With adequate preparation needle aspiration also offers the possibility of diagnosis for clear-cell or dark-cell carcinoma, for cribrous carcinoma even with mucus formation, and for solid anaplastic carcinoma.

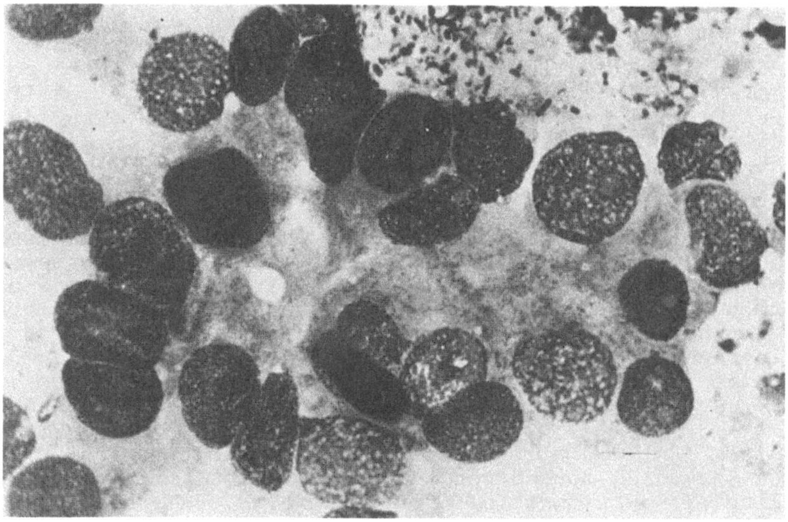

*Fig. 4. Poorly differentiated adenocarcinoma of prostate. Severe swelling of nuclei with increased proliferation. (Aspiration biopsy, dry fixation, May-Grünwald-Giemsa) Patient aged 66. x 600 (cf. Fig. 5)*

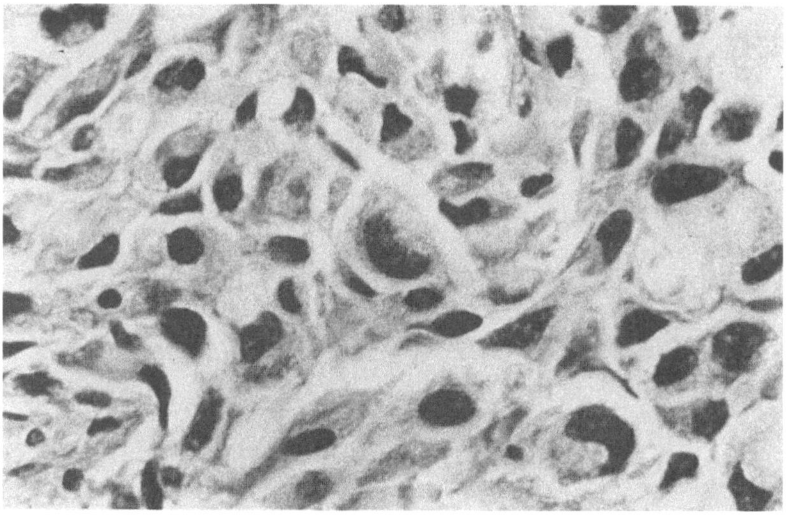

*Fig. 5. Poorly differentiated adenocarcinoma of prostate; polymorphic cell pattern after histologic preparation. (Formalin, paraffin, H & E) Same patient as in Fig. 4. x 600*

In fact it would be inexpedient to use needle aspiration techniques for nothing more than the five Papanicolaou gradings of probability; that would never utilize the whole of its diagnostic potential. Aspiration biopsy cytology provides facilities for cytologic classification which may substantially supplement the usual histologic description of various types of carcinoma.

Like other epithelial organs prostate epithelium shows a certain polarity between undifferentiated reserve cells, some kind of basal cells, and the functionally differentiated cells of acinus type (19) (see Figs. 3 and 4). The carcinomas of different types seem to repeat the developmental sequence either correctly or with skipping over or stopping at certain stages (13).

Atraumatic needling of biopsy material may be repeated as often as necessary without inconvenience or damage to the patient (7, 14). Punctures of the tumor and of the adjacent tissue make it possible to define the outline and growth rate of circumscribed carcinomas. Sequential punctures may also help to monitor therapeutic effects on tumor tissue. Hormone-sensitive carcinomas, for example, will show marked cellular dystrophy after a short period of estrogen therapy (Fig. 6), occasionally with emphasis on metaplasia of squamous epithelium or with glycogen storage (1-3, 9). Autoradiography and ferment-cytochemical examination have successfully contributed to the diagnosis of these cases (8, 20).

ZAJICEK (24) was at first reluctant to adopt aspiration biopsy cytology as a screening method for the detection of latent prostate carcinomas. His opinion was plausible for carcinomas of merely focal manifestation inside an organ of great volume and otherwise normal appearance. On the other hand, the occasion for "screening" the prostate is given whenever minimal palpatory findings require diagnostic assessment. The prostate is in fact a small organ to be readily covered by aspiration biopsy in most of its parts. Unlike the so-called cell-constant organs, the prostate is under endocrine control, with enhanced cell regeneration and generalized reactions. Here carcinomatous development allows the definition of characteristic prestages, and this organ appears to be an adequate model for a well-trained team to study aspiration biopsy as a screening technique.

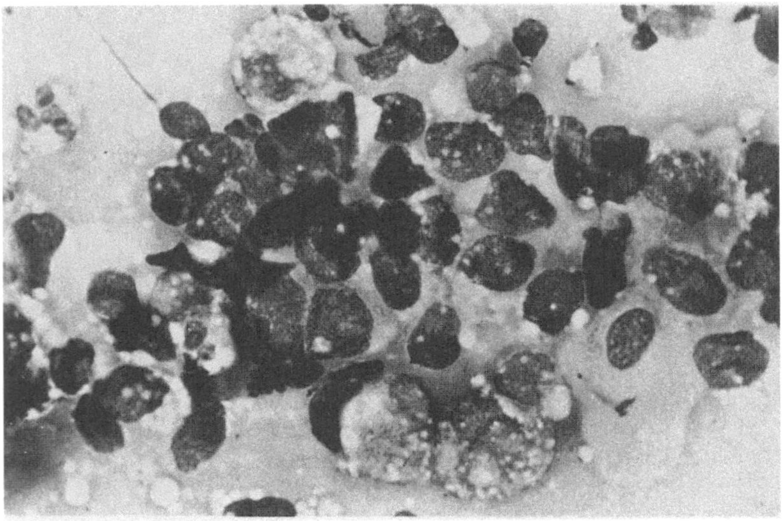

*Fig. 6. Carcinomatous epithelium of prostate. Severe dystrophy after estrogen therapy. (Aspiration biopsy, dry fixation, May-Grünwald-Giemsa) Patient aged 55. x 600*

We found that aspiration biopsy techniques could be mastered satisfactorily by urologists after some 50 test punctures; from that point on, even negative results would be reliable. Correct interpretation of aspiration cytologic preparations requires the histodiagnostic experience of several years and calls for close cooperation with the clinician.


## SUMMARY

Fine needle aspiration biopsy cytology allows safe morphologic tumor diagnosis in the prostate based on cytologic and histologic criteria. Specific technical difficulties of the procedure are not greater than in surgical pathology. The standardized equipment developed by FRANZÉN is recommended. Aspiration biopsy is atraumatic and without complications. The method introduces a new clinical approach to the application of recent advances in cell research. Among other improvements, aspiration biopsy may falicitate cytologic classification of prostate carcinoma. The method should be adapted to screening programs.


## REFERENCES


1. Alken, C.E., Dhom, G., Hohbach, M., Sachse, D., Schröder, F.H., Straube, W.: Therapie des Prostatacarcinoms und Verlaufskontrolle. Urologe A 11, 216-220 (1972)
2. Alken, C.E., Dhom, G., Straube, W., Braun, J.S., Kopper, B., Rehker, H.: Therapie des Prostata-Carcinoms und Verlaufskontrolle (III). Urologe A 14, 112-116 (1975)
3. Alken, C.E., Dhom, G., Straube, W., Schmidt-Hermes, H.J., Moormann, J.G., Moeller, J.F.: Therapie des Prostata-Carcinoms und Verlaufskontrolle (II). Urologe A 12, 191-197 (1973)
4. Altman, H.W., Müller, H.A.: Grundlagen der Karyologie. Verh. dtsch. Ges. Path. 57, 2-33 (1973)
5. Andersson, L., Jönsson, G., Brunk, U.: Puncture biopsy of the prostate in the diagnosis of prostatic cancer. Scand. J. Urol. Nephrol. 1, 227-234 (1967)
6. Ekmann, H., Hedberg, K., Persson, P.S.: Cytological versus histological examination of needle biopsy specimens in the diagnosis of prostatic cancer. Brit. J. Urol. 39, 544-548 (1967)
7. Engzell, U., Esposti, P.L., Rubio, C., Sigurdson, A., Zajicek, J.: Investigation on tumor spread in connection with aspiration biopsy. Acta radiol. {Ther.} (Stockh.) 10, 385-398 (1971)
8. Esposti, P.L.: Cytologic diagnosis of prostatic tumors with the aid of transrectal aspiration biopsy. A critical review of 1,110 cases and a report of morphologic and cytochemical studies. Acta cytol. (Baltimore) 10, 182-186 (1966)
9. Esposti, P.L.: Cytologic malignancy grading of prostatic carcinoma by transrectal aspiration biopsy. A five-year follow-up study of 469 hormonal treated patients. Scand. J. Urol. Nephrol. 5, 199-209 (1971)
10. Faul, P., Klosterhalfen, H., Schmidt, E.: Erfahrung mit der Feinnadelbiopsie (Saug- bzw. Aspirationsbiopsie nach Franzén) der Prostata. Urologe A 10, 120-126 (1971)
11. Faul, P., Praetorius, M.: Die cytologische Diagnose des Prostatacarcinoms und seine verschiedenen Malignitätsgrade. Urologe A 12, 259-267 (1973)

12. Franzén, S., Giertz, G., Zajicek, J.: Cytological diagnosis of prostatic tumours by transrectal aspiration biopsy: A preliminary report. Brit. J. Urol. 32, 193-196 (1960)
13. Kastendieck, H., Altennähr, E., Burchardt, P.: Elektronenmikroskopische Untersuchungen zur Zelldifferenzierung in Prostatacarcinomen. Virchows Arch. A 361, 241-256 (1973)
14. Kaulen, H., Davidts, H.H., Albrecht, K.F., Liebegott, G.: Die besonderen Vorteile der Aspirationszytologie beim Prostatacarcinom aus klinischer Sicht. Verh. dtsch. Ges. Path. 57, 313-314 (1973)
15. Linsk, J.A., Axilrod, H.D., Solyn, R., Delaverdac, C.: Transrectal cytologic aspiration in the diagnosis of prostatic carcinoma. J. Urol. (Baltimore) 108, 455-459 (1972)
16. McNeal, J.E.: Age related changes in prostatic epithelium associated with carcinoma. In: Some Aspects of the Aetiology and Biochemistry of Prostatic Cancer. Griffiths, K., Pierrepoint, C.G. (eds.) Third Tenovus Workshop, Cardiff, 1970
17. Miller, A., Seljelid, R.: Cellular atypia in the prostate. Scand. J. Urol. Nephrol. 5, 17-21 (1971)
18. Müller, H.A.: Das Erscheinungsbild des Prostatacarcinoms in succedanen Saug- und Stanzbiopsien. Verh. dtsch. Ges. Path. 57, 329-333 (1973)
19. Okada, K.: Ultrastructural changes of the prostatic cancer cells by castration. Jap. J. Urol. 57, 803-821 (1966)
20. Rabes, H., Faul, P.: Bestimmung der Proliferationsaktivität von menschlichen Prostatapunktaten durch Thymidin-$^3$H-Autoradiographie. Verh. dtsch. Ges. Path. 57, 318-322 (1973)
21. Staehler, W., Ziegler, H., Völtert, D., Schubert, G.E.: Zytodiagnostik der Prostata. Grundriß und Atlas. Stuttgart-New York: Schattauer, 1975
22. Thoenes, W.: Zytoplasmatische Aspekte der Onkozytologie. Verh. dtsch. Ges. Path. 57, 61-81 (1973)
23. Zajicek, J.: Transrectale Aspirationsbiopsie der Prostatatumoren. Verh. dtsch. Ges. Path. 57, 148-150 (1973)
24. Zajicek, J.: Aspiration Biopsy Cytology. Part 1, Cytology of Supradiaphragmatic Organs. Basel: Karger, 1974

# Prognosis of Prostatic Carcinoma

G. T. Mellinger

Approximately 15 years ago the Veterans Administration Cooperative Urological Research Group began a controlled, randomized, prospective study and comparison of various treatments for prostatic carcinoma. Our staging system is shown below (Table 1):

Table 1. VACURG staging system

| Stage | Rectal examination | Serum prostatic Acid phosphatase | Distant metastases (X-ray or biopsy) |
|---|---|---|---|
| I | No palpable tumor | Normal[a] | None |
| II | Palpable nodule | Normal | None |
| III | Local extension outside prostate | Normal | None |
| IV | Any findings | Elevated and/or | Present |

[a] Normal ≤ 1.0 King-Armstrong units/100 ml.

<u>STAGE I</u> - Normal prostatic acid phosphatase level (≤10.0 King-Armstrong units); no X-ray or bone scan evidence of metastases; rectal examination showing no positive evidence of carcinoma of the prostate. Diagnosis is made only on the basis of tissue removed during biopsy or prostatectomy.

<u>STAGE II</u> - Normal prostatic acid phosphatase level (≤1.0 King-Armstrong units); no X-ray or bone scan evidence of carcinoma, but without evidence of extension beyond the boundaries of the prostate or into the seminal vesicle, as determined by rectal examination.

<u>STAGE III</u> - Normal prostatic acid phosphatase level (≤1.0 King-Armstrong); no X-ray or bone scan evidence of osseous metastases, but with evidence of spread to contiguous tissues, as determined by rectal examination.

<u>STAGE IV</u> - An elevated prostatic acid phosphatase level (>1.0 King-Armstrong units) and/ or X-ray or bone scan demonstration of osseous metastases, or positive biopsy of any distant tissue. This group also may or may not show evidence of local extension beyond the prostate.

Study I admitted 2313 patients from 1960 through 1967. In stage I and II patients we compared radical prostatectomy plus placebo with radical prostatectomy plus 5.0 mg of stilbestrol daily.

Stage III and stage IV patients were randomized into four treatment groups: those given 5.0 mg of stilbestrol per day, those treated by orchidectomy alone, those receiving 5.0 mg of stilbestrol per day plus orchidectomy, and those given a placebo. Analysis of response to therapy (3, 8, 9) showed that 5.0 mg of stilbestrol daily reduced the cancer death rate significantly (Fig. 1), but was associated with a significant increase in cardiovascular deaths which more than offset the reduced mortality. Cardiovascular deaths included those due to myocardial infarction, congestive heart failure, pulmonary embolism, and cerebrovascular accidents. Biopsy specimens of prostatic tissue from 1294 patients in Prostatic Carcinoma Study I were graded histologically for analysis.

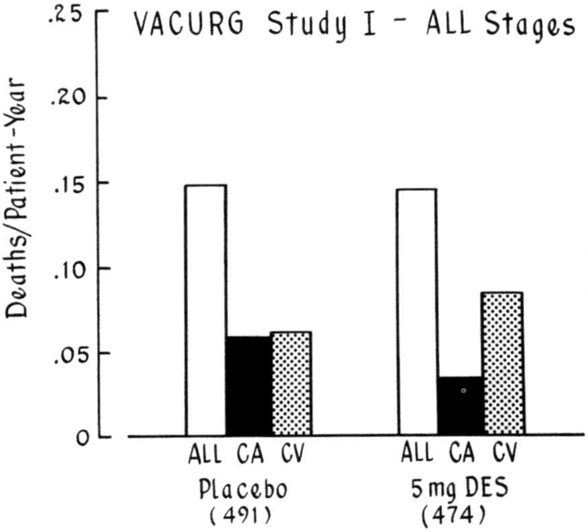


*Fig. 1. Deaths/patient year: Study I - all stages*

Study II admitted 561 patients from 1967 to 1969 and in this study patients with stage I or stage II carcinomas were randomized between treatment with radical prostatectomy or no treatment. There has been no significant difference in the survival of these two groups, but the groups are small and the length of follow-up has been relatively short.

In stage III and stage IV patients, 1.0 mg of stilbestrol daily seemed as effective as 5.0 mg daily in controlling cancers (Fig. 2) without the disadvantages incurred with the larger dosage. The cardiovascular death rate was no higher among the patients receiving 1.0 mg of stilbestrol daily than it was among patients on placebo or 0.2 mg of stilbestrol. However, 1.0 mg of stilbestrol daily was much more effective in reducing cancer mortality (5)

Of 561 patients admitted to study II, 541 tumors were graded histologically.

Prostatic Carcinoma Study III was begun in 1969, and at present patients are still being admitted into this study. Stage I and stage II patients are randomized to no treatment or to radical prostatectomy as they were in study II, if they are judged able to tolerate radical prostatectomy. However, if patients are either too old or too ill to tolerate the operation, or if they refuse surgery, then they are assigned at random to placebo or to 1.0 mg of stilbestrol daily.

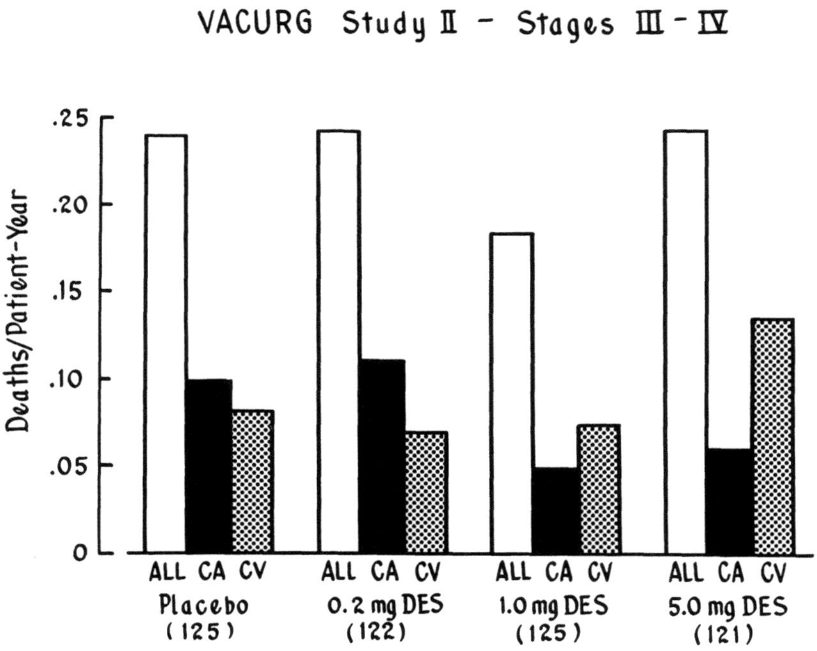


*Fig. 2. Deaths/patient year: Study I - stages III and IV*

For stage III and stage IV patients, therapy is randomized to 1.0 mg of stilbestrol per day, or 2.5 mg of Premarin per day, or 30 mg of Provera per day, or 30 mg of Provera plus 1.0 mg of stilbestrol per day.

At present, the period of observation has been too short for significant differences in survival to be noted. Histologic grading is available for all 1077 patients from this continuing study III, and for approximately 2911 patients from all studies combined, for correlation with follow-up data. A rotating evaluation committee determines the cause of each patient's death on the basis of the clinical record, and evaluation summary by the local investigator, the death certificate, and an autopsy, when such is performed. In all cases the original histologic diagnosis is made by the local pathologist and is confirmed by the research group's referee pathologist, Dr. Donald GLEASON of Minneapolis, Minn.

The histologic grading system which the Veterans Administration Cooperative Urological Research Group uses was devised by GLEASON (1, 6). This grading system considers only the degree of glandular differentiation and the growth pattern of the tumor in relation to the prostate stroma. The grading is performed under low magnification and can be performed rapidly on small biopsy specimens. Approximately 60% of the cases were graded on the basis of needle biopsy only. This system separates cancer of the prostate into five patterns.

Pattern 1 (Fig. 3a) is very well differentiated, the tumor consisting of single, separate, round to oval glands which are quite uniform in size. They grow abnormally in closely packed, roughly rounded masses with definitely limited edges. Pattern 1 was seen in 3.5% of the cases.

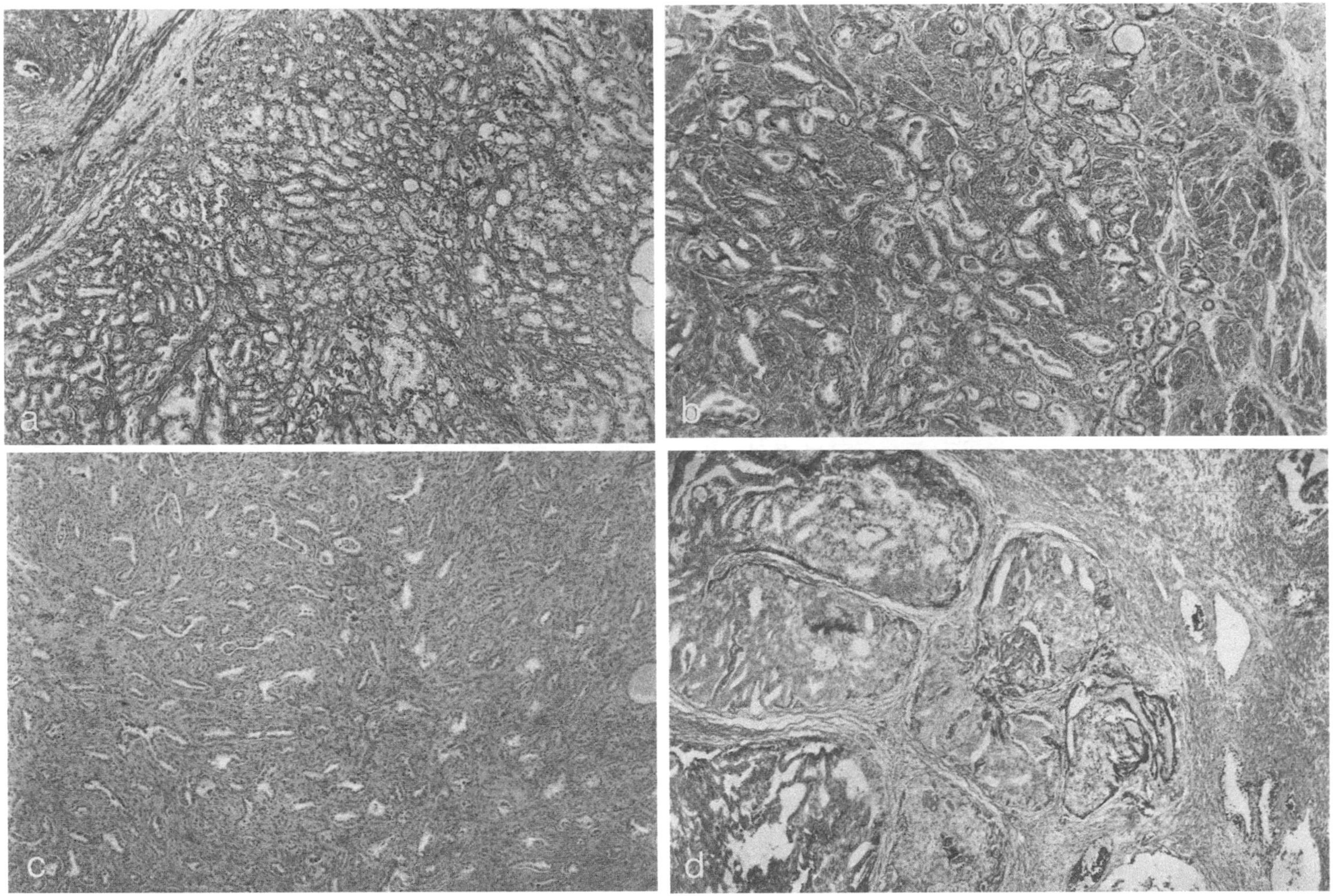

*Fig. 3a-d.* (a) Category 1; (b) Category 2; (c) Category 3; (d) Category 3

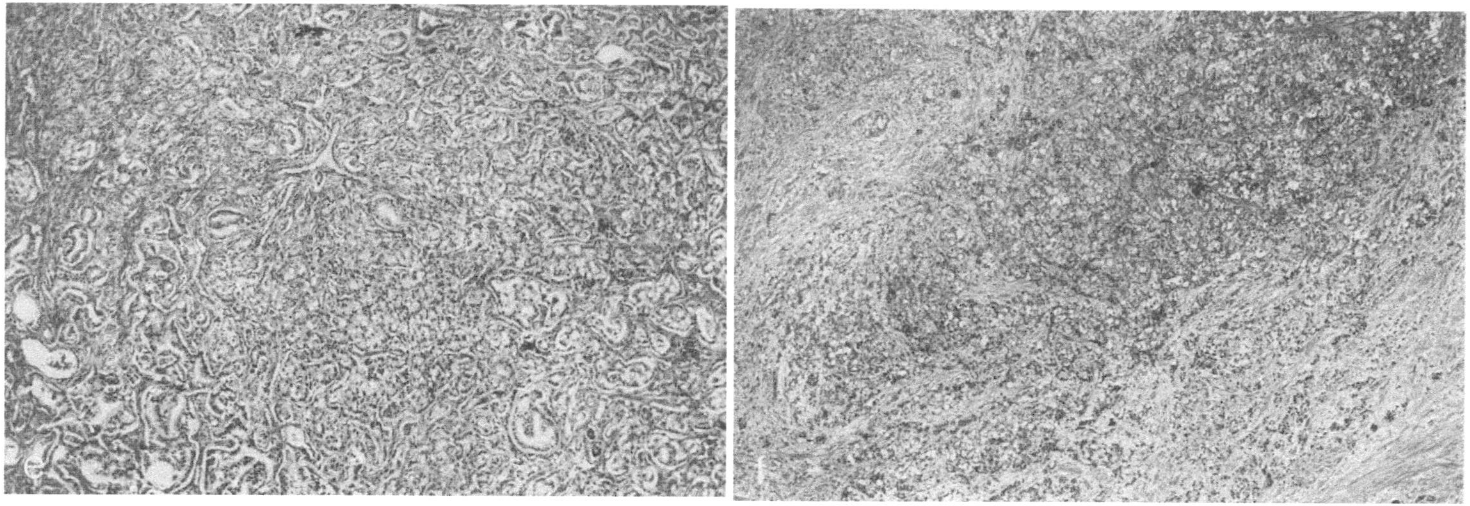

*Fig. 3e and f. (e) Category 4; (f) Category 5*

Pattern 2 (Fig. 3b) is well differentiated and consists of single, separate, round to oval glands which are similar in size and shape to those in pattern 1, but with more variation. Also, there is more stromal spacing between the glands in pattern 2, and the tumor masses are less well circumscribed and are not as definitely rounded as in pattern 1. Pattern 2 was seen in 24.4% of the cases.

Pattern 3 is moderately differentiated. This is the most common pattern, and includes two distinctive appearances. The first (Fig. 3c) is an extension of patterns 1 and 2, with single, separate glands which may be much smaller than those in patterns 1 and 2. Some of the glands may be much larger, or about the same size as those in patterns 1 and 2. The individual glands are much more irregular in size and shape than in patterns 1 and 2, many being more elongated or angular. They may be more closely packed together, but more commonly they are separated by stroma. The areas of tumor are usually quite irregular in outline, without a clearly definable boundary. Larger glands may have some papillary infoldings or a thick epithelium containing tiny glandular lumina. These latter appearances provide the transition to the second distinctive appearance observed in pattern 3 (Fig. 3d), which is the occurrence of sharply circumscribed masses of papillary and cribriform tumor. These vary in size and may be quite large, but the essential feature is the smooth and usually rounded edge around all the circumscribed masses of tumor. Any or all of these patterns may appear in one patient. They may be tiny glands, large irregular glands, and sharply circumscribed papillary and cribriform masses. All are included under the designation of pattern 3, which was seen in 87.7% of the tumors.

Pattern 4 is poorly differentiated. This tumor consists of irregular masses of fused glands (Fig. 3e). That is, the glands are not single and separate, but coalesce and branch. The fusion may be so extreme that it appears as solid masses of epithelium containing multiple glandular lumina lined by poorly oriented layers of polygonal cells. Some cells may have two areas facing separate rounded gland spaces. The multiple glandular lumina are usually of small or medium size. In contrast to the sharply circumscribed and smoothly rounded masses in pattern 3, the pattern 4 tumors grow in very raggedly outlined masses which seem to infiltrate the stroma very aggressively. Also included are similar tumors closely resembling hypernephroma. Pattern 4 was noted in 12.1% of cases.

Pattern 5 (Fig. 3f) is very poorly differentiated. Here the tumor shows minimal glandular differentiation and consists of raggedly infiltrating masses of epithelial cells with only poorly-formed, tiny, glandular lumina appearing something like the comedocarcinoma of the breast. Pattern 5 was seen in 22.6% of cases. The percentages here add up to 150% because about 50 per cent of the tumors showed at least two different patterns. Since the classification does not consider cytologic details, these patterns can be shown schematically in a samplified drawing (Fig. 4) made by GLEASON. It is based entirely on the microscopic outline of the tumor tissue and its relation to the uninvolved prostate. All of the black in the drawing represents tumor glands and tumor tissue with all of the cellular detail obscured.

When two different patterns were definitely present, they were recorded as two different patterns, with the pattern most extensive in area being described as the primary pattern, and the less extensive in area being described as the secondary pattern. The two patterns were recorded as two digits: for example, 2-3 indicated a tumor with more than 50% of pattern 2 and less than 50% of pattern 3. Likewise, a tumor designated 5-4 contained more than 50% of pattern 5 and less than 50% of pattern 4.

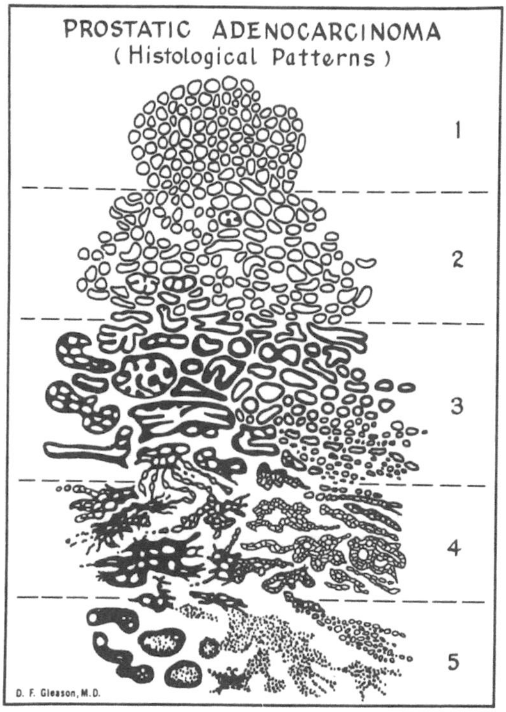


*Fig. 4. Diagram of histologic patterns of prostatic adenocarcinoma*

For uniformity, two digits were recorded for tumors with only one histologic pattern, so that a tumor showing only pattern 3 was recorded as 3-3. To measure biological malignancy, the death rate was employed i.e., deaths per patient year of follow-up. The total follow-up time for the 2911 patients who were studied histologically is 9730.4 years, ranging from zero to 14 years per patient. Mortality rates were calculated for patient groups according to their primary histologic patterns, and then calculated according to their secondary histologic patterns. Strong correlation was found between the mortality rates and the primary pattern, and there was a very similar, although somewhat weaker, correlation with the secondary patterns. Of course, both correlations were stronger when only deaths due to cancer included in the numerators. Then we added together the primary pattern and the secondary pattern numbers, and this was designated as the patient's pattern score. Stronger and more regular correlation was found between mortality rate and this pattern score than between mortality rate and any other histologic scale. In addition, we found that the observed death rate correlated well with the tumor grades and various tumor-related clinical findings noted in the initial pretreatment examinations of the patients. For example, there was strong correlation between the histologic score and the presence of identifiable metastases, pain due to cancer, dilation of the upper urinary tract, and abnormal elevation of the serum prostatic acid phosphatase level. When the patients were grouped according to their clinical stages (Fig. 5), histologic grading still showed strong correlation with mortality rates within the clinical stages, and the death rates associated with the histologic pattern scores showed overlapping of death rates between the clinical stages. As an example, stage I and stage II patients with high histologic scores had higher death rates than stage IV patients with low histologic scores. This indicated that histologic grading had predictive

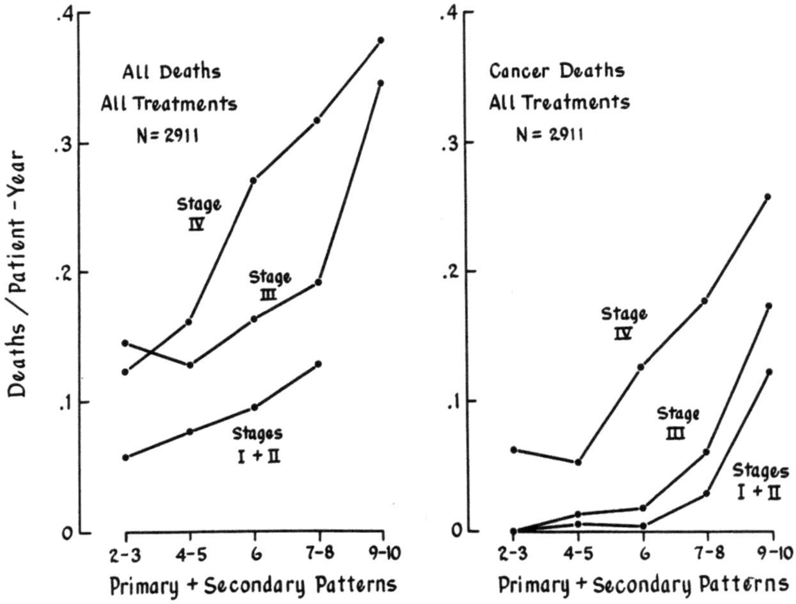


*Fig. 5. Deaths/patient year classified by primary and secondary histologic pattern and clinical stage*

power additional to that provided by clinical staging and suggested that combining grading and staging would given even stronger predictive discrimination. Therefore, the numerical values of the primary and secondary patterns and the values of the clinical stage were simply added together. However, stage IV required a weighting value of 5 rather than 4. This combined grading and staging score was designated as the "category", which could be from 3 to 15. For example, stage I, value 1, plus primary pattern 1, value 1, plus secondary pattern 1, value 1, equals 3. Again stage IV (weighted as 5), value 5, plus primary pattern 5, value 5, plus secondary pattern 5, value 5, equals 15.

Calculation of mortality rates for each category (Fig. 6) yielded very strong correlations for all deaths, and particularly for cancer deaths. It is noteworthy that no cancer deaths occurred in categories 3, 4, and 5, and that the cancer death rates were very slow in categories 6 and 7.

Categories formed by combining grading and staging also revealed differences in response to stilbestrol therapy (Fig. 7). The patients in category 9 and higher showed a definite reduction in cancer death rates if they had received 1.0 mg or more of stilbestrol daily, in comparison with patients who had received placebo or only 0.2 mg of stilbestrol per day.

Some information on the natural history of untreated carcinoma of the prostate is provided by the total death rates and the cancer death rates for patients on placebo or 0.2 mg of stilbestrol. The very low death rates and the absence of any response to treatment in the lower categories suggest that some of the patients in these groups should not be subjected to any hazardous treatment. Certainly patients in categories 3, 4, and 5, who had no cancer deaths, fall into such a

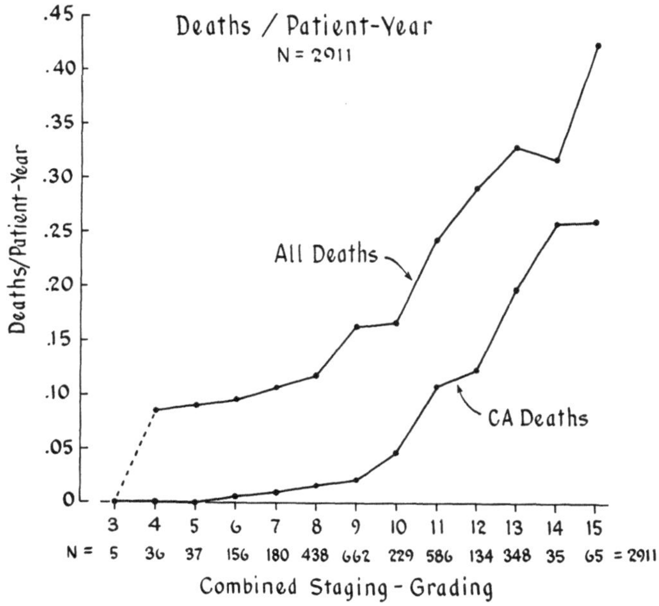


*Fig. 6. Deaths/patient year as related to combined staging and grading*

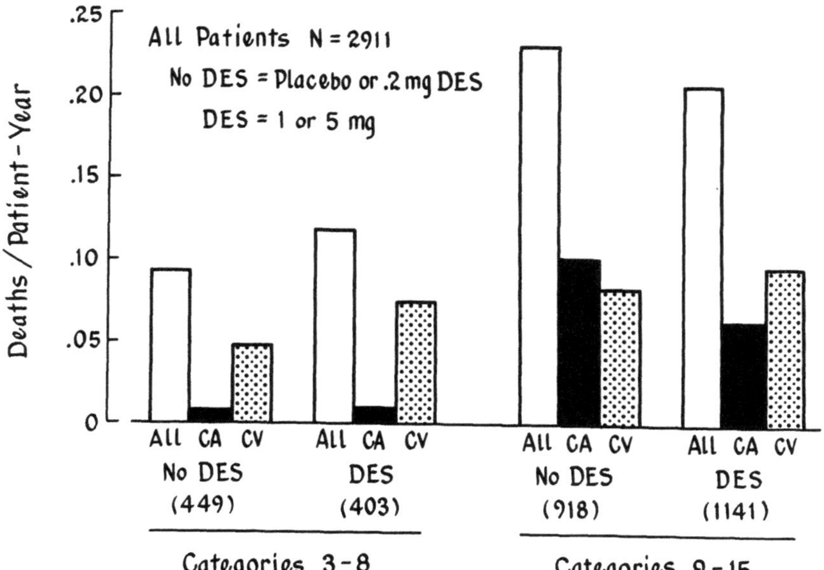


*Fig. 7. Causes of death and treatment separated by histologic categories*

group, and we feel that these limits of that group can be extended (Fig. 8). Cancer death rates and total death rates show a definite upward slope in categories 8, 9, and 10. There were no detectable benifits from stilbestrol therapy in 29% of the patients who were in categories 3 to 8. Also, in categories 3 to 8 the cancer death rate was about 1 cancer death per 111 patients as compared with a death rate 9 times as cancer death in 12 patients, per year, for patients in categories 9 to 15.

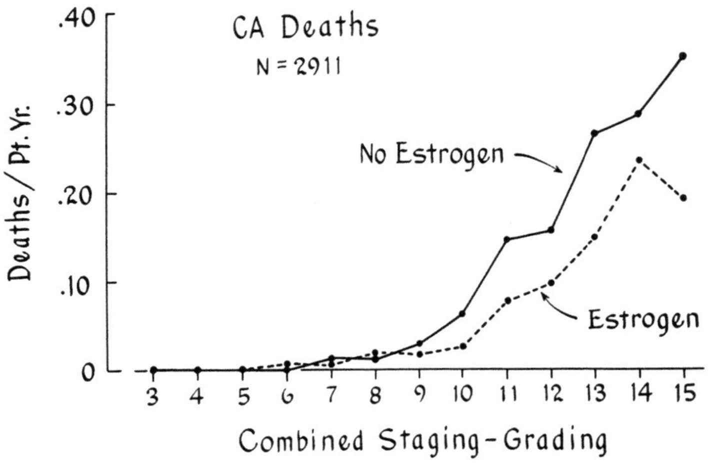


*Fig. 8. Cancer deaths/patient year and combined staging and grading*

Separation of patients into two groups (categories 3 to 8, and categories 9 to 15) emphasizes the lower death rates and the absence of any response to therapy in the group comprised of the lower categories. The increased cardiovascular mortality and total mortality in the treated group probably would be greatly lessened by giving no treatment at all. In the group made up of the higher categories, the cancer death rate of the patients on placebo or 0.2 mg of stilbestrol is 9 times as high as that of the comparable group of lower categories, but the cancer death rate is still significantly reduced in the higher-category group which received 1.0 mg or 5.0 mg of stilbestrol daily.

These data confirm conclusively that the spectrum of histologic patterns in adenocarcinoma of the prostate is strongly correlated with its spectrum of biological malignancy. Our data show that the histologic grades of the tumors are strongly correlated with the incidence of metastases, with elevated serum prostatic acid phosphatase, with pain due to cancer, and with the subsequently observed death rates. The question as to whether tumor histology changes over a period of time is important, but we cannot answer that question now. Our studies did not include systematic re-biopsies. However, the small number of repeat biopsies which is available suggests that many of the tumors retain their initial microscopic appearance for long periods of time, even though these biopsies are heavily biased toward those patients whose cancers are progressive clinically. Our data suggest, but do not prove, that the majority of prostatic carcinomas have a definite pattern of histology and a definite pattern of malignancy, and that these are maintained for long periods of time. The long survivals and rare cancer deaths found in the presence of the low-grade tumors would not be expected if there were frequent and inexorable progression to higher grades of malignancy.

There are other variables which seem to relate to the patient's prognosis, and a few will be mentioned briefly. The 17-hydroxycorticosteroids, like the corticosteroid-binding globulins, show a dose-related response to diethylstilbestrol (2, 4). A detailed analysis has shown that the initial value of the 17-hydroxycorticosteroids provides useful information as to prognosis. In general, the higher their initial value, the worse is the prognosis. The 17-hydroxycorticosteroid levels do not predict the cause of death; instead they are useful in predicting death from all causes combined. From this, and for many other reasons, it appears that the serum level of the 17-hydroxycorticosteroids represents a generalized measure of stress. Cholesterol levels have been measured quite carefully, but have not been found useful in forecasting prognosis. However, serum triglycerides have shown the paradoxical result that the prognosis is worse if the levels are in the normal range than if they are either above or below normal. We are trying to study this peculiar finding in more detail.

Another variable which affects survival is the extent of metastases detectable by X-ray. The extent of metastases in each of eight major sites was estimated on a four-point scale. Analysis of data recorded (7) in that manner for 103 patients with metastases demonstrable at the time of diagnosis showed that these eight sites were involved in this order: ilium, 83%; pubis and ischium, 78%; lumbosacral spine, 71%; thoracic spine, 60%; rib, 53%; femur, 48%; shoulder, 39%, and lung, 24%. In addition, there was positive correlation between the height of the serum prostatic acid phosphatase level and the number of sites involved. Because the various sites correlated highly with the presence of metastases, prognostic groups could be constructed, using the extent of involvement in only three sites with little loss of information. Those chosen to yield the best predictions were lung, pubis and ischium, and femur. Based on the findings at these three sites, risk groups were constructed and theoretical curves were drawn. These were compared to the actuarial curves observed for these patients, and these curves were in good agreement with the mathematical model for samples of these sizes, and showed remarkable differences pointing to the probability of death due to prostatic cancer as a function of the extent of metastatic involvement.

## SUMMARY

A 15-year controlled, randomized, prospective study of 2911 patients by the Veterans Administration Cooperative Urological Research Group compares various treatments for prostatic carcinoma, and employs a staging system that separates the carcinomas into five patterns. Values are assigned to specific patterns, and stronger correlation is found between these pattern scores and mortality than with any other histologic scale. Strong correlation exists between pattern score and clinical stages yielded categories with numerical values of 3 through 15, which give even higher predictive discrimination. In categories 3 through 8, low mortality and lack of response to therapy suggest increased cardiovascular and total mortality might be less with no treatment at all. In categories 9 through 15, the use of 1.0 mg of stilbestrol daily is accompanied by a significantly lower cardiovascular death rate, thus reducing the disadvantages encountered with a dose of 5.0 mg of stilbestrol per day.

The spectrum of histologic patterns in adenocarcinoma of the prostate is strongly correlated with its spectrum of biological malignancy and its manifestations. Long survivals and rare cancer deaths found in the presence of low-grade tumors suggest that tumors possibly may retain their initial microscopic appearance over long periods of time. Others variables relating to prognosis are discussed briefly. Prognostic groups contructed on the basis of metastases at three sites, and theoretical and actuarial curves drawn, show differences pointing to the probability of death due to prostatic carcinoma as a function of the extent of metastatic involvement.

REFERENCES


1. Bailar, J.C., Mellinger, G.T., Gleason, D.F.: Survival rates of patients with prostatic cancer, tumor stage and differentiation - preliminary report. Cancer Chemother. Rep. 50, 129-136 (1966)
2. Blackard, C.E., Byar, D.P., Seal, U.S., Doe, R.P., Veterans Administration Cooperative Urological Research Group: Correlation of pretreatment serum non-protein bound cortisol and total 17-hydroxycorticosteroid values with survival in patients with prostatic cancer. New Engl. J. Med. 291, 751-755 (Oct., 1974)
3. Blackard, J.C., Doe, R.P., Mellinger, G.T., Byar, D.P.: Incidence of cardiovascular disease in patients receiving diethylstilbestrol for carcinoma of the prostate. Cancer (Philad.) 26, 249-256 (1970)
4. Blackard, J.C., Byar, D.P., Seal, U.S., Doe, R.P., Veterans Administration Cooperative Urological Research Group: Correlation of pre-treatment serum 17-hydroxycorticosteroid values with survival in patients with prostatic cancer. J. Urol. (Baltimore) 113, 517-520 (April, 1975)
5. Byar, D.P.: The Veterans Administration Cooperative Urological Research Group's studies of cancer of the prostate. Cancer (Philad.) 32, 1126-1130 (1973)
6. Gleason, D.F.: Classification of prostatic carcinomas. Cancer Chemother. Rep. 50, 125-128 (1966)
7. Hovsepian, J.A., Byar, D.P., Veterans Administration Cooperative Urological Research Group: Carcinoma of the prostate: Correlation between radiologic quantitation of metastases and patient survival. Urology 6, 11-16 (1975)
8. Veterans Administration Cooperative Urological Research Group: Carcinoma of the prostate: Treatment comparisons. J. Urol. (Baltimore) 98, 590-594 (1964)
9. Veterans Administration Cooperative Urological Research Group: Treatment and survival of patients with cancer of the prostate. Surg. Gynec. Obstet. 124, 1011-1017 (1967)

# Estramustine Phosphate Therapy in Carcinoma of the Prostate

L. ANDERSSON, F. EDSMYR, G. JÖNSSON, and I. KÖNYVES

Estramustine phosphate in the treatment of prostatic carcinoma was introduced in 1966. The substance is an estradiol-17-β-phosphate which is esterified with nor nitrogen mustard as a carbamate. It has become known under the trade name Estracyt.

Nitrogen mustard in the therapy of carcinoma was used for the first time in 1942. Due to the systemic toxicity of this category of substances, mainly in the bone marrow and the gastrointestinal epithelium efforts have been made to link the nitrogen mustard with some carrier substance with could direct the drug to the tumour tissue where it could hopefully exert its effect locally. Estrogen receptors have been demonstrated in the cytoplasm of prostatic cells in various species, including man. By linking nitrogen mustard with an estrogen, it was hoped to direct the compound to the prostate, to achieve a tumoricidal effect locally without too severe systemic reaction and possibly even an additional estrogenic effect on the carcinoma.

By giving $^{3}$H- and $^{14}$C-labelled estramustine phosphate to patients about to undergo prostatectomy and then analyzing tissue specimens removed during the operation it has been demonstrated that an accumulation of the substance occurs in the prostate.

The mode of action of estramustine phosphate is incompletely elucidated. Epithelial proliferation and activity in the prostate are known to be dependent on dihydrotestosterone. Estramustine phosphate has been found to inhibit the activity of 5α-reductase and thereby the transformation of testosterone to dihydrotestosterone in the prostate in the rat (4) and in the dog (1).

There is preliminary evidence that estramustine phosphate blocks steroid hormone receptors in the prostate (4). The implication of this on the treatment of carcinoma is not known so far.

Estramustine phosphate has also been proved to give systemic effects. JÖNSSON et al. (3) observed a marked decrease of FSH and LH in plasma as well as of plasma testosterone in patients on estramustine therapy. However, the drug has been found to have weak estrogenic properties with a uterotropic effect about 100 times weaker than estradiol (2).

## DOSAGE

Estramustine phosphate was first used in a methyl glucamine salt solution for intravenous injection, but is now also available in a disodium salt compound for oral administration.

The usual dosage for intravenous therapy has been 300-600 mg per day for 3 weeks. If the patient improved treatment was continued with the same dose once or twice weekly for about 2 months. After this initial treatment period the patients received injections once or twice weekly for periods of 4-8 weeks by treatment-free intervals of various lengths.

Estracyt capsules were, as a rule, given in a total daily dose of 560-840 mg, divided in two doses.

## SELECTION OF PATIENTS

In the majority of cases estramustine phosphate was used as a kind of last resort therapy. JÖNSSON and coworkers, who introduced this kind of treatment, have recently (7) listed their criteria for starting estramustine phosphate therapy as follows:

1. Prostatic carcinoma not responsive to conventional therapy
2. Far-advanced tumor growing rapidly and most often undifferentiated
3. A life expectancy of less than 6 months.

## CLINICAL MATERIAL

Until March 1975, 23 publications had appeared reporting on 466 patients treated with estramustine phosphate for carcinoma of the prostate in open clinical trials (Table 1). As is seen from the table the majority of the patients had had previous estrogenic hormone therapy, but had either been nonresponsive or had developed so-called secondary resistance to this form of therapy. The number of patients on intravenous and on oral treatment was about equal. Fifty of the patients on oral treatment had an initial 3-week course of intravenous injections.

Of the 466 patients 82% were in stage IV according to the Veterans Administration Cooperative Urological Research Group classification (1964), i.e., they had skeletal and/or soft tissue metastases or increased acid phosphatase activity or both. Many of the patients were in a very bad condition and bedridden because of skeletal pain and sometimes uremia.

Table 1. Clinical results of Estracyt on prostatic carcinoma

| Route of administration | Previous estrogen-therapy | | Previously untreated | | Total | |
|---|---|---|---|---|---|---|
| | No of patients | Positive responses | No of patients | Positive responses | No of patients | Positive responses |
| Intravenous | 217 | 135 | 28 | 24 | 245 | 159 |
| Oral | 185 | 88 | 36 | 29 | 221 | 117 |
| Total | 402 | 223 (55%) | 64 | 53 (83%) | 466 | 276 (59%) |

## RESULTS

The clinical response to therapy was considered satisfactory if the patients noticed disappearance of metastatic pain, and definite improvement of performance status, and if there was regression of metastases and/or significant reduction of the primary tumor mass with consequent relief of urinary tract obstruction.

As seen in Table 1 there was an overall favourable response in 59% of the 466 patients. The frequency of positive results was significantly higher (83%) in the 64 patients who had estramustine phosphate as the initial therapy than in those 402 patients (55%) who had been on previous estrogen therapy.

Regression of pulmonary or other kind of soft tissue metastases was reported to occur more often than regression of skeletal lesions (7). In our material we observed a number of patients who had a remarkable disappearance of skeletal pain and simultaneous recalcification of osteolytic bone lesions, which should be considered a slowing up of the tumor progression in the bone tissue.

As with other forms of therapy in carcinoma of the prostate, a relationship was observed between normalization of an increased acid phosphatase activity and good clinical response (6).

In all objective responders there was a good subjective improvement. In an additional group of patients there was a subjective response with pain relief and increased well-being without it being possible to record any objective change.

If a patient had a favourable reaction to estramustine phosphate this usually occurred within 2-3 weeks or in any case within 2 months. MITTELMAN et al. (5) observed no relationship between positive response to estramustine phosphate and previous response to estrogen therapy or orchidectomy nor to duration of the disease prior to estramustine phosphate therapy. In their material more than half of the responders benefited for 6 months or more.

## SIDE-EFFECTS

The side-effects in the total material of 466 patients are reported in Table 2. Most common were gastrointestinal troubles, nausea and vomiting, mainly following oral administration, bone-marrow suppression and disturbance of liver function. The bone-marrow suppression was reversible in all cases except one. As a rule treatment was continued with a lower dosage. In the categories thrombophlebitis, liver disturbance, and gastrointestinal symptoms, treatment was interrupted in some of the cases.

### The Stockholm Estracyt Oral Clinical Trial

In the joint material of 466 patients on estramustine phosphate the frequency of positive response in the previously untreated group was not only higher than in the other group but also higher than has been reported in most series on ordinary estrogen therapy. For this reason

Table 2. Side-effects of Estracyt administration

| Side-effects | Route of administration | | Total (466 patients) |
|---|---|---|---|
| | Intravenous (245 patients) | Oral (221 patients) | |
| Suppression of bone marrow | 18 | 8 | 26 |
| Thrombophlebitis | 20% | 1 | |
| Venous thrombosis | - | 1 | 1 |
| Liver disturbances | 9 | 20 | 29 |
| Precordial pains | - | 2 | 2 |
| Gastrointestinal symptoms | 17 | 48 | 65 |
| Gynecomastia | few | 5 | |
| Drug allergy | 4 | 1 | 5 |
| Oedema | 1 | - | 1 |

we decided to start a randomized, prospective study comparing oral estramustine phosphate with estrogenic hormones in the primary treatment of prostatic carcinoma. Four hospital departments in Stockholm are participating in the investigation.

The trial includes patients in tumor stages II-IV and carcinoma of high and medium differentiation. The poorly differentiated carcinomas are excluded, because they are at present involved in another clinical trial.

The patients are randomized for one of the following alternatives of therapy.

1. Oral estramustine phosphate 840 mg/day
2. Intramuscular polyestradiol phosphate 80 mg monthly + oral ethinyl estradiol 2 mg/day for two weeks and thereafter 150 µg/day.

The trial started in October 1974. At present 21 patients have been observed for 6 months or more. The material is too small and the observation period too short to permit any conclusions as to the results of treatment. One observation, however, has already been striking. The frequency of gynecomastia is different in the two groups. Gynecomastia was observed in 5/11 patients on polyestradiol phosphate and ethinyl estradiol, but in none of the 10 patients given estramustine phosphate.

SUMMARY

Estramustine phosphate, a nor nitrogen mustard derivative of estradiol-17-β-phosphate, was introduced in the treatment of prostatic carcinoma in 1966. Until March 1975, 466 patients have been reported on this treatment in open clinical trials: 82% of the patients were in stage IV. In 402 patients, nonresponsive to previous estrogen therapy, significant improvement occurred in 55%. In 64 previously untreated patients there was a favourable response in 83%.

Side-effects were mainly bone marrow suppression, liver disturbance, thrombophlebitis following intravenous injection, and gastrointestinal troubles, mainly following oral administration.

A prospective, randomized study comparing oral estramustine phosphate and conventional estrogen therapy in carcinoma of the prostate is in progress.

## REFERENCES


1. Farnsworth, W.E.: Personal communication
2. Fredholm, B., Jensen, G., Lindskog, M., Müntzing, J.: Effects of estramustine phosphate (Estracyt®) on growth of DMBA-induced mammary tumours in rats. Acta pharmacol. (Kbh.) 35 (1974) (abstract)
3. Jönsson, G., Olsson, A.M., Luttropp, W., Cekan, Z., Purvis, K., Diczfalusy, E.: Treatment of prostatic carcinoma with various types of estrogen derivatives. II Steroid levels. Vitam. and Horm. 33, 351 (1975)
4. Kirdani, R.Y., Müntzing, J., Verkarakis, M.J., Murphy, G.P., Sandberg, A.A.: Studies on the antiprostatic action of Estracyt, a nitrogen mustard of estradiol. Cancer Res. 34, 1031-1037 (1974)
5. Mittelman, A., Shukla, S.K., Welwaart, K., Murphy, G.P.: Oral estramustine phosphate (NSC-89199) in the treatment of advanced (Stage D) carcinoma of the prostate. Cancer Chemother. Rep. Part 1, 59, 219-223 (1975)
6. Nillius, A., Könyves, I.: Oral Estracyt® (estramustine phosphate) in the treatment of advanced carcinoma of the prostate. In press (1975)
7. Nilsson, T., Jönsson, G.: Clinical results with estramustine phosphate (NSC-89199): A comparison of the intravenous and oral preparations. Cancer Chemother. Rep. Part 1, 59, 229-232 (1975)
8. The Veterans Administration Cooperative Urological Research Group: Carcinoma of the prostate: A continuing co-operative study. J. Urol. (Baltimore) 91, 590-594 (1964)

# The Conservative Treatment of Prostatic Carcinoma

H. KLOSTERHALFEN

The treatment of prostatic carcinoma has been one of the subjects of almost every urological meeting in the recent years and will probably continue to be so in the future.

This is mainly due to the high incidence of this disease, which is second to carcinoma of the bowel among malignant deseases of males and first among those who are 50 and older.

Conservative treatment of prostatic carcinoma includes:

1. Antiandrogenic therapy
2. Cryosurgery
3. Radiation therapy

## 1. ANTIANDROGENIC THERAPY

Antiandrogenic therapy is a result of Huggin's findings 30 years ago, who demonstrated the stimulating effect of androgens on prostatic carcinoma cells and the inhibiting effect of estrogens. His results, which are still accepted, form the basis for the different types of modern treatment.

The ideal therapy would be a radical elimination of those organs where androgens can be produced. The question how to do this is highly controversial, and has resulted in a worldwide discussion as to whether orchidectomy or estrogen therapy is better for those patients.

There are arguments for both types of therapy. Some of them are based on psychological and emotional aspects rather than on data, which is understandable, since orchidectomy as well as estrogen therapy are not only local treatments but interact with the hormones of the whole body and may influence the personality of the patient.

Regarding this question, whether orchidectomy or estrogen therapy is preferable in the conservative treatment of prostatic carcinoma, I have the following opinion: Since 90% of the androgens are produced in the testes it is consequential to remove these organs by an orchiectomy or, as we do, by a subcapsular orchiectomy. Both are simple and minor surgical procedures with almost no risk for the patient. Especially in the American literature it is pointed out that this operation might result in psychological distress for the patient. We cannot accept this argument. In our experience no patient ever refused an orchiectomy, when the physician took the time to explain why an orchiectomy was important and necessary for his health. Here it is much easier to explain a subcapsular orchiectomy, leaving the epididymus and the tunica albuginea inside the scrotum, than to talk about castration.

To summarize the most important points of our present policy regarding endocrine therapy of prostatic carcinoma:

1. Orchiectomy is the most effective endocrine therapy.
2. Orchiectomy has no side-effects as, e.g., estrogen therapy.
3. The results of estrogen treatment are no more effective than those of orchiectomy. But estrogen therapy has significant cardiovascular complications such as edema.
4. Estrogens stimulate pituitary prolactin secretion, which potentiates adrenal testosterone activity.
5. Adrenal testosterone activity can be completely blocked by cortisone therapy (Fig. 1) (4). In a prospective study one group of 56 prostatic cancer patients received long-term cortisone therapy following orchiectomy. In comparison to other groups it is evident that they are in better physical and psychological condition.
6. If orchiectomy is refused, we recommend treatment with diethyl-dioxy-stilben-diphosphate (Honvan). A diuretic should be added to prevent edema.

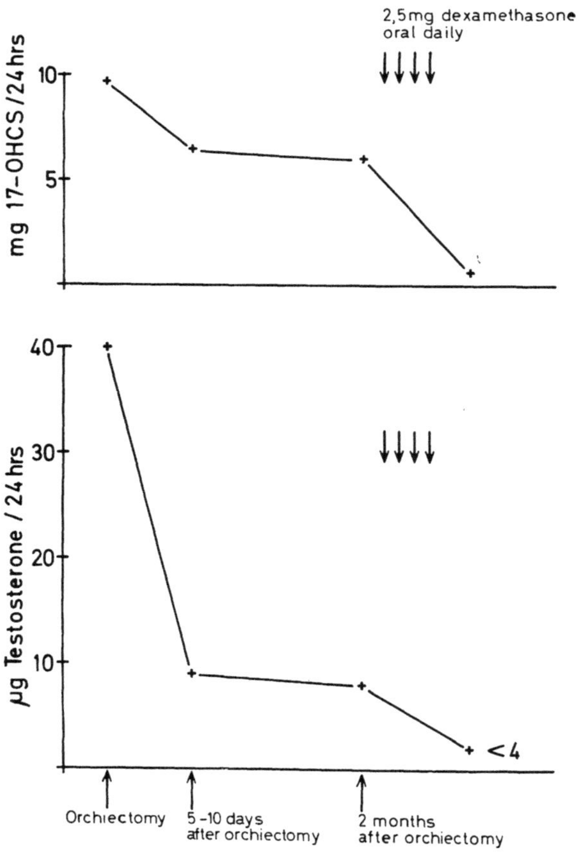


*Fig. 1. Blocking of testosterone and 17-OHCS excretion by cortisone*

Therapy with so-called antiandrogens (e.g. cyproterone acetate) is a new type of treatment, which needs further investigation. Treatment with cyproterone acetate results in an androgen resistance in those organs that otherwise are stimulated by testosterone. To our knowledge the same theoretical justification exists for treatment with cyproterone acetate in prostatic cancer as for estrogens, except that further investigation seems necessary to find out the right dosage, side-effects, and amount of reabsorption. In our prospective study we treated 61 patient with this type of drug and have controlled them for about 6 years.

Therapy resistance might develop during conservative treatment. If, after a remission, prostatic cancer progresses again, you might consider hypophysectomy. To date, we have performed it in 18 patients, of whom 13 have been followed up. Six of them had an objective remission after surgery. Our neurosurgeons do this as a microsurgical procedure by a transsphenoidal approach. There is no high surgical risk and it can be done even in sick patients. The immediate relief of pain caused by metastases can be very impressive. Furthermore, there can be a direct influence on the tumor (Fig. 2).

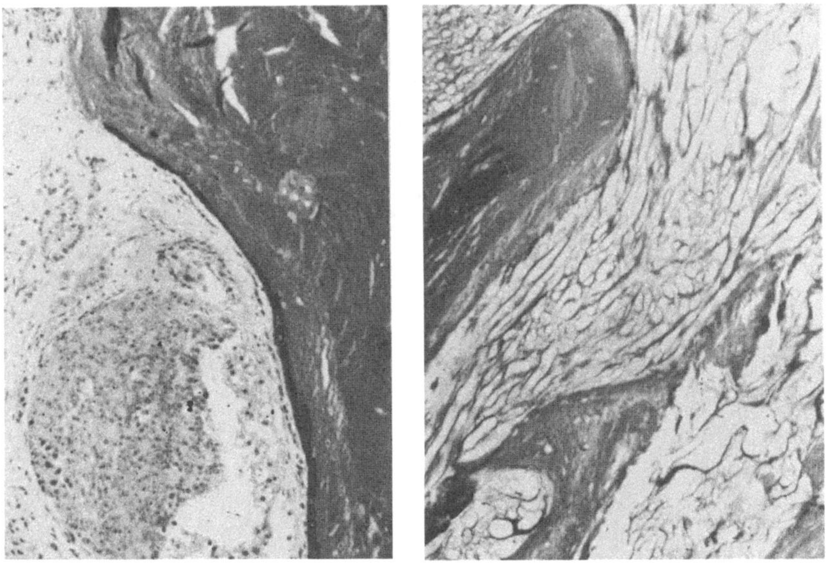

*Fig. 2. Biopsy specimen of bone before (left) and after (right) hypophysectomy*

We know little about who is a good candidate for this procedure, which means we cannot predict who will benefit from this operation. Only those prostatic cancers might respond that proved to be "hormone-dependent" after orchiectomy or during estrogen therapy, or its effect might be due to the blocking of the pituitary prolactin. An unpublished finding of our department is that the serum prolactin level is significantly higher in patients with prostatic carcinoma than in controls.

Beta-emitting strontium-89 is a further possibility for treating generalized bone metastases and their symptoms. It requires infusion. Since it is a beta-emitting agent, there is no need for special protection, and 50% of the radioactivity will be eliminated by the kidneys within 2 weeks. The blood count should be controlled weekly. This treatment can be done where there is an equipment for scintigraphy. It is quite impressive to see the immediate pain relief following this treatment which is effective for weeks.

## 2. CRYOSURGERY

A new therapy of prostatic cancer is cryosurgery. This is effective in the treatment of local tumors and also can influence metastases using the technique of repeated local freezing (4) of the prostate , a finding which was recently described again by Ablin (1973). The possible explanation is that this is due to antibody formation following cryosurgery. And in fact some investigators were able to demonstrate an increase of immune globuline in those patients. Cryosurgery may become part of the standard treatment in prostatic carcinoma.

We have a two-step cryosurgical approach:

1. The perineal approach using a special probe, when the prostate is exposed
2. The transurethral approach with the standard probe

We hope to destroy most of the primary tumor using this external and internal procedure.

## 3. RADIATION THERAPY

For a long time radiation therapy received little attention in the treatment of prostatic carcinoma, because conventional radiation therapy was ineffective and had severe side-effects on the bladder and rectum.

These conditions changed with the advent of modern high voltage therapy. We are now managing 350 radiated patients with almost no severe complications. Using a dosage of 6000 rad in 6 weeks by telecobalt radiation, it is our impression that this therapy is quite effective in treating prostatic cancer with no or little harm to bladder and rectum (Fig. 3). However, a dosage of 8000 rad, increases significantly the incidence of complications, as BAGSHAW (2) has emphasized. It is evident by microscopic investigation of the tumor tissue that radiation results in regression of the cancer cells but on the other hand some cancer cells can still be detected. It is not known if they still have the same vitality and activity.

Today radiation therapy is part of the classic treatment of localized prostatic cancer. It is quite effective but may not cure the patient. I recommend radiation therapy alone only in those patients who refuse other treatments mainly to preserve their potency.

Though one cannot deny some progress and new findings in the conservative treatment of prostatic carcinoma, there is no question that all types of treatment, even if they seem to be striking in the beginning, fail to cure the patients. This is no argument against conservative treatment, which at least has proved to be effective in prolonging and improving life in advanced prostatic cancer.

Most important for further investigations is the question: Is it possible to demonstrate specific androgen receptors in prostatic cancer

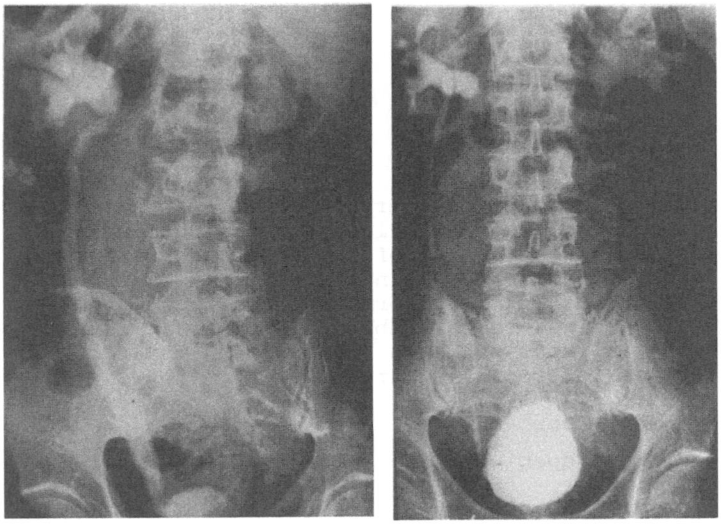

*Fig. 3. Urography before and after high voltage irradiation of prostate*

cells? It has been possible to demonstrate estrogen receptors in breast cancer, a fact which became important for therapy. It seems reasonable to expect androgen receptors in prostatic cancer, since it is comparable in many aspects to breast cancer. It would change our therapy in that we would not attempt any sort of hormone therapy in those patients in whom androgen receptors cannot be detected. A lot of work and investigation needs to be done.

## SUMMARY

### Conservative Treatment of Prostatic Carcinoma

With regard to conservative therapy of prostatic carcinoma it is still a disturbing fact that everybody seems to have his own interpretation of the subject, and quite often the type and dosage of medication are prescribed according to the subjective impression of the attending physician. At this moment it seems to be necessary to stop the present confusing and arbitrary practice of conservative therapy and give clear guidelines based on accepted experimental and clinical data. This needs to be done for the types of medication as well as for their dosage.

Conservative treatment is indicated whenever the tumor has infiltrated beyond the prostate so that radical removal is not possible. Conservative therapy includes

1. Antiandrogenic therapy
2. Cryotherapy
3. Radiation therapy.

1. Orchiectomy is the most effective antiandrogenic treatment. Estrogen therapy, frequently used instead of orchiectomy, has no better results. It has side-effects not seen after orchiectomy including cardiovascular reactions (e.g., edema) and the stimulation of pituitary

prolactin secretion, which results in increased adrenal testosterone activity. Cortisone, given in the right dosage, is effective in blocking adrenal testosterone, which influences tumor growth. In case orchiectomy is refused we recommend diethyl-dioxy-stilben-diphosphate (Honvan) and add saluretics to prevent edema. Estradiol (Estramustin phosphate) has a high incidence of severe side-effects and should be given only in advanced cases, when other types of treatment prove to be ineffective. Antiandrogens (cyproterone acetate) are still the subject of clinical investigations. So far one can say that they seem to be a good alternative to estrogens, though there are slight side-effects. Pituitary prolactin inhibitory agents are now being investigated. They are indicated when there is an elevated prolactin serum concentration in patients with prostatic cancer.

In case there is further tumor progress after a primary remission, hypophysectomy can be considered: 50% of hypophysectomized patients have another remission; others have at least relief of pain. Another way to achieve pain relief is treatment with beta-emitting $^{89}Sr$.

2. Cryosurgery is gaining an accepted place in the treatment of prostatic carcinoma. The cryosurgical approach is indicated whenever the tumor has infiltrated beyond the prostate, and in patients with metastases. A few but well-documented findings have shown a good effect of local cryosurgery on distant metastases on the basis of antigen-antibody reaction.

3. Radiation therapy is an accepted standard therapy. It has proved to be effective but not curative.

Each type of conservative therapy is only effective for a certain period of time - sometimes even in the advanced stage of the disease. On the other hand, it offers the patient a few more years of worthwhile life.

## REFERENCES


1. Ablin, R.J.: In: Cryosurgery in Urology. Ed. H.J. Reuter, p.4. G. Thieme, Stuttgart 1973
2. Bagshaw, M.A.: Carcinoma of the prostate: the place of radiotherapy. In: Proc. XIII Int. Congr. Radiol. Madrid 1973, Vol. II, pp. 67-72
3. Firusian, N., Mellin, P., Schmidt, C.G., Kierfeld: Eigenes Verfahren der Therapie der Knochenmetastasen des Prostata-Carcinomas mittels des Beta-strahlenden Strontium 89. Verh. dtsch. Ges. Urol, 24 359-364 (1973)
4. Gursel, E.: Regression of prostatic cancer following sequential cryotherapy to the prostate. J. Urol. (Baltimore) 108, 928-932 (1972)
5. Klosterhalfen, H., Voigt, K.D., Tamm, J.: Die Wirkung der Orchidektomie auf die Ausscheidung von Testosteron, 17-Ketosteroiden, Oestrogenen, Pregnandiol, 17 - OH-Corticosteroiden und Gonadotropinen im Urin. Urol. int. (Basel) 20, 364-375 (1965)
6. Soanes, W.A., Ablin, R.J.: Remission of metastatic lesions following cryosurgery in prostatic cancer: immunogic considerations. J. Urol. (Baltimore) 104, 154-159 (1970).

# Palliative Cryotherapy in Inoperable Prostate Carcinoma

G. SESIA, U. FERRANDO, G. FONTANA, M. LAUDI, and F. CAUDA

## INTRODUCTION

In previous papers we examined cryotherapy in detail, including its history, physical principles, pathogenesis, histologic alterations, technique, indications, and contraindications. This previous work showed that the best indication for cryotherapy, other than inoperable adenoma with retention, was prostate carcinoma with urinary retention. Cryotherapy does not require an anaesthetic, it does not give rise to hemorrhage, it does not lead to dissemination, it can be repeated, the patient need not take to his bed, only brief hospitalization is required, it is easy to perform, it has an antalgic effect, and it does not lead to fibrinolytic attacks. The purpose of the present paper is: (1) to report our results in 8 years of palliative cryotherapy in prostate carcinoma; (2) to emphasize the immunologic interest of cryotherapy; and (3) to lay down a program for the future.

## MATERIALS AND METHODS

We have reviewed 91 cases of carcinoma of the prostate treated with cryotherapy and estrogens between 1967 and 1974. For comparison purposes, the results obtained in a further 113 patients subjected to hormone treatment (estrogens and/or castration) are reported. All the patients, whether treated with cryotherapy or not, were suffering from inoperable carcinoma of the prostate (stage III-IV). Cryotherapy was employed for palliative, disobstruction purposes, and was therefore confined to one session only (on the average, two 15-min periods of nitrogen protoxide at - 90°C); applied exclusively to patients with urinary retention; applied practically to all prostate carcinomas with retention even though the general condition was very poor, a fact which affected mortality; and was associated with estrogens. The usual criteria were employed for diagnosis (clinical examination, rectal palpation, radiologic examinations, phosphatase, etc.). Biopsy, preferably using perineal route, was done in doubtful cases. Follow-up was carried out on the occasion of further patient admittances (12%); by submitting patients to check-ups (47%); and on the basis of replies to a questionnaire (41%).

## DISCUSSION

A total of 91 patients (44.6%) treated with cryotherapy were considered. Their ages ranged from 67 to 74; average age was 70.33 years ($\pm$ 7.50).

We were only able to collect data in 67% of the patients treated, which limits the value of our results. At the same time hormonal therapy was used to treat 113 patients (55.4%) (average age 69 ± 8.6 years). Of this second group, follow-up was possible in 59 cases (52.2%).

The first indication to emerge from our studies is that survival is equal in all cases treated with cryotherapy (plus estrogens) and in the cases which only received hormonal treatment. More precisely, in the first group, survival is 17.8 months and in the second 17.5 months, with no statistically significant difference.

Cryotherapy-treated cases of carcinoma and adenoma for the period 1967-1974 are shown in Tables 1 and 2 respectively.

Table 1. Cryotherapy-treated cases of carcinoma 1967-1974

| Year | Patients admitted | No. of cryotherapies (%) |
|---|---|---|
| 1967 | 29 | 7 (31.8) |
| 1968 | 39 | 21 (53.8) |
| 1969 | 28 | 14 (50.0) |
| 1970 | 39 | 7 (17.9) |
| 1971 | 27 | 10 (37.0) |
| 1972 | 28 | 8 (28.5) |
| 1973 | 21 | 13 (61.9) |
| 1974 | 30 | 14 (46.6) |
| Total | 241 | 94 |

Table 2. Adenomas treated with cryotherapy 1967-1974

| Year | Patients operated | No. of cryotherapies (%) |
|---|---|---|
| 1967 | 180 | 19 (10.5) |
| 1968 | 210 | 75 (35.7) |
| 1969 | 130 | 26 (20.0) |
| 1970 | 170 | 23 (13.5) |
| 1971 | 190 | 3 ( 1.5) |
| 1972 | 163 | 16 ( 9.6) |
| 1973 | 150 | 21 (14.0) |
| 1974 | 94 | 12 (12.7) |
| Total | 1287 | 195 |

The percentage difference between the two groups is evident. In the carcinomas, more than 44% of the cases were treated, whereas in the adenomas the percentage is much lower, e.g., 3 cases out of 190 in 1971, 12 out of 95 in 1974, etc.; thus a very low percentage in accord with our indications, which are precise but limited. Furthermore, whereas in inoperable carcinoma cryotherapy is in our opinion the best indication where obstruction exists, the opposite is the case in adenoma (i.e., cryotherapy should only be employed when no other therapy is possible). The frequency with which we have used cryotherapy in adenoma in the last 3 years has been 12%.

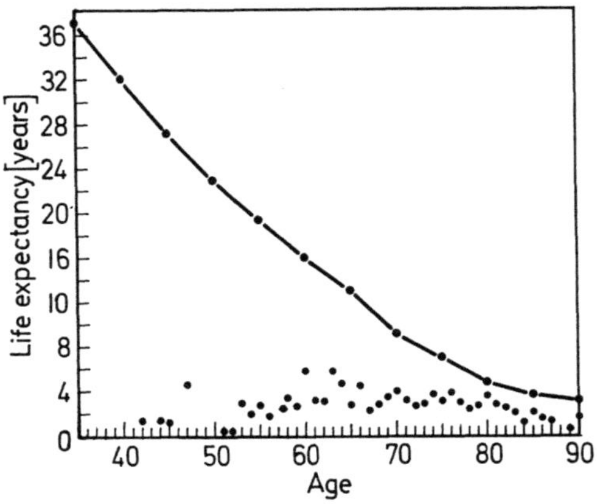


*Fig. 1. Life expectancy in carcinoma of the prostate (by Flocks (2))*

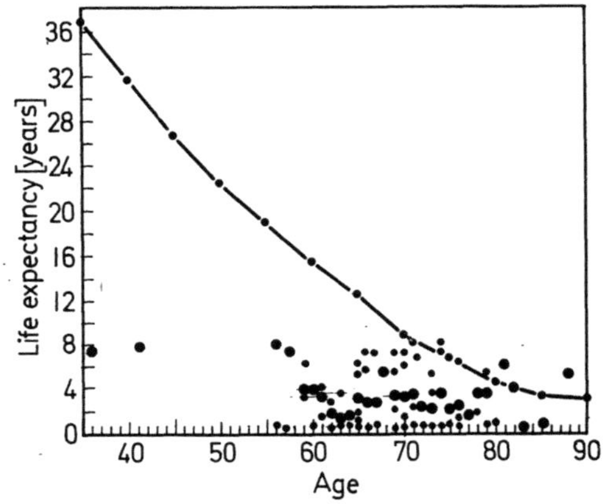


*Fig. 2. Life expectancy in prostate cancer*

Fig. 1 shows survival in cases of carcinoma of the prostate according to FLOCKS (18) compared with the average life span of citizens of the New York metropolitan area.

Figure 2 summarises survival in our patients submitted to cryotherapy.

Survival from the date of intervention in 61 cases of carcinoma of the prostate (stage III-IV) treated with cryotherapy plus estrogens was 17.8 months on the average. The collapse in the survival rate within the first 2 years is evident (Fig. 3). The high mortality is not due to cryotherapy because the other 59 patients suffering from carcinoma of the prostate and undergoing other treatment did not have a significantly higher survival (17.5 months on the average). In the first 2 years a slightly better survival percentage is seen in patients treated with cryotherapy, but the difference is not statistically significant. Figure 4 shows survival according to BYAR (1, 2) in patients suffering from carcinoma of the prostate at stage III-IV treated with 1 mg of diethylstilboesterol. The results are much better than ours.

The explanation for these differences can be laid at the door of the deplorable custom in Italy to diagnose carcinoma of the prostate in the out-clinic, patients immediately commencing treatment with estrogens.

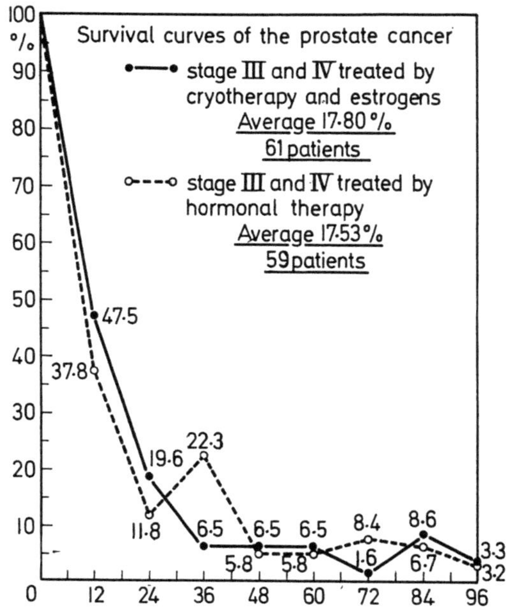


*Fig. 3. Survival months - post operative day*

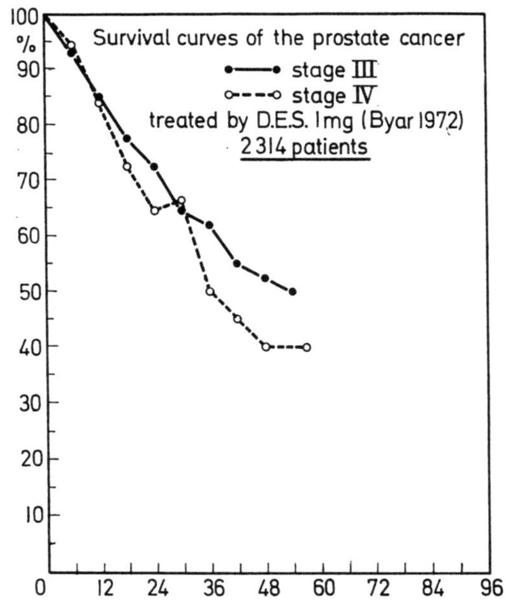


*Fig. 4. Months for diagnosis*

Patients are not hospitalized at diagnosis but later, when complications appear (of which urinary retention is one of the latest).

If we examine (Fig. 5) the survival of our patients starting not from admission but from the moment diagnosis is made, the results are similar to those reported by BYAR in the Veterans group report.

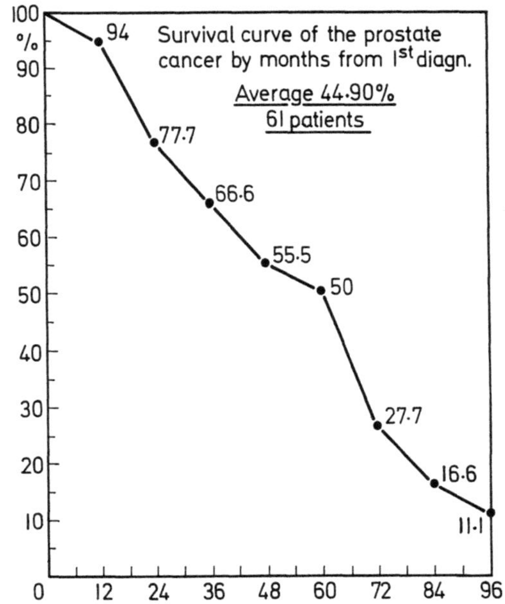


*Fig. 5. Survival of prostate cancer treated by cryotherapy in 61 patients followed from initial diagnosis*

Operating deaths (occurring prior to discharge) numbered 6 (6.5%). One of the deaths was due to sepsis following aggravation of a chronic preexisting infection. Two were caused by uremia (preexisting renal insufficiency which worsened after cryotherapy). The other three deaths involved vascular accidents (one infarct and two cardiac failures).

So in at least three cases, infection either directly (sepsis) or indirectly (pyelonephritis leading to increased catabolism and a worsening of renal function) caused death. While agreeing with other workers that cryotherapy is a modest operation, almost always well tolerated, examination of our series shows that infection is the greatest risk, every effort must therefore be made to limit the dangers (guided antibiotic therapy, continuous vesical washing, etc.).

Of the 59 patients who underwent hormonal therapy during the same period, 7 died in hospital (6.1%), 1 for unknown reasons, 2 from neoplastic cachexia, 1 from infection, and 1 from intestinal occlusion. Percentages are therefore similar to deaths due to cryotherapy.

During the 8 years of our investigation, 23 patients (37.7%) died. In carcinomas of the prostate submitted to other treatment, mortality was 42% with no statistically significant difference. In other words, palliative cryotherapy neither lengthens nor shortens the life of patients suffering from prostate carcinoma.

It would almost seem that the tumor's natural course is not influenced by the treatment and a similar conclusion emerges from the Veterans group report.

We have seen that infection is the major risk of cryotherapy. It might therefore be thought that in patients so treated, urologic causes (pyelonephritis, uremia) of death would be the most frequent. In fact, urologic causes of death were lower (47.8%) than the figure of 64% encountered in patients not given cryotherapy.

In the patients treated with cryotherapy, metastases were present in 30.5% of cases at follow-up. In those who underwent other treatment, they were present in 35% of cases. We cannot comment on this difference at this time because much of the data are still being processed.

The disobstructive result was good in 87% of cases - i.e., it was possible for these patients suffering from urinary retention to resume normal micturition.

Micturition remained stable in time, as is shown by the low frequency or reoperations which included two iteral cryotherapies, two surgical enlargements of the neck, three cystolithectomies, three vasectomies, and one endoscopic resection.

In the adenomas, the success percentage was slightly lower (83%). To summarise our results, I would say that palliative cryotherapy (1) has a disobstructive effect in most cases (87%) of prostate carcinoma with retention; (2) that this disobstructive effect permits satisfactory micturition and is stable over time; and (3) there is no evidence of an increase in the survival of treated patients. It should, however, be borne in mind that we always employed cryotherapy as a palliative and in association with traditional therapies.

## IMMUNOLOGIC ACTION OF CRYOTHERAPY

From the very beginning of research into the use of cryotherapy in urology, a group of workers headed by ABLIN pointed out that cryotherapy induced immunologic alterations.

In 1970 ABLIN et al.'s report of regression in three cases of histologically identified metastasis in patients treated with cryotherapy repeated at 30-day intervals aroused enormous interest.

Recently (November 1974), ABLIN chaired a round table in Turin on the immunologic reponse to cryotherapy. The following facts emerged:

1. Specific prostate antigens exist.
2. Cryotherapy applied to the seminal vesicles of the rabbit releases antigens with formation of antibodies that are also specific for prostate tissue.
3. Cryosurgery repeated 2-3 times increases the quantity of antibodies.
4. Age reduces the immunologic response of cell mediators.
5. Estrogens diminish immunologic response.
6. Antigens are nonneoplastic prostatic, indeed, the presence of carcinomatous tissue slightly reduces the quantity of specific antigens.

During the round table it was decided to form a study group, chaired by Ablin, to assess immunosensitivity in prostatic carcinoma (i.e., previous immunologic diseases, previous immunosuppressive therapy, present humoral immunity, present cell, especially lymphocyte, immunity).

As far the authors, we have decided: (1) to cooperate with the above program as far as possible; (2) to continue to confine cryotherapy to cases of urinary retention, with repeated applications so as to increase the immune response; and (3) to avoid, in patients treated with cryotherapy, all therapeutic measures (estrogens, irradiation, cortisone, cytotoxics, etc.) that might lead to a reduction in antitumoral response.

SUMMARY

Cryotherapy was applied by us as a palliative in 91 cases of carcinoma of the prostate.

1. Disobstruction was achieved in 87% of patients.
2. Results proved stable over time.
3. Operating mortality, survival curve, number of deaths, etc. was not statistically different in patients treated with cryotherapy compared with patients undergoing other treatments.
4. Precutions are required to combat infection in cryotherapy patients in the first few weeks.

We feel authorized to pursue cryotherapy in the future exploiting all its immunologic possibilities.

REFERENCES

1. Byar, D.P., and Veterans Administration Cooperative Urological Research Group: Survival of patients with incidentally found microscopic cancer of prostate. J. Urol. 108, 908-913 (1972)
2. Flocks, R.H., Nelson, C.M.K., Boatman, D.L.: Perineal cryosurgery for prostatic carcinoma. J. Urol. 108, 933-935 (1972)

# Follow-up of Prostate Carcinoma with Serial Bone Scanning Using Cyclotron-Produced 18-Fluorine

A. C. Buck, G. D. Chisholm, and M. V. Merrick

## INTRODUCTION

Carcinoma of the prostate presents one of the major problems in urology. It has the highest incidence of all urogenital neoplasms in the male and is responsible for over 4000 deaths annually in the United Kingdom. Even when the diagnosis has been established there remain two important considerations in the management of these patients: (1) assessment of the extent of the disease to enable precise staging and (2) a reliable and accurate method of evaluating the progression of the disease or response to treatment in the absence of clinical symptoms and signs.

The use of radioisotope scintigraphy has become an important means of detecting osseous metastases in malignant disease. They are, however, no reports of the long-term follow-up of bone scan examinations. This report concerns our experience with 18-fluorine ($^{18}F$) bone scanning in patients with carcinoma of the prostate and our observations made from serial follow-up studies over the past 5 years.

## PATIENTS AND METHOD

Seventy-four patients with carcinoma of the prostate were studied. Their ages ranged from 51 to 82 years (mean 71.5 years). In 68 patients the diagnosis was confirmed by histology of primary or metastatic lesions. In the remaining 6 patients diagnosis was based on raised serum acid phosphatase, a clinically hard gland, and the radiological demonstration of bone secondaries. All patients were seen at the time of diagnosis and at subsequent visits at 3 monthly or 6 monthly intervals in a special clinic. Forty-one patients are alive and 33 have died.

A combined radiological survey and $^{18}F$ bone scan was initiated at the time of diagnosis and repeated annually. The X-rays and scans were examined together by an experienced radiologist. The clinical observations, biochemical, radiological and scan results were entered on prepared data sheets.

Initially bone scans were performed 1 h after an i.v. injection of 2 mCi of $^{18}F$ using 17 fields of the Nuclear Chicago Pho Gamma II scintillation camera collecting fifteen to twenty thousand counts per field. Since 1971 imaging was carried out 2 h after a dose of 5-10 mCi of $^{18}F$ with the rectilinear scanner (Ohio Nuclear Model 84 fitted with twin 5 x 2 NaI detectors) set to collect 1200 counts per square cm from the area of interest. In some patients 111-indium bleomycin has been used to distinguish metastases from non-malignant bone lesions. Where possible, bone biopsies were taken from accessible scan positive areas. Post-mortem examinations were performed in patients dying in hospital and the positions of secondary lesions in these cases compared with those diagnosed ante-mortem.

Sixty-three patients were treated with stilbestrol and/or castration from the time of diagnosis. It is now our policy not to treat patients with incidentally diagnosed tumours confined to the enucleated specimen of the prostate. Hypophysectomy was carried out in three patients with widespread painful metastases.

## RESULTS

140 scans with their corresponding X-rays were available for study (Table 1). The large number of patients with a single scan is due to a considerable proportion of patients with advanced disease already being followed at the beginning of the study. Forty patients have been followed for more than 2 years and eight of these for up to 5 years.

Table 1. Number of patients with carcinoma of prostate followed with annual $^{18}F$ bone scan and skeletal radiological surveys

| Follow-up | Patients | Alive | Dead |
|---|---|---|---|
| 4 years | 8 | 6 | 2 |
| 3 years | 10 | 6 | 4 |
| 2 years | 22 | 12 | 10 |
| 1 year | 34 | 17 | 17 |
| Total | 74 | 41 | 33 |

All of the 30 patients with radiological metastases have had a positive abnormal bone scan. Scan abnormalities were more extensive than the lesions seen on X-ray in the majority of cases.

Of the 44 patients with no evidence of metastatic disease on conventional radiological bone surveys, 11 patients (25%) had a positive bone scan. In this study there were no false negative bone scans. However, in a further 17 patients the scans showed abnormal uptake of $^{18}F$ which was due to non-malignant lesions (osteoarthritis in 13 and Paget's bone disease in 4). The areas of increased uptake of isotope corresponded with lesions seen on X-ray and the diagnosis was confirmed by biopsy or at autopsy (Table 2).

Table 2. Correlation between bone scans and X-ray in 74 patients showing that 11/44 (25%) patients were X-ray negative but scan positive

| | | X-ray | |
|---|---|---|---|
| | | Positive 30 | Negative 44 |
| $^{18}$Scan | Negative | 0 | 33 |
| | Positive | 30 | 11 |

Of the 11 patients who had a positive scan and negative X-rays; 5 are alive and 6 have died. Histologically proven metastases became evident on X-ray up to 3.5 years after the initial positive bone scan in half these patients.

Of the 33 patients with neither radiological nor scan evidence of metastases only one patient has become scan positive but remains X-ray negative, while one patient has become scan and X-ray positive.

A comparison of indium-labelled bleomycin with $^{18}F$ scan in patients with radiological abnormalities in shown in Figures 1 and 2.

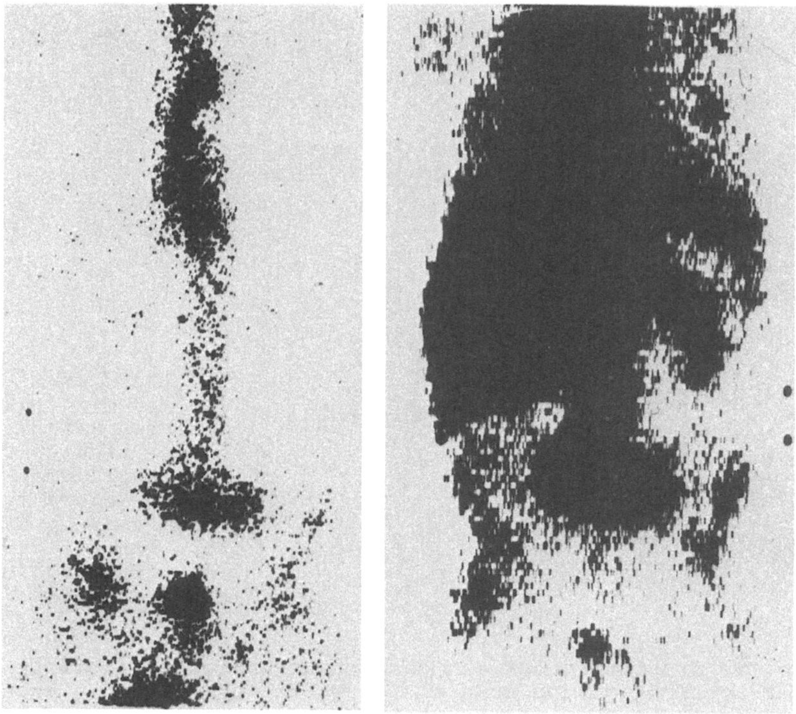

*Fig. 1. Case 1. T.L. Fluorine-18 bone scan (left) shows abnormal uptake of isotope in the vertebrae and right side of the pelvis. Indium-111 Bleomycin scan (right) shows corresponding increased uptake in pelvis. Bone biopsy confirmed metastatic deposits*

## DISCUSSION

It is now well established that scintigraphy with bone seeking radioisotopes is superior to conventional radiology in the detection of skeletal metastases in carcinoma of the prostate (2, 4, 8, 10). Since the introduction of $^{18}F$ into clinical practice (1) it has become accepted as the best available radio-pharmaceutical for the detection of skeletal secondary deposits (6). Direct comparison with $^{87m}Sr$ (3) and $^{85}Sr$ (7) indicate its superiority over these agents. Bone scanning also has its limitations but increasing experience has enabled the place of this test to be defined. A critical evaluation of the scan and X-rays is essential to enable a correct interpretation of the scan,

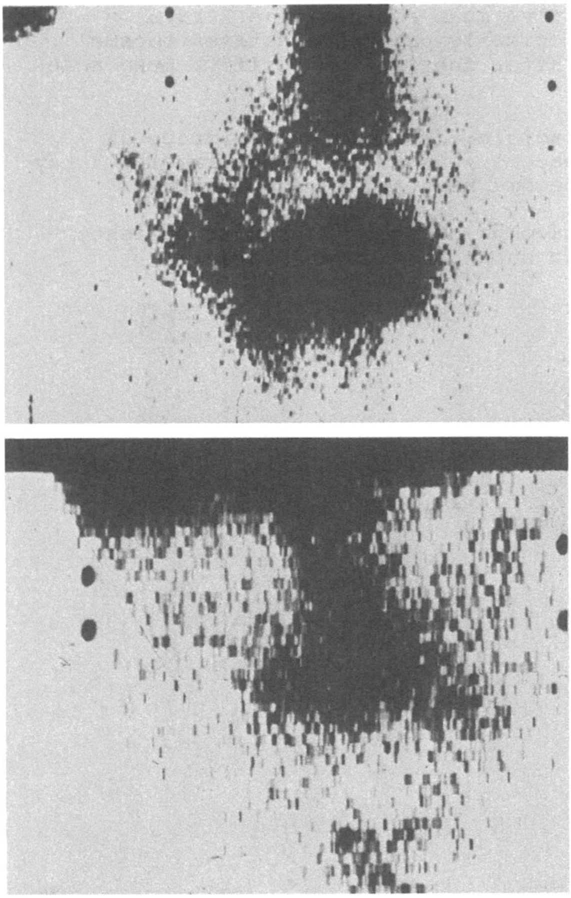

*Fig. 2. Case 2. S.J. Fluorine-18 scan (above) shows abnormal uptake of isotope on the right side of pelvis. Indium-111 Bleomycin scan (below) shows reduced uptake of isotope by the marrow in this area. Bone biopsy from ilium and ischial tuberosity confirmed Paget's disease*

since the distiction between metastases and other forms of bone disease is not apparent on the scan alone. Where possible bone biopsy should be performed to confirm the diagnosis and to eliminate false positive lesions.

Information obtained from bone scanning may be helpful in deciding treatment policy in two ways: firstly, it may help in the assessment of new cases for radical prostatectomy or curative radiotherapy. Secondly, it may be helpful in the follow-up of cases to determine healing or progression of metastases. It has been suggested that the possibility of cure in patients with carcinoma of the prostate can only apply to patients with a stage 1 or 2 lesion and a life expectancy of 10 years or more (5, 9). It is realized that few new cases fulfil these criteria. However, the use of $^{18}F$ bone scanning allows the policy of radical treatment to be considered more rationally.

The object of this study has been to follow up the scan appearances over a period of several years. It is now evident that the change from X-ray negative-scan positive to X-ray positive-scan positive indicates progress of the disease rather than healing bone lesions. Our results have shown that half these patients have developed proven metastases while on estrogen/castration therapy. Every case with radiological abnormalities had an abnormal scan. In many instances the scan showed more extensive involvement than the X-rays. In following the progress of patients treated with hormonal manipulation a favorable response was indicated by clinical improvement and in some cases radiological evidence of healing or regression of bone lesions, but the bone scan remained unchanged. This is not surprising as uptake of isotope reflects osteoid activity. The majority of patients with a normal bone scan initially have remained so. However, it is expected that more patients in this group will develop abnormalities as they continue to be followed up for longer periods.

During this study the possibility of obtaining more accurate tumor localization using indium-labelled bleomycin, known to give clinically useful tumor to background ratios, has been explored. The preliminary results are encouraging in the small number of patients studied. Clearly, a soft tissue tumor-seeking radio-pharmaceutical will be greatly welcomed in the screening of these patients.

## SUMMARY

Seventy-four patients with carcinoma of the prostate were studied annually by combined radiological and $^{18}F$ scintigraphy over a 5-year period.

Of the patients who have no radiological evidence of bone metastases, 25% have a positive $^{18}F$ bone scan. Follow-up of these patients has shown that scan abnormalities preceded X-ray changes from between 1 to 4 years.

False negative scans were not seen with $^{18}F$ which allows for greater accuracy in the detection of skeletal metastases. The accurate staging of carcinoma of the prostate cannot be made without bone scanning.

Preliminary results with $^{111}In$ bleomycin as an adjunct to $^{18}F$ have shown this to be a useful radio-pharmaceutical to distinguish metastases from benign lesions, and further studies are warranted.

## REFERENCES

1. Blau, M., Nagler, W., Bender, M.A.: Fluorine-18: a new isotope for bone scanning. J. Nucl. Med. 3, 332-334 (1962)
2. Faber, D.D., Wahman, G.E., Baily, T.A., Flocks, R.H., Culp, D., Morrison, R.T.: An evaluation of the Strontium 85 scan for the detection and localization of bone metastases from prostate carcinoma. J. Urol. (Baltimore) 97, 526-532 (1967)
3. Galasko, C.S.B., Westerman, B., Sellwood, R.A., Li, J., Burn, J.I.: Use of the gamma camera for early detection of osseous metastases from mammary cancer. Brit. J. Surg. 55, 613-615 (1968)
4. Kontturi, M., Kivinitty, K.: Radiostrontiumin the early diagnosis of bone metastases in patients with prostatic carcinoma. Scand. J. Urol. Nephrol. 5, 210-214 (1971)
5. Lehman, T.H., Kirchheim, D., Braun, E., Moore, R.: An evaluation of radical prostatectomy for incidentally diagnosis carcinoma of the prostate. J. Urol. (Baltimore) 99, 646-650 (1968)

6. Merrick, M.V.: Detection of skeletal metastases: a comparison of three radioisotopic techniques using $^{18}F$ and radiology. Brit. J. Radiol. 46, 968-971 (1973)
7. Ronai, P., Winchell, H.S., Anger, H.O.: Skeletal survey for metastatic tumours of bone using 18-F and 85-Sr with the scintillation camera and whole-body scanner. J. Nucl. Med. 9, 517-522 (1968)
8. Shearer, R.J., Constable, A.R., Girling, M., Hendry, W.F., Fergusson, J.D.: Radioisotopic bone scintigraphy with the gamma camera in the investigation of prostatic cancer. Brit. med. J. ii, 362-365 (1974)
9. Veenema, R.J., Lattimer, J.K., Gursel, E.: Prostate cancer treated by retropubic prostato-vesiculectomy. 16th Congr. Soc. Int. Urol. Amsterdam, 1973, Vol. I
10. Williams, D.F., Blahd, W.H., Wetterau, L.: Radioactive fluorine-18 photoscanning: a diagnostic evaluation in carcinoma of the prostate. J. Urol. (Baltimore) 100, 675-679 (1968)

## II. Penis Carcinoma

# Epidemiology of Cancer of the Penis

L. PERSKY

## INTRODUCTION

Cancer of the penis is a serious health problem in many parts of the world. Most penile cancers (Fig. 1) are epidermoid or squamous cell (Fig. 2) carcinomas of the glans or prepuce (17, 19, 69, 70). Rarer types include melanoma (9, 31), basal cell carcinoma (28) (Fig. 3), sarcomas (35, 39, 41), endotheliomas (5, 21), and metastases from other parts of the body (1, 71, 73). Verrucous carcinoma, or Buschke-Löwenstein giant condyloma (Fig. 4) may represent an intermediary stage between penile condyloma (Fig. 5) and epidermoid carcinoma (10). Erythroplasia of Queyrat (Fig. 6), leukoplakia, and Bowen's disease (Fig. 7) have been considered precancerous lesions (11, 33, 36, 42, 50, 62, 67, 70, 72).

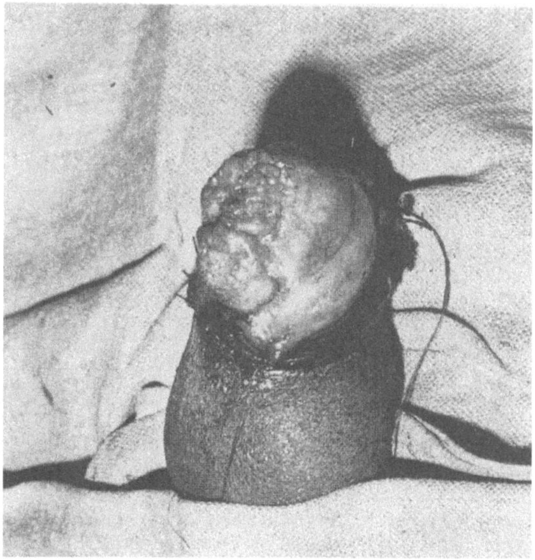

*Fig. 1. Gross specimen of epidermoid penile carcinoma*

## INCIDENCE

Obtaining accurate incidence data presents problems, especially in developing countries. Comparison of incidences is also difficult in age-related diseases such as cancer, due to varying age distributions

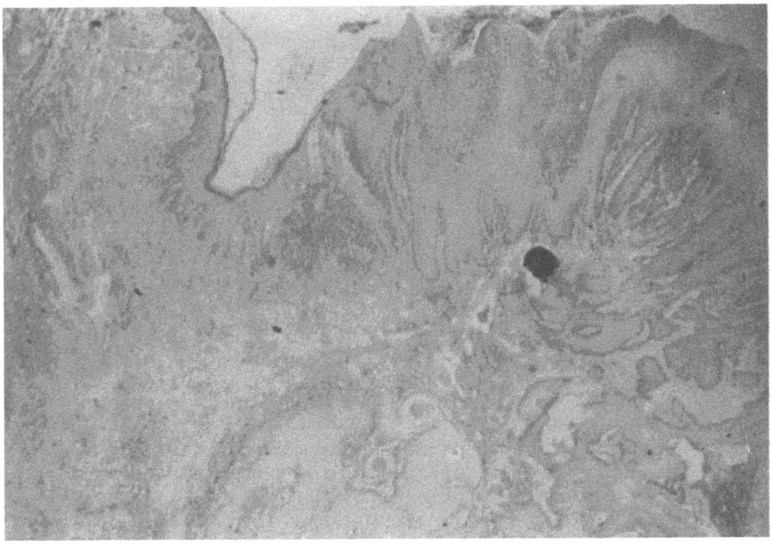

*Fig. 2. Microscopic section of squamous penile carcinoma*

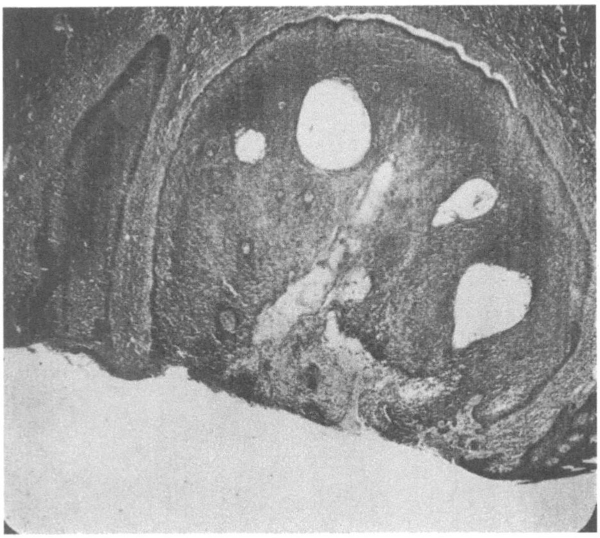

*Fig. 3. Basal cell carcinoma of penis*

in different countries. Age-standardizations have been attempted, but none are universally employed. Further comparison problems result from the many ways incidence of penile cancer is reported and from the combining of rates for penile cancer with those for cancer of the scrotum and other male organs.

United States

Incidence of penile carcinoma in the United States is low. In recent years, it has made up only 0.3 to 0.4% of malignancies in males (78, 79)

In the San Francisco area 0.6 cases per 100,000 males were recorded in 1972 and 0.8 in 1970 (81). A study covering over 10% of the US population from 1969 to 1971 showed a rate of 0.9/100,000 males (78). In Connecticut in 1968 and 1969, it was 0.4 and 0.8 respectively (82). From 1960 to 1962 the incidence was 0.8 in New York and 0.9 in Connecticut (25). Age-adjusted rates in large American cities was 1.1 in 1955-1959 and 1.2 in 1950-1954 (17).

Canada

Canada reported 0.7 cases per 100,000 males in 1971 and 0.9 from 1960 to 1962 (25, 31).

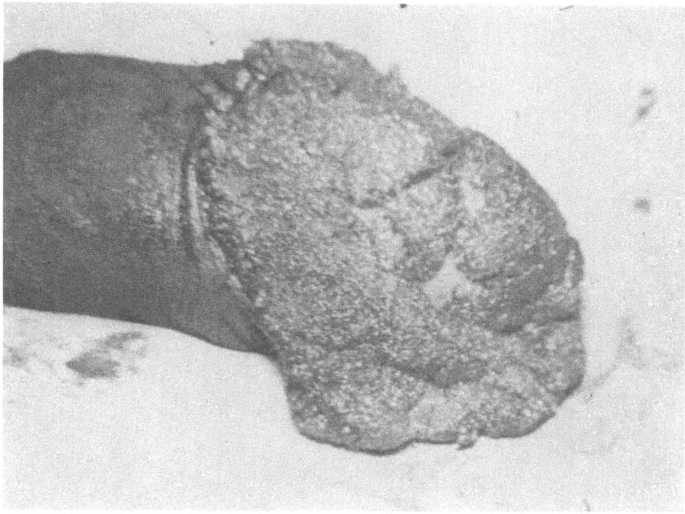

*Fig. 4. Buschke-Löwenstein giant condyloma*

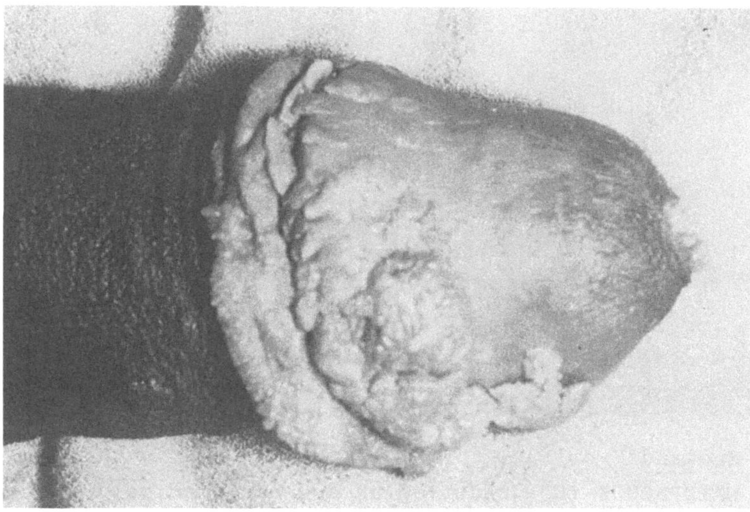

*Fig. 5. Simple penile condyloma*

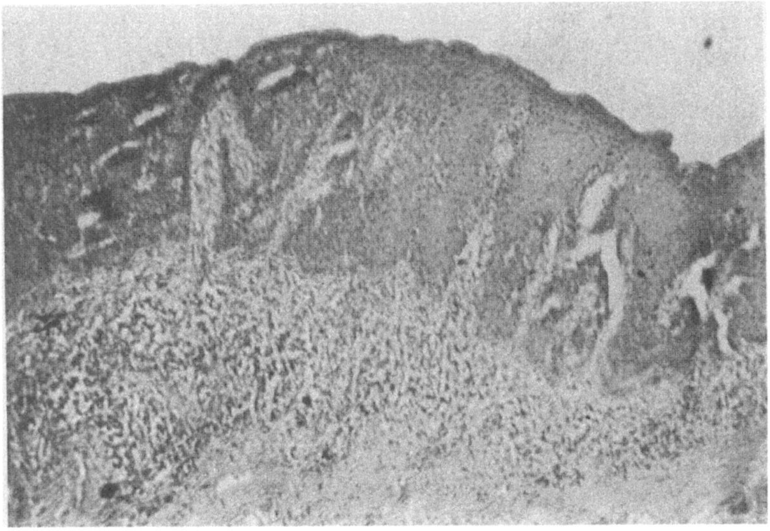

*Fig. 6 Erythroplasia of Queyrat*

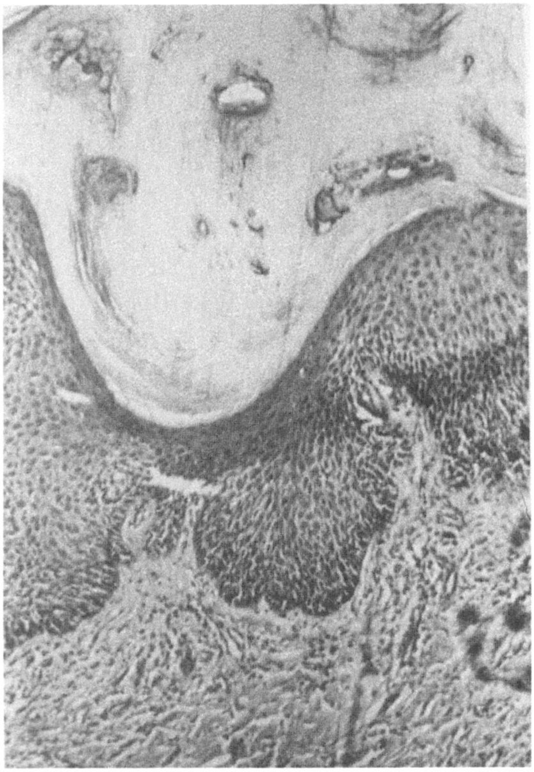

*Fig. 7. Carcinoma in situ or Bowen's disease*

England

WATERHOUSE (80) reported an age-adjusted rate of 1.2/100,000 males in the Birmingham area of England with an increasing trend over a recent 10-year period. GRIFFITHS (34) reported an overall decreasing trend over the past 50 years.

An approximate rate of 1.0/100,000 males was reported for England and Wales for 1968-1969, 1.3 for 1964, and 1.2 for 1960-1962 (25, 81-83).

France

The Anticancerous Centres in France registered 43 cases in 1967 (82).

Norway

The incidence in Norway from 1959 to 1961 was 1.0/100,000 males (25).

Denmark and Sweden

A fairly consistent rate of around 1.3/100,000 males was reported in Denmark from 1943 to 1967 (15, 25). The same rate was registered in Sweden in 1967 and in 1959-1961 (25, 82).

Finland

Finland had 0.8 cases/100,000 males in 1970, 0.5 in 1967, 0.4 in 1966 and 1963, and 0.7 from 1959 to 1961 (25, 81-83).

Iceland

Iceland reported a rate of 1.0/100,000 males from 1955 to 1963 (25).

Belgium

Belgium's Mutual Sickness Insurance Funds registered 33 cases in 1970, 27 in 1969, and 24 in 1968 (81, 82).

Netherlands

In 1969, The Hague reported a rate of 0.8/100,000 males, Rotterdam 2.1, and the Province of Friesland 0.9 (82). In 1960-1962, the combined incidence in the Netherlands was 1.1 (25).

Italy and Bulgaria

The Sickness Insurance Fund in Italy registered a rate of 0.5/100,000 males in 1969 (81). The same rate was reported for Bulgaria in 1968 (82).

Portugal

The Oncological Hospital in Lisbon reported 31 cases in 1969 (82).

Poland and Yugoslavia

A rate of 0.7/100,000 males was reported for Poland in 1970 and for Yugoslavia from 1956 to 1960 (25, 81).

Hungary

Hungary had rates of 0.7, 0.8, and 0.9 during 1971, 1969, and 1966 respectively (81, 82).

Union of Soviet Socialistic Republics

SHABAB (67) reported penile cancer to make up 0.5-1% of cancers in males in the USSR in recent years.

Israel

A very low incidence is seen in Israel. Only one case was reported in 1969 and three cases from 1960 to 1963 for an incidence of 0.1/100,000 males (25, 81).

Puerto Rico

Incidence in Puerto Rico is high, comprising almost 20% of cancers in males (44). Rates of around 4.5-5/100,000 males were reported during the 1950s and 1960s (25, 51, 53).

Mexico

RIVEROS (63) reported carcinoma of the penis to comprise almost 10% of cancers in males at the Institute of Cancer in Mexico City.

Brazil

From 1950 to 1960 4.5% of cancers in males at the Cancer Clinic of Recife were reported to be of the penis (63).

Columbia

A rate of 2.3/100,000 males was reported at Cali from 1962 to 1964 (25). Five percent of persons examined at the National Institute of Cancer in Bogota from 1950 to 1960 had penile malignancies (63).

Paraguay and Venezuela

RIVEROS (63) reported that about 6% of tumors in males examined at the Institute of Pathological Anatomy at Ascuncion, Paraguay, and 3% of all cancers at the Caracas Cancer Institute in Venezuela from 1941 to 1960 were of the penis.

China

In a 1919 study in Hainan, China, cancer of the penis made up 22% of all cancers and 12.6% in a study covering the period 1919-1939 (7, 8).

India

In different parts of India, frequency has varied from 2.8 to 22% of all neoplasms in males (9, 46, 58, 77). Tata Memorial Hospital alone recorded 1553 cases from 1941 to 1972 (69).

Ceylon

Cancer of the penis has also been common in Ceylon. SPITTEL (72) said he personally operated on 91 cases from 1911 to 1915. COORAY (16) reported penile carcinoma to be the most frequent cancer in Ceylonese males, comprising 13.7% of all cancers.

Malaya

Incidence in Singapore from 1950 to 1961 was only 0.8/100,000 males, but the 1957 census showed 54% of the population to be under 21 years of age (25). In 1958, MARSDEN (52) reported 91 cases in 4650 total malignancies.

Burma

In 1936, NATH (56) reported cancer of the penis to comprise about 15% of cancers in males in Rangoon, Burma.

Vietnam

MUIR (55) reported that 11.5% of tumors in South Vietnamese males in 1957 were of the penis.

Thailand

A study covering the years 1964-1967 showed penile cancer to make up 6.6% of cancers in males in North Thailand (54), and a Bangkok study showed it to comprise 6.3% of cancers in males from 1951 to 1952 (60).

Kenya

In the early 1960s, 1.9% of cancers in Kenya males were of the penis (22).

Mozambique

The rate in Lourenco Marques, Mozambique, from 1956 to 1960 was 1.9/100,000 males (25).

Nigeria

Low rates have been reported in Nigeria. In Ibadan the rate was 0.2/100,000 males (based on a standard African population) from 1960 to 1965 and 0.1 from 1960 to 1962 (25, 26).

South Africa

A rate of 4.6/100,000 males was reported in Natal from 1964 to 1966 (76). Tribal rates at a hospital near Johannesburg varied from 0.3 to 1.0 per 1000 admissions from 1960 to 1964 (64), and 1.7% of cancers in Johannesburg Bantu males from 1953 to 1955 were of the penis (40).

Uganda

Penile carcinoma is the most frequently diagnosed cancer in Ugandan males (23). In 1968-1970, it made up 6.3% of tumors seen in Kyadondo County males or 3.3/100,000 (75). From 1964 to 1968, it was the second most frequently diagnosed of all tumors in Uganda, accounting for 12% of cancers in males or 2.2/100,000 (23, 76). From 1947 to 1960, it comprised 12.2% of cancers in males recorded by the Kampla Cancer Registry with an age-specific incidence of 3.75/100,000 males in Kyadondo County (22). From 1897 to 1965, it constituted 7-10% of cancers diagnosed in Ugandan males (23).

## INTERPRETATION OF INCIDENCES

### Circumcision

Low rates of penile carcinima are found in Moslems or Mohamedans, who routinely circumcise young males (46, 52, 56, 58, 72). Extremely low rates are found in Jews, who practice infant circumcision (4, 48). In a rare instance where circumcision did not markedly reduce rates, it was done by rural or village "quacks" without sterile technique and with much of the prepuce remaining (74).
In Kenya, where most tribes circumcise in childhood or at puberty, incidence is low with most cases found in the two noncircumcising tribes (22-24). In Uganda, where circumcision is not generally practiced, incidence is high (23). Very low rates are seen in Nigeria and Ethiopia, where circumcision is routine (23, 76).
MENAKANIT (54) found penile cancer to rank second among cancers in Thailand, where circumcision is not common. A high rate has been reported in Puerto Rico, where male infants are not routinely circumcised (53). None of 61 cases in Jamaica nor the 168 cases in Paraguay has been circumcised at an early age (3, 63). In Brazil, where circumcision is uncommon, death rates from penile carcinoma are much higher than in England or the United States (12).

Low rates in the United States and England have been attributed in large part to high rates of infant circumcision (20, 37, 47). Among cases that have occurred, circumcision in infancy have been rare (6, 11, 18, 19, 29, 30, 37, 43).

## Hygiene

NGAI (57) implicated poor hygiene in the high incidence of penile carcinoma in China, as did RIVEROS (63) in Latin America. In Ceylon, where incidence is high, perineal binders have interfered with cleanliness (16, 17). Thai males, who have high rates, bathe frequently but often in semipublic places vearing sarongs which make it difficult to cleanse the genital area (54).

Great variation in incidence among noncircumcising tribes in Uganda suggests social and hygienic factors (12, 23). The Lugbara, who do not circumcise but have high standards of cleanliness, have lower rates than the nearby Nyoro (65). Sensitivity of carcinoma of the penis to social habit changes has been noted in Kyadondo County (75). High rates in East Africa have been attributed to poor hygiene practices (38).

The low incidence in the United States and Great Britain has been attributed to high standards of sexual hygiene along with high rates of infant circumcision (20, 34). In Sweden, where personal standards of hygiene are high, penile carcinoma is rare even though circumcision has not been routinely practiced (45).

## Phimosis

Phimosis further complicates good genital hygiene and has been called the most common precancerous condition (17). High rates of congenital phimosis have been associated with high rates of penile cancer (8, 12, 16, 54, 63, 67, 77). In Sweden, phimosis was found in about half of 229 cases of penile cancer (27). It was noted in 69% of cases at the Mayo Clinic (36). Tumerous changes in glans and prepuce have been reported to be more frequent in rabbits with artificial phimosis (67).

## Smegma

Some authors blame the irritating or inflammatory effects of retained smegma for carcinoma of the penis (30, 34, 57, 72, 77). Some suggest it may contain chemical carcinogens (17, 32, 67), while others say such carcinogens have not been conclusively demonstrated (19, 45, 61). The cancer-inducing potential of smegma (which begins to be produced during the first days of life) has been suggested to possibly account for the reduced effectiveness of circumcision done after the neonatal period in preventing penile carcinoma (34, 67).

## Infection

Infection that may result from retained smegma has been cited as a major predisposing factor in cancer of the penis (34, 37, 63, 70). In Malaya, 90% of cases diagnosed by MARSDEN (52) had had chronic suppuration. Frequent infection was noted in cases with poor and incomplete circumcision in Indonesia (74). FREW (29) found evidence of infection in 45 of 46 cases reviewed.

## Venereal Disease

TEMPLETON (76) found venereal disease widespread in Uganda, where incidence of penile cancer is high. RIVEROS (63) found that patients with carcinoma of the penis often had a history of venereal disease while ECKSTROM did not find venereal disease to play an important role in the 229 cases he analyzed.

GOLDBERG (32) discussed a possible relationship between granuloma inguinable and penile carcinoma. ANNAMUNTHODO (3) found about half of Jamaican cases had gonococcal infections but was unable to assess their role in the etiology of the cancers. Some feel carcinoma of the penis and venereal disease are probably simply "fellow travelers" (36).

## Viruses

SHAW (68) reported that human foreskin cells infected with adenovirus showed certain characteristics of transformation, and PIENTA (59) described viral transformation of rhesus foreskin cells. BRUNS (10) suggested that viral interaction might cause verrucous carcinoma of the penis.

## Socioeconomic Factors

Studiesin various countries have shown carcinoma of the penis tends to be found most often in persons of low income whose living conditions are poor (2, 3, 53, 57, 63). Other studies have been unable to draw conclusions as to social or occupational pre ponderance (37, 77).

## Racial Factors

Incidences have been higher in non-whites than in whites in the United States (26, 49, 78, 79); however, these and other racial tribal variations are probably due to extrinsic factors such as circumcision and hygiene practices.

## Immunologic Defenciency

CATALONA (14) reported subnormal immunologic responses in about 50% of patients with penile carcinoma.

## Environment

Hot humid climates seem to favor development of penile carcinoma (5, 12, 17). GRIFFITHS (34) suggested a possible environmental factor from cohort analyses in England and Wales.

Substantial differences in incidence have been noted in various geographic locations in Uganda with tribes living in different districts having varying incidences while those living in one area tend to have similar incidences (65, 66). Migrants into an area were found to have an incidence closer to the one for that area than to the one from which they came. DODGE (23) suggested that some factors such as herpes genitalis might be more common in high incidence areas.

## Paget's Disease

Paget's disease may be a predisposing factor in some cases (11, 36, 50).

## Trauma

Trauma has been suggested as a possible factor in the high incidence among the Zulus (45). It has also been noted in a small percent of cases in various studies but is probably coincidental (4, 6, 36).

## Age

Carcinoma of the penis is rarely seen in males under 25 and incidence rises rapidly with age (25, 34, 80-83).

## CONCLUSION

Although many factors seem to influence the epidemiology of penile cancer, emphasis on circumcision or exposure of the preputial cavity along with good genital hygiene probably provides the best means of control at the present time.


## ABSTRACT

World-wide incidences of penile cancer are reviewed and epidemiologic factors including circumcision, hygiene, phimosis, smegma, irritation, infection, venereal disease, viruses, environment, race, immune response, trauma, and age are discussed. The lowest rates appear in groups practicing infant circumcision and in areas where standards of sexual hygiene are high.


## REFERENCES


1. Abeshouse, B.S.: Metastatic tumors of the penis: A review of the literature and report of two cases. J. Urol. 86, 99-112 (1961)
2. Ackerman, L.V., Del Regato, J.A.: Cancer: diagnosis, treatment, and prognosis, 4th ed. St. Louis: Mosby, 1970, pp. 684-690
3. Annamunthodo, H.: Carcinoma of the penis in Jamaica. J. Inter. Coll. Surg. 35, 21-31 (1961)
4. Auster, L.S.: Genital cancer in Jews. New York State J. Med. 65, 266-280 (1965)
5. Badenoch, A.W.: Manual of Urology, 2nd ed. Chicago: Year Book Medical Publishers, 1974, pp. 314-323
6. Beggs, J.H., Spratt, J.S.: Epidermoid carcinoma of the penis. J. urol. 91, 166-172 (1964)
7. Bercovitz, N.: Cancer in Hainan, China: a preliminary statistical study of 131 operations with special reference to age, incidence, anatomical distribution, and etiology. China Med. J. 34, 119-123 (1920)
8. Bercovitz, N.: Cancer in Hainan, China: a supplemetary statistical study of 451 cases with special reference to age, anatomical distribution, and etiology. Cancer Res. 1, 154-157 (1941)
9. Bracken, R.B., Diokno, A.C.: Melanoma of the penis and the urethra: two cases reports and review of the literature. J. Urol. 111, 198-200 (1974)

60. Piyaratn, P.: Relative incidence of malignant neoplasms in Thailand. Cancer (Philad.) 12, 693-696 (1959)
61. Reddy, D.G., Baruah, I.K.S.M.: Carcinogenic action of human smegma. Arch. Path. (Chicago) 75, 414-420 (1963)
62. Rege, P.R., Evans, A.T.: Erythroplasia of Queyrat. J. Urol. (Baltimore) 111, 784-785 (1974)
63. Riveros, M., Lerron, R.F.: Geographical pathology of cancer of the penis. Cancer (Baltimore) 16, 798-811 (1963)
64. Robertson, M.A., Harington, J.S., Bradshaw, E.: The cancer pattern in Africans at Baragwanath hospital, Johannesburg. Brit. J. Cancer 25, 377-384 (1971)
65. Schmauz, R., Jain, D.K.: Geographical variation of carcinoma of the penis in Uganda. Brit. J. Cancer 25, 25-32 (1971)
66. Schmauz, R.: Correlates of histologic differentiation of carcinoma of the penis: results from a five year survey in Uganda, 1964-68. Recent Results Cancer Res. 39, 157-164 (1972)
67. Shabad, A.L.: Some aspects of etiology and prevention of penile cancer. J. Urol. (Baltimore) 92, 696-702 (1964)
68. Shaw, G.J., McFarlane, E.S.: Adenovirus-12 transformation of human foreskin cells. Canad. J. Microbiol. 15, 811-812 (1969)
69. Shrikhande, S.S., Sirsat, M.V.: Muco-epidermoid carcinoma of the penis: re-ort of an unusual case. Brit. J. Urol. 46, 233-235 (1974)
70. Smith, D.R.: General Urology. Los Altos: Lange Medical Publications, 1972, pp. 292-294
71. Smith, M.J.V., Bonacarti, A.F.: Malignant priapism due to clear cell carcinoma: a case report and review of the literature. J. Urol. (Baltimore) 92, 297-299 (1964)
72. Spittel, R.L.: Betal chewing and cancer. Brit. med. J. 2, 632 (1923)
73. Spreen, S.A., Keys, R.H., Richard, H., Jr., Evans, A.T.: Acute urinary retention secondary to metastatic prostatic carcinoma to the penis: a case report. J. Urol. (Baltimore) 113, 59 (1975)
74. Tan, R.E.: Observations on frequency of carcinoma of the penis at Macassar and its environs (South Celebes). J. Urol. (Baltimore) 89, 704-705 (1963)
75. Templeton, A.C., Buxton, E., Bianchi, A.: Cancer in kyadondo County, Uganda, 1968-70. J. nat. Cancer Inst. 48, 865-874 (1972).
76. Templeton, A.C., Hutt, M.S.R.: Distribution of tumors in Uganda. Recent Results Cancer Res. 41, 1-22 (1973)
77. Thomas, J.A., Small, C.S.: Carcinoma of the penis in Southern India. J. Urol. (Baltimore) 100, 520-526 (1967)
78. U.S. National Cancer Institute. Biomatry Branch. The Third National Cancer Survey: Advanced Three Year Report: 1969-1971 Incidence (Excluding Carcinoma in situ). Bethesda, Md.: 1974 DHEW Pub. No. (NIH) 74-637
79. U.S. National Institutes of Health Report No. 4: End Results in Cancer. Bethesda, Md.: 1972 DHEW Pub. No. (NIH) 73-272

# On the Classification of Penis Carcinoma and Its 10-Year Survival *

P. LICHTENAUER, H. SCHEER, and T. LOUTON

Penis carcinoma is a relatively uncommon tumor. In Europe and North America it consists of only 0.3-05% of all malignant tumors. The experience of one clinic or one person is an inadequate basis on which to judge the merits of the various classification systems. The BRD-Journal " Der Urologe" (4) on the other hand cited more than 670 cases of penis carcinoma treated in Germany between 1960 and 1970. In the Far East and other tropical regions penis carcinoma is apparently much more frequent, attaining 18-20% of all malignant tumors. We managed to assemble histories of 509 cases of penis carcinoma with the intention of comparing the various classification systems.

In the past, the description and classification of penis carcinoma was derived solely from the viewpoint of the particular therapist. Valid interdisciplinary comparisons were very difficult to obtain.

In 1967 the International Union Against Cancer (UICC) proposed the TNM classification of penis carcinoma shown in Table 1 (5). This classification has much to offer since penis carcinoma is a superficial carcinoma which predominantly invades lymph nodes and whose first region for spreading is in the flexures of the groin. The UICC suggests that the primary tumor of penis carcinoma should be classified according to size.

This UICC scheme seems to us theoretical and of little practical value in the clinic. The actual size of a carcinoma cannot often be determined on initial inspection but only after operative treatment. Also, during this initial inspection one may not have the necessary calipers avaiable with which to determine the diameters of the carcinoma.

In 1968 OTT and KOCH (1, 3) of the surgical clinic of the University of Heidelberg suggested a modification of the TNM system. In their scheme the primary tumor is classified from the viewpoint of localization and its degree of infiltration (Table 2).

Using our colleted data we compared these two systems. Originally we used the 5-year survival rate as the criterion by which the comparison would be made (Fig. 1). Table 3 compares the 5-year survival rates between the UICC and Heidelberg classifications.

There were no real differences in the survival rates regarding the corresponding T forms. Especially surprising is the similar survival rate for the T1 group of this tumor between the two classifications since UICC T1 encompasses all tumors up to 2 cm in diameter, regardless of localization, whereas the Heidelberg T1 classification consists only

* In part taken from the running dissertation of H. SCHEER.

Table 1. UICC classification for carcinoma of the penis

| | | |
|---|---|---|
| T | - | Primary tumor |
| TIS | = | Preinvasive carcinoma (carcinoma in situ) |
| TO | = | No evidence of primary tumor |
| T1 | = | Tumor 2 cm or less in its largest dimension, strictly superficial or exophytic |
| T2 | = | Tumor more than 2 cm but not more than 5 cm in its largest dimension with minimal infiltration |
| T3 | = | Tumor more than 5 cm in its largest dimension, or tumor of any size with deep infiltration, including the urethra |
| T4 | = | Tumor infiltration neighboring structures |
| N | - | Regional lymph nodes |
| NO | = | No palpable nodes |
| N1 | = | Movable unilateral nodes: |
| | | N1a = nodes not considered to contain growth |
| | | N1b = nodes considered to contain growth. |
| N2 | = | Movable bilateral nodes: |
| | | N2a = nodes not considered to contain growth |
| | | N2b = nodes considered to contain growth. |
| N3 | = | Fixed nodes |
| M | - | Distant metastases. |
| MO | = | No evidence of distant metastases |
| M1 | = | Distant metastases present. |

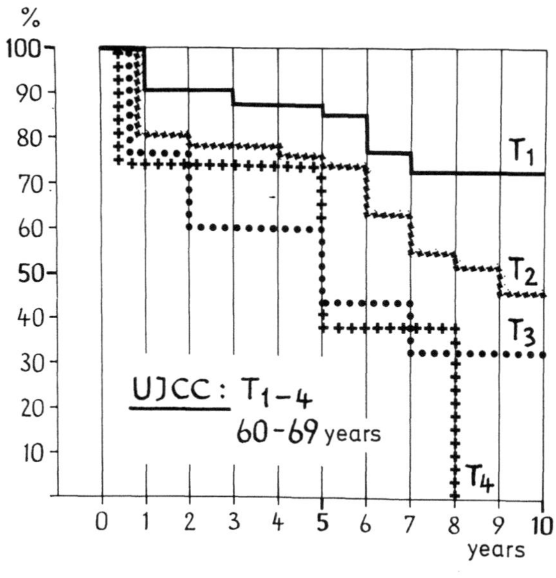


*Fig. 1. Survival rate curves over a 10-year period of primary tumor of UICC system without consideration of possible spreading to lymph nodes*

Table 2. Heidelberg proposal for classification of penis carcinoma

| | | |
|---|---|---|
| T | - | Primary tumor |
| TO | = | No primary tumor to be found |
| T1 | = | Tumor of the preputium |
| T2 | = | Tumor of the glans penis |
| T3 | = | Tumor which has infiltrated the penis shaft |
| T4 | = | Tumor which has crossed the boundary of the penis |
| N | - | Regional lymph nodes |
| NO | = | Nonpalpable lymph nodes |
| N1 | = | Novable and palpable lymph nodes on one or both sides |
| N2 | = | Packed and/or fixed lymph nodes in one or both sides |
| N3 | = | Parailiacal or other lymph nodes of the pelvis or paraaortal area are invaded (which cannot be initially considered in the clinic) |
| N4 | = | Tumor infiltration of lymph nodes without specified location |
| M | - | Distant metastases |
| MO | = | No evidence of distant metastases |
| M1 | = | Distant metastases present |

Table 3. Five-year survival rate by primary tumor

| TNM stage | UICC classification | Heidelberg classification |
|---|---|---|
| T1 | 53% | 54% |
| T2 | 43% | 46% |
| T3 | 27% | 37% |
| T4 | 10% | 10% |

of preputial tumors. Purely from clinical experiences one would think, that one suffering from a preputial carcinoma would have a much better chance of survival than one with even a small tumor of the glans penis. Both of these cases would be included under T1 of the UICC system.

Statistically we were unable to find a real difference in our data between these groups.

More and more people think the 5-year survival rate an inadequate method for judging the progress of carcinoma. Instead of this we have used a 10-year survival rate computed according to CUTLER and EDERER (2). In addition, the case were grouped into decades according to the patient age at the time of diagnosis. Thus comparisons were made only of people who had about the same life expectancy.

Using this 10-year-survival-rate we then compared the two classification systems with respect only to the primary tumor; lymph nodes conditions were not considered. The single tumor forms of the UICC scheme vary proportionally in their behavior (Fig. 1). The small carcinomas, those less than 2 cm in diameter, have a 5-year survival rate of ca. 85%, after 10 years about 75%. Of the T2 tumors the 5-year survival rate is about 75% and after 10 years barely 50% of these patients survive. The T3 tumor behave similarily: after 5 years only 50% survive; after 10 years 70% of these patients have died. Of the further advanced penis carcinomas (T4 patients), i.e., those whose tumors extend the bounds of the penis, none survived 10 years; indeed after 5 years 50% of these patients have died. The data from this group of patients indicate that the deviation of this material is extensive.

For the Heidelberg classification the results are approximately similar. One notices here that the T2 and T3 survival curves lie very close to one another. The reason for this lies with the difference in defining primary tumor. In the UICC scheme, the T3 group measures more than 5 cm in diameter with extended infiltration, whereas in the Heidelberg scheme T3 also includes tumors which have just begun to infiltrate, e.g., those still small carcinomas in the sulcus coronarius glandis. After penis amputation and irradiation therapy for those smaller forms of penis carcinoma, the life expectancy will be higher than with those extensive carcinomas, which would be grouped under T3 according to the UICC. In comparing both schemes one can clearly see that (with respect to penis carcinoma at any rate) the 5-year limit is not a sufficient basis on which to study the progress of carcinoma. After 10 years about twice as many patients died as after 5 years.

As with many malignant tumors, the size and localization of the primary penis carcinoma seldom have a direct relation to the survival of the patient. What is important is the degree of tumor spreading. The first stations of the lymph system for penis carcinoma are to be found in the groin and are thus clinically accessible. In a large number of cases lymph nodes in the groin are already palpable at the first visit of a patient suffering from this disease. The percentage relation between the different sizes of primary tumor to the corresponding palpable lymph nodes is similar in both classifications in spite of the different definitions of primary tumor. Also, if the status of lymph nodes in the groin region is histologically verified, the percentage relation between primary tumor and its actual metastases is similar.

The classification of lymph node invasion is very differentiated in the UICC proposal (Table 1). First, lymph nodes are differentiated according to whether they are palpable on one or both sides; second, lymph nodes that are unspecified are distinguished from those specific with respect to actual metastases; third, palpable and still movable lymph nodes are distinguished from those that are fixed in the surrounding tissue. This system has many weak points. For example, the judgment, whether a clinically palpable lymph node is suspected of having been invaded by malignant tissue, is highly subjective and would most likely differ from examiner to examiner. We also think there is no reason to believe that the difference between a uni- or bilateral invasion is important with respect to this tumor; rather what really is important is whether or not the carcinoma has reached its first point of entry or perhaps even gone past it. When the corresponding life tables are graphed, one sees that there is no difference in the corresponding life expectancy of those patients, neither 5 nor 10 years after the initial one-sided or two-sided palpation results. However, there is a distinctly different life expectancy between nonpalpable lymph nodes and palpable, movable lymph nodes, that is, for those nodes which clinically show the beginning signs of tumor spread, and also for those lymph nodes which are palpated as fixed within the surrounding groin area, that is, where there is a strong clinical suspension of actual carcinoma spreading which has already moved beyond the actual lymph nodes into the neighboring tissues.

This simplication of the state of the lymph system and its invasion is incorporated in the Heidelberg-scheme (Table 2).

N3 and N4 are of little interest from a statistical point of view, since they are uncommon and not well known. In N0, N1 and N2 the simplified N classification results in the 10-year curves shown in Figure 2a. Of these patients who initially had nonpalpable lymph nodes in the groin, i.e., those for whom there was no suspicion of lymph invasion, 85% were alive after 5 years and 80% after 10 years. Of those patients in whom a beginning invasion of the lymph system was suspected, i.e., N1, 65% were alive after 5 years and 45% after 10 years. Of those patients in whom there was a strong suspicion of a progressive invasion of the lymph system i.e., N2, 40% were alive after 5 years, 30% after 10 years. We have calculated the standard deviation for each group of data and recorded it at 5 and 10 years as an illustration of the expected variance. Seventy percent of all of our corresponding data fall in this area. When this standard deviation is doubled, one can generate a confidence interval in which one would expect about 95% of such samples to fall. The bands for this are relatively narrow and the expected prognosis is determined. On the other hand, the bands of N0 and N1 intersect one another at the 10-year point. Thus, a differentiated prognosis for the next 10 years remains from a clinical point of view a point of discussion. Too often unpalpable nodes actually have been invaded and up to 50% of the palpable nodes are of an unspecific origin without direct relation to the carcinoma.

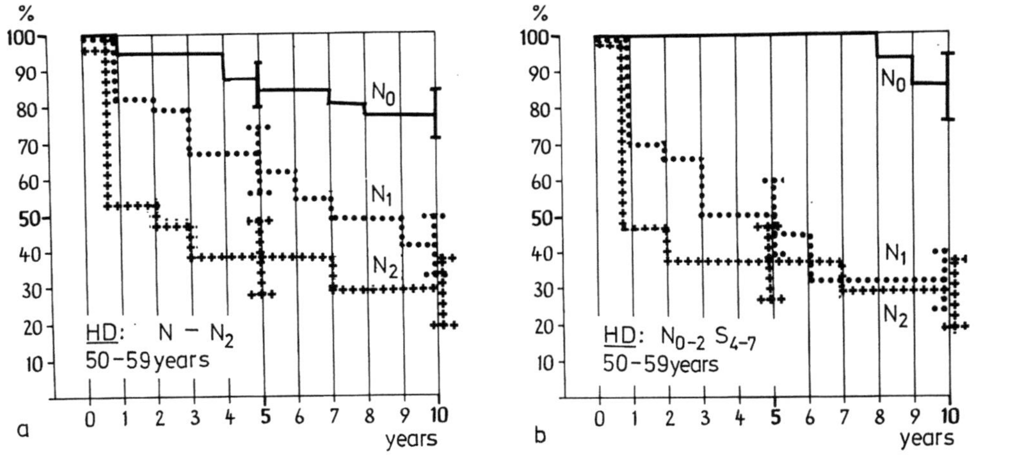


*Fig. 2a and b. Different 10-year survival rate curves of penis carcinoma with; (a) only clinical evaluation of spreading to lymph nodes, and (b) histologic examination of the lymph nodes*

Only when the status of the lymph system of the groin is determined histologically (Fig. 2b) (C code in TNM nomenclature) a definite prognosis is possible. It can be seen, that those patients with negative histologic results have practically a 100% chance of surviving the next 10 years - especially with respect to the tumor. Of those patients who have positive histologic results, only 50% will survive the next 5 years, even though they would be intensively treated. After 10 years only 30% of this group of patients will still be alive. Thus, the overall survival chances for those patients with verified metastases of penis carcinoma have a poorer prognosis as well as a clearer prognosis than those classified under N1 after only a clinical examination. On the other hand, the 10-year curves for the N2-patients (i.e., those patients, who have fixed palpable lymph nodes in the groin) show little difference between the clinical determination and an additional histologic verification. The results of palpation are so typical for actual tumor spreading, that an additional histologic examination of these nodes can only confirm, and but seldom contradict, this suspicion. After 5 years fewer than 40% of the patients are alive. He who lives that long, however, seems to have good prospects of surviving to the 10th year after initial diagnosis and therapy. The possible, if rare spread to distant lymph nodes from penis carcinoma are classified in both schemes as MO (no evidence of distant metastases) and M1 (distant metastases present). There is no point in computing a life table for these cases, as there are very few of them.

When one has only a relatively small sample to evaluate, one is forced to group some of the single TNM classifications together. In order to avoid the problem posed by considerable differences in patients' ages and in life expectancy, we have divided the cases of each tumor class according to age of patient at time of diagnosis. The classification is by decades, starting at 50 years. The life table was computed as per the method of CUTLER and EDERER for each decade and tumor class. The criterion was again 10-year survival rate and this could then be compared with a control population of the Federal Republic of Germany. These latter data came from abbreviated life tables for Germany for the years 1971-1972 from the German statistical yearbook for 1974.

The main and important object in grouping the patients with penis carcinoma was lymphogenic tumor spreading since the determines further progress of the carcinoma. The size and localization of the actual tumor and its degree of local infiltration are of lesser importance as long as the primary tumor remains within the bounds of the penis (Table 4).

Table 4. Penis carcinoma

| | | | |
|---|---|---|---|
| Stage I | T1 - 3 | NO | MO |
| Stage II | T1 - 3 | N1 | MO |
| Stage III | T1 - 3 | N2 | MO |
| Stage IV | T4 | NO - 2 | M1 |
| | | NO - 2 | MO - 1 |

In Table 4 the first three forms of the primary tumor are brought in the so-called stage I of penis carcinoma. This applies as long as there is no evidence of tumor spreading into the regional lymph nodes and as long as there are no distant metastases.

In stage II we grouped those patients whose primary tumor was still within the bounds of the penis, and whose regional lymph nodes had a beginning invasion, but in whom there was no sign of distant metastases.

In stage III we are grouped those patients whose primary tumor was still within the bounds of the penis, but who showed a progressive state of tumor invasion of the regional lymph nodes; distant metastases were still unknown.

In stage IV are grouped those patients, in whom the primary tumor has escaped the bounds of the penis or that it has invaded distant lymph nodes.

We divided these single stages into groups by decades and compared the corresponding 10-year curves with a control group (all citizens of this age).

A calculation of the life table for the patients between 40 and 49 years of age was not appropriated, since there were too few cases, at least in Europe.

The computation for the group of patient between 50 and 59 years of age may be seen in Figure 3 where 95% of the control group (<u>thick back line above</u>) is still living after 10 years. In comparison with the stage I patients, i.e., those who presumably have no lymph system invasion, 85% survived 5 years and at 10 years the survival rate is 20% lower than in the control group. On the other hand it should be borne in mind that when the invasion of the lymph system is definitely negated by histologic findings, their survival rate is logically as good as that of the control group. The patient group with a clinical possibility of a beginning tumor spreading into the lymph system (stage II) has a lower survival rate in spite of intensive care and therapy. At 5 years the rate is lower by 30% than the control group, and at 10 years 50% them of have died.

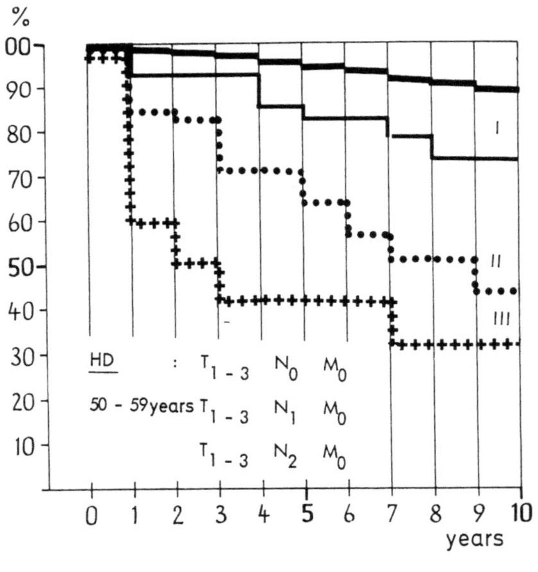


*Fig. 3. Ten-year survival rate curves according to status of patients between 50 and 59 years of age*

In the stage III of penis carcinoma, where the regional metastases are already spreading into the surroundings, the survival rate is considerably lower: at 5 years only 50% and at 10 years only 40% of these patients are still alive.

Stage IV, at least in our collection, contains so few cases that there was no point in computing the corresponding life table.

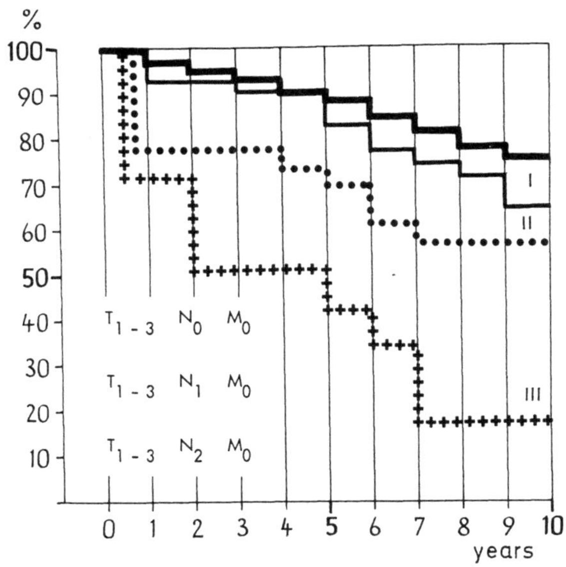


*Fig. 4. Ten-year survival rate curves according to status of patients between 60 and 69 years of age*

The 10-year curves for patients 60-69 years of age are shown in Figure 4. Here the expected survival rate after 10 years is only 80%. The first stage of penis carcinoma (no invasion of the lymph nodes) shows a 5-10% lower curve, whereby the standard deviation of the data was so large that the expected survival rate for patients who clinically belong to stage I have roughly the same expected survival rate as a sample of the healthy population of this age (assuming, of course, that they have received proper treatment).

Survival rates for the second stage of this disease are after 5 years about 15-20% lower than the expected survival rates. After 10 years only 60% of this group are still living.

In stage III of this cancer the patient's chances for survival are drastically reduced, from 40 to 50% less than normal. Thus, at the end of 10 years, only 20% of this group is still living.

The 10-year curves for patients 70-79 years old in Figure 5. During this decade so many factors influence the life expectancy of the patient that the actual tumor will lead to death in only a few cases. All curves show a 45° downward slope. The life expectancy of a person having penis carcinoma is roughly the same as the control. Here the four stages of penis carcinoma no longer need to be considered separately; the patients will most likely die of their tumor but not necessarily because of it.

## SUMMARY


With respect to the primary tumor there is no difference between the proposal of the UICC and the Heidelberg version for TNM classification of the penis carcinoma. Clinically the Heidelberg scheme seems more practical, but there were no statistical differences between them.

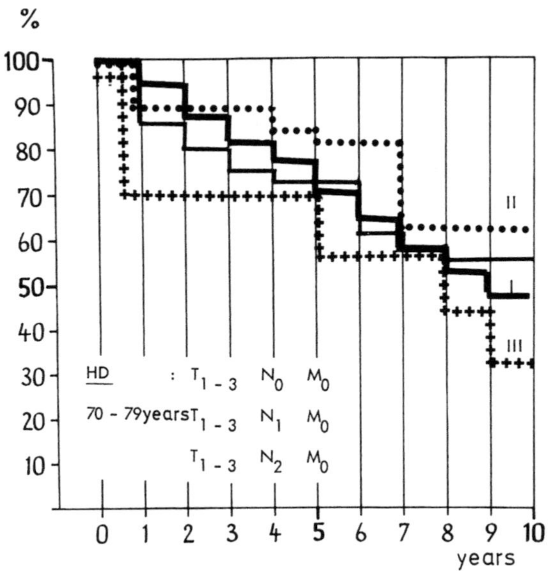


*Fig. 5. Ten-year survival rate curves according to status of patients between 70 and 79 years of age*

With respect to the prognosis for the patient, the size and localization of the primary tumor are of secondary importance. What is important is the degree of tumor spreading in the lymph system. From this point of view, one needs only to differentiate between T1 (tumor restricted to the penis) and T2 (tumor extending the bounds of the penis).

On the other hand, size, localization, and degree of infiltration of penis carcinoma do have different therapeutic consequences, so from this point of view the differentiation of the primary tumor from T1 up to T4 should be retained.

With respect to the classification of the state of the corresponding lymph system it is our opinion that the UICC proposal is too differentiated and has little meaning. In its stead, the Heidelberg scheme is clear and simple. Any examiner can complete it.

With the help of life tables extending beyond 10 years after diagnosis we were able to determine that 5 years is not a sufficiently long time to close a case of penis cancer. Even with proper treatment, the patient may suffer up to 10 years or more from the disease. In patients aged between 50 and 59 years of age the cancer seems to grow faster; in spite of proper and intensive treatment those patients had a clearly limited life expectancy. In patients aged 60-69 and more so in those between 70 and 79 years of age the tumor seemed to grow slowly and often had no effect on the survival rate.

## REFERENCES

1. Arnal, M.L., Dold, U., Ehlers, C.Th., Gögler, E., Ott, G.: Dtsch. med. Wschr. 93, 694 (1968)
2. Cutler, F.J., Ederer, F.: J. chron. Diseases 8, 699 (1958)
3. Koch, K.H.: Über das Penis-Carcinom und seine Einteilung nach dem TNM-System. Diss. Heidelberg 1968

4. Lichtenauer, P., Ott, G., Dröge, K.H.: Urologe A 12, 66 (1973)
5. UICC: Clin. Trial 9, 72 (1968)
6. UICC: The TNM system (General Rules)
Research Commission committee on clinical stage classification on applied statistics. Geneva 1952

# Problems of Therapeutic Surgery in Penis Carcinoma

P. BRÜHL *

Carcinoma of the penis occurs rarely, and among our patients it takes with a frequency of 0.6% last place among the malignant diseases of the male urogenital tract after carcinoma of the kidney, prostate, bladder, and testicles. It originates mostly in the inner part of the prepuce of the penis or the inner part of the glans, and, sparing the corpus spongiosum urethrae, spreads within the corpus cavernosum. In our department, in the period from 1928 to 1974, 124 penile cancers were observed. In 69 of these cases the histologic diagnosis could be reviewed and the further process could be surveyed. In 95.7% a squamous cell carcinoma had been found (Table 1).

Table 1. Histologic statements in 69 penile cancers eligible for evaluation (University of Bonn, 1928-1974)

| Histology | Patient | (%) |
|---|---|---|
| Squamous cell carcinoma with cornification | 51 | (73.9) |
| Squamous cell carcinoma without cornification | 15 | (21.7) |
| Total squamous cell carcinoma | 66 | (95.6) |
| Malignant epithelioma | 1 | (1.4) |
| Malignant fibroepithelioma | 1 | (1.4) |
| Poorly differentiated rhabdomyo-sarcoma | 1 | (1.4) |

The treatment of carcinoma of the penis is based on a combination of radiation therapy and surgery and the modalities of the treatment depend on the stage of the tumor. In every suspicious macroscopic case we demand a test excision with a subsequent histologic examination before entering into therapy, because there are many differential diagnostic possibilities in carcinomas of the penis (5, 9).

A small lesion, confined to the prepuce, is mostly managed by circumcision alone. Local radiation is added to circumcision when the lesion is in the glans and biopsy shows it to be limited to the superficial

* Department of Urology, University of Bonn, GFR.

surface of the epithelium. In these cases radiation of the regional lymph nodes is not necessary.

When the tumor involves both the prepuce and the glans and also extends into the shaft of the penis for a short distance, partial amputation is recommended. But it should be noted that today possibilities of applying supervoltage rays in this stage of carcinoma of the penis apparently show at least the same results as surgery, thus avoiding mutilation (7). Resection of the prepuce is obligatory for an adequate radiotherapy.

This may be of extreme importance in the younger patient where normal sexual and urinary function are psychologically important. In the older patient this loss of normal function may not carry the same psychological consequences. The average age of our patients was 65; the youngest patient was 38 years old.

For the purpose of partial amputation the skin of the penis is cut 3 cm proximal to the macroscopic edge of the carcinoma. The corpora cavernosa are cut slightly further up in order to obtain a good covering of the penile stump at the end of the operation (Fig. 1) (17). Carcinomas extending higher and attacking the proximal part of the corpora cavernosa, demand total amputation of the penis with perineal implantation of the urethra (Fig. 2a) (4). Splitting of the skin above the symphisis, mobilization of the bulbus and the roots of the penis, and their resection after separating the urethra. The urethra and the corpus spongiosum are brought through a median incision in the perineal skin and implanted there. For functional reasons VAHLENSIECK recomends implantation of the urethra into the scrotal skin (Fig. 2b). Carcinomas that are far more extended and also have attacked the scrotum demand the total amputation of penis, scrotum, and testicles.

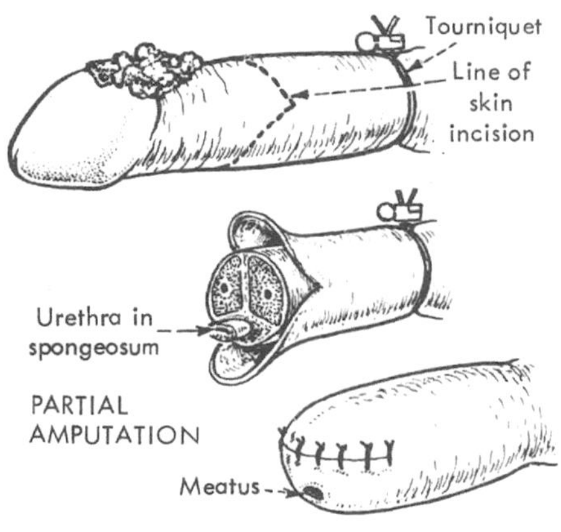


*Fig. 1. Partial amputation of the penis*

The indications for removal of the regional lymph nodes (Fig. 3a) (15) in carcinoma of the penis are contested. Lymphangiography may be helpful in assessing the extent of the lymphatic spread but the possibility of false negative node involvement should be remembered. Good technique and great practice are the most important prerequisites for satisfactory results (Fig. 3b) (14). Some authors recommend observation of the lymph system after amputation of the primary affection and they demand bilateral lymphadenectomy of the regional nodes only when an adequate suspicion is given. In many cases the enlarged lymph nodes are caused by inflammable reactions and disappear after excision of the tumorous

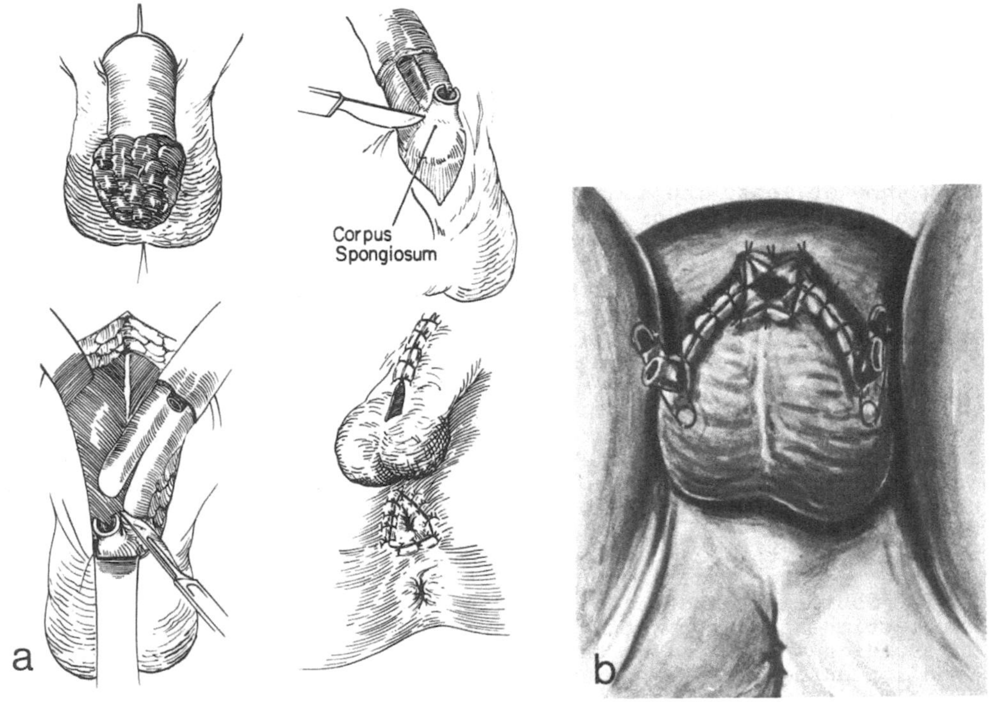


*Fig. 2a and b. (a) Total amputation of penis; (b) Implantation of urethra into scrotal skin*

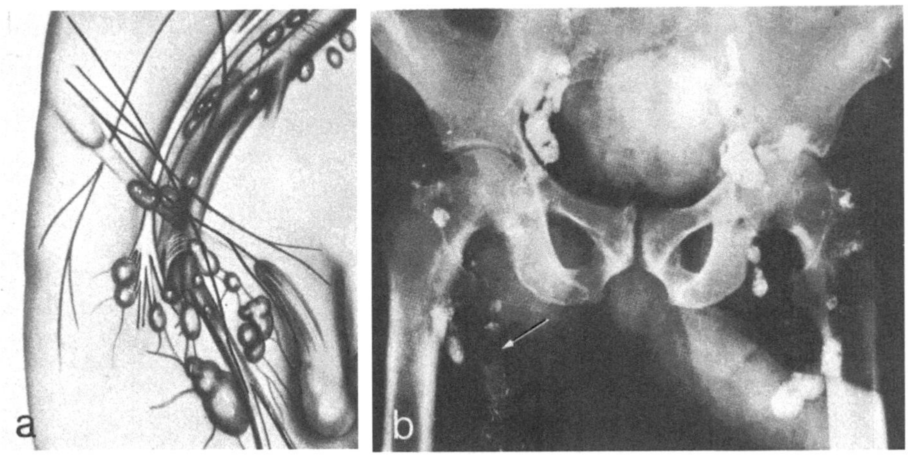


*Fig. 3a and b. Carcinoma of penis; involvement of right femoral node; lymphagiogram (b) and line of section (a) in inguinal lymphadenectomy*

part of the penis. In such cases lymphadenectomy would be unnecessary. Moreover, lymphadenectomy is frequently accompanied by complications in the healing process and may cause an edema of the lower extremities. In 14% of our cases showing enlarged lymph nodes only histologic signs of inflammation were found. According to SKINNER et al. (18) 20% of cases with palpable inconspicious lymph nodes show micrometastases. Prior to such exploration, extirpation and multiple microscopic sections of all regional lymph nodes are indispensable. Other authors do not distinguish between a prophylactic lymphadenectomy and a therapeutic one and in any case plead for a regional lymphadenectomy to be carried out either simultaneously or in two stages (6). It is also recommended that postoperative supervoltage-therapy be applied and lymphadenectomy be made only on condition that the nodes are really palpable.

For a better understanding of the problems of treatment of penile cancer the anatomy of the lymph system must be outlined (Fig. 4) (8): the first lymphatic region for the efferent lymphatic vessels of the skin of the penis and scrotum is the medial group (5) of the superficial inguinal lymph nodes (Fig. 4a). The efferent lymph vessels of the corpus and glans penis (Fig. 4b) also have their drainage in those lymph nodes (6).

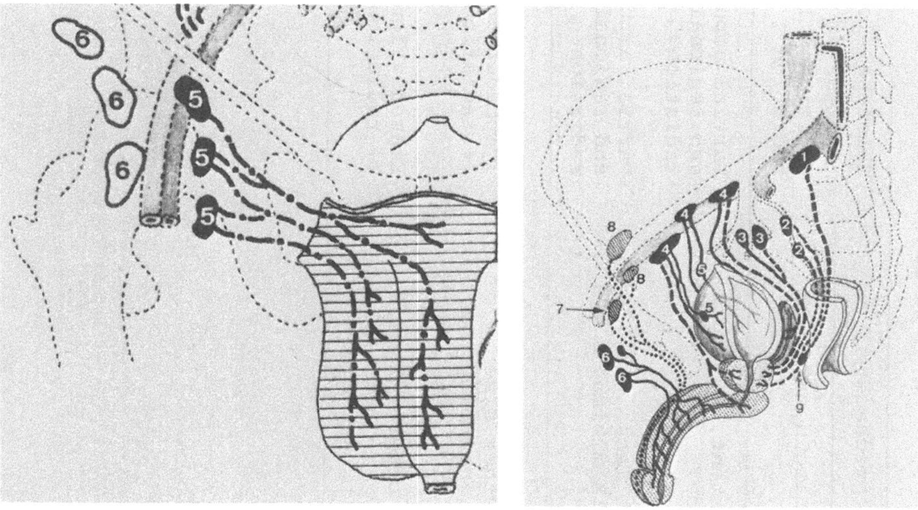


*Fig. 4. Efferent lymph vessels of genital skin and of corpus and glans penis to medial group of superficial inguinal lymph nodes*

Accessory vessels from the glans may end in the nodus lymphaticus inguinalis profundus (7) and in the nearby lower nodi lymphatici iliaci interni (8) (the so-called nodi lymphatici lacunaris medialis et lateralis). Some rare variants may be connections with the paravesical and other parailiacal lymph nodes (8). So there is no real indication for removal. On the one hand the indications are not in proportion to the operative complications. On the other hand, no patient, having metastases in those nodes has lived longer than 2 years (10, 11).

We conform our therapeutic modalities to the stage of the carcinoma (Table 2). In stage TO (precancer) we restrict ourselves to excision of the suspicious areas. In some cases local treatment with thiotepa

Table 2. Five-year survival according to clinical stage of tumor (UICC) and treatment of patients with carcinoma of penis

| | Clinical stage | No of patients | Treatment | | 5-year survival (%) |
|---|---|---|---|---|---|
| TO | No primary tumor found (precancer) | 4 | Thiotepa, local | | No recurrence |
| TIS | Preinvasive carcinoma (carcinoma in situ) | O | Excision + local radiation | | |
| T1 | Tumor 2 cm or less in extent, superficial or exophytic | 28 | Partial amputation and regional radiation | Lymphadenectomy in enlarged lymph nodes (previous biopsy) | 58 |
| T2 | Tumor more than 2 cm but less than 5 cm in extent, with minimal infiltration | 36 | Partial amputation and regional radiation | | 41 |
| T3 | Tumor more than 5 cm in maximum extent or a tumor of another size with deep infiltration, including the urethra | 2 | Total amputation + lymphadenectomy (+ radiation) | | 1 Patient |
| T4 | Tumor infiltration into other tissue | 2 | Emasculation (+ radiation) | | O |

(triethylene phosphoramide) was carried out successfully. When histologically a stage TIS has been found, excision is followed by local radiation. If there are no palpable lymph nodes in stages T1-T2 we carry out only partial amputation and following radiation with supervoltage rays. We have no experience with exclusive primary radiation in these stages. This is recommended by ENGELSTAD (2) and recently used with good results by LULE (13) who works with high speed electrons. Above all, this way of treatment must be discussed with the younger patient. In stage T3 we treat patients under 65 years with total amputation and regional lymphadenectomy, carried out simultaneously or, if the patient's condition is reduced and if the carcinoma is infected, carried out in two stages. In cases with histologic lymph node participation postoperative supervoltage therapy must be done. If the patient is over 65 years old we carry out regional lymphadenectomy only in cases suspicious for lymph node metastases and for the rest we restrict ourselves to postoperative regional supervoltage therapy. In stage T4, which nowadays' is seen rarely, a lymph node affection seems to be the rule. In this case emasculation is followed by other mostly palliative treatments (lymphadenectomy and radiation). Of course the internal situation (operability) and age of the patient are decisive for choice of therapy. With patients under 65 years regional lymphadenectomy should be done. Radiation follows on principle. With older patients we restrict ourselves to further surgical treatments. If the metastases have proceeded (N2) the 5-year survival will be high reduced. If the patient presents with clinically inoperable fixed (N3) inguinal nodes or distant metastases the prognosis is extremely poor. But generally the prognosis of adequately treated carcinoma of the penis is good (Table 2).

In this context the necessity of preventive circumcision for the purpose of facilitating genital hygiene should be pointed out, since the etiologic cause of phimosis in the formation of carcinoma of the penis is generally recognized (3, 6, 20).

## SUMMARY

Very often penile cancer occurs histologically as a squamous cell carcinoma. Its treatment is based on radiation therapy and surgery and depends on the stage of the tumor, age of patient, and anatomy and pathology of the lymph system of the male genitalia. In an evaluation of 69 cases, the problems of therapy and prognosis are discussed. Preventive circumcision for the purpose of facilitating genital hygiene is reputed to be the operative prophylaxis.

## REFERENCES

1. Czembirek, H., Lichtenauer, P.: Lymphographie vom Dorsum penis. Röfo. 113, 494-497 (1970)
2. Engelstad, R.B.: Treatment of cancer of the penis at the Norwegian Radium Hospital. Amer. J. Roentgenol. 01, 60, 801 (1948)
3. Feustel, A., Zochert, G., Bellmann, H.: Beitrag zur Ätiologie und Prognose des Peniskarzinoms. Z. Urol. 9, 688-694 (1972)
4. Glenn, J.F., Boyce, W.H.: The penis and urethra. In: Urologic Surgery. New York and Evanston: Hoeber-Harper, 1969, p. 493
5. Gödde, St.: Das Peniskarzinom. Dtsch. med. J. 19, 725-729 (1968)

6. Hardner, G.J., Bhanalaph, T., Murphy, G.P., Albert, D.J., Moore, R.H.: Carcinoma of the penis: Analysis of therapy in 100 consecutive cases. J. Urol. (Baltimore) 108, 428-430 (1972)
7. Kärcher, K.H.: Die Strahlentherapie des Peniskarzinoms. In: Krebsbehandlung als interdisziplinäre Aufgabe. Kärcher, K.H. (ed.) Berlin-Heidelberg-New York: Springer-Verlag, 1975, p. 728
8. Kubik, S.: Anatomie des Lymphsystems. Radiol. clin. biol. 42, 243-257 (1973)
9. Kuchenbuch, H.S., Jung, H.D.: Beitrag zur Epidemiologie, Erfassung, Diagnose und Therapie des Peniskarzinoms. Arch. Geschwulstforsch. 39/2, 128-136 (1972)
10. Lichtenauer, P., Ehlers, P., Gödde, St., Koch, W., Ott, G.: Die TNM-Klassifizierung und die Bedeutung der Diagnosesicherung (C) beim Penis-Carzinom. Z. Krebsforsch. 77, 83-90 (1972)
11. Lichtenauer, P., Ott, G., Dröge, K.H.: Zur Klassifizierung, Verlauf und Behandlung des Penis-Karzinoms (Statistische Auswertung von 317 bioptisch nachgewiesenen Penis-Karzinomen) Urologe A 12, 66-70 (1973)
12. Ludvik, W., Jentzsch, K.: Peniskarzinom. In: Krebsbehandlung als interdisziplinäre Aufgabe. Kärcher, K.H. (ed.). Berlin-Heidelberg-New York: Springer-Verlag, 1975, p. 724
13. Lule, E.: Die Strahlentherapie des Peniskarzinoms. In: Krebsbehandlung als interdisziplinäre Aufgabe. Kärcher, K.H. (ed.). Berlin-Heidelberg-New York: Springer-Verlag, 1975, p. 728
14. Miller, E.M.: Lymphography. In: Clinical Urography, erd ed. Emmet, J.L., Witten, D.M. (eds.). Philadelphia: W.B. Saunders, 1971, Vol. III, p. 2036
15. Roen, P.R.: Atlas of Urologic Surgery. New York: Meredith Publishing, 1967, p. 387
16. Schindler, E., May, P.: Das Peniskarzinom. Med. Welt 24, 1205-1207 (1973)
17. Scott, R., Deane, R.F., Callander, R.: Penis tumours. In: Urology Illustrated. Edinburgh, London, New York: Churchill Livingstone, 1975, p. 299
18. Skinner, D.G., Leadbetter, W.F., Kelley, S.B.: The surgical management of squamous cell carcinoma of the penis. J. Urol. (Baltimore) 107, 273 (1972)
19. Vahlensieck, W.: Penis und Harnröhre. In: Spezielle Chirurgie für die Praxis. Baumgärtl, F., Kremer, K., Schreiber, H.W. (eds.). Stuttgart: Thieme, 1972, p. 474
20. Vary, L., Karatson, A., Bochkor, B., Wabrosch, G., Gyarmathy, F., Bard, R., Pânykó, E., Sallai, Zs., Asztalos, L., Balogh, F.: Das Klinikum des Peniskarzinoms. Urol. int. (Basel) 26, 171-183 (1971)

# Treatment of Penis Carcinoma with Interstitially Administered Iridium; Comparison with Radium Therapy

Z. DAŃCZAK-GINALSKA

From 1947 up to 1971, 48 patients with penis carcinoma have undergone preventive brachycurietherapy at the Institut of Oncology in Warsaw.

In Poland, the index of morbidity in respect of penis carcinoma is 0.7 per 100,000 population (10), i.e., approximately 130 persons per year are taken ill.

Only 10% of these patients undergo radiotherapy in oncological institutes. The remaining patients, suffering from various degrees of the disease, undergo surgical treatment (amputations) in urological clinics.

## MATERIAL

The paper compares the results of treatment of 30 patients suffering from penis carcinoma treated by radium therapy in the period 1947-1960 and 18 patients treated by Iridium-192 by the period 1968-1971.

The age of the patients ranged from 22 to 77 years. Seventy-five percent of the patients were under 60 years of age, and almost 50% were under 50 years of age. The mean age in both groups was 53 years. In all cases the diagnosis was confirmed by microscopic examination, which established carcinoma planoepitheliale spinocellulare, usually with a high degree of cancer maturity (keratoblasticum). In two cases a very immature, highly malignant form of tumor was found.

All patients were follow up for a minimum of 3 years. The TNM grading system, accepted by UICC, was used for the evaluation of the degree of clinical progression of the tumor (2).

No distant recurrences were observed (Mo).

The clinical progression of the tumor for the compared groups of patients is shown in Table 1.

In patients treated with $^{192}Ir$, the penis carcinoma was locally more advanced, while the invasion of the tumor process in the lymph nodes was similar.

Table 1. Clinical progression of the tumor for the compared groups of patients

| | $^{192}Ir$ | | | | | $^{226}Ra$ | | | | |
|---|---|---|---|---|---|---|---|---|---|---|
| | $N_0$ | $N_1$ | $N_2$ | Total No. | % | Total % | No. | $N_2$ | $N_1$ | $N_0$ |
| $T_1$ | 1 | 1 | 0 | 2 | 11 | 40 | 12 | 5 | 3 | 4 |
| $T_2$ | 2 | 3 | 1 | 6 | 33 | 33 | 10 | 5 | 5 | 0 |
| $T_3$ | 1 | 0 | 5 | 6 | 33 | 24 | 7 | 2 | 3 | 2 |
| Recurrence postoperation | 1 | 2 | 1 | 4 | 23 | 3 | 1 | 0 | 0 | 1 |
| Total | 5 | 6 | 7 | 18 | 100 | 100 | 30 | 12 | 11 | 7 |
| % | 28 | 33 | 39 | 100 | | | 100 | 40 | 37 | 23 |

METHODS OF TREATMENT

Radium therapy was conducted by the mold technique, according to Paterson (12). The doses ranged from 1100 to 8700 mgh, which was equivalent to doses of approximately 6000-8000 rad. The overall treatment time was 22-60 h, and treatment took 4-6 days. In the case of mold work, from 30 to 160 mg of radium-226 were used.

The $^{192}Ir$ therapy was conducted by afterloading methods, elaborated by Pierquin (13, 14). Initially, directional interstitial needles and then intradermal wires were used (Fig. 1).

From two to six source lines were used. The activity of $^{192}Ir$ was 0.7-2 mCi/cm. The T-minimum dose was 7000 rad, the T-maximum dose approximately 9000 rad. In two cases, the T-minimum dose was lowered to 6000 rad.

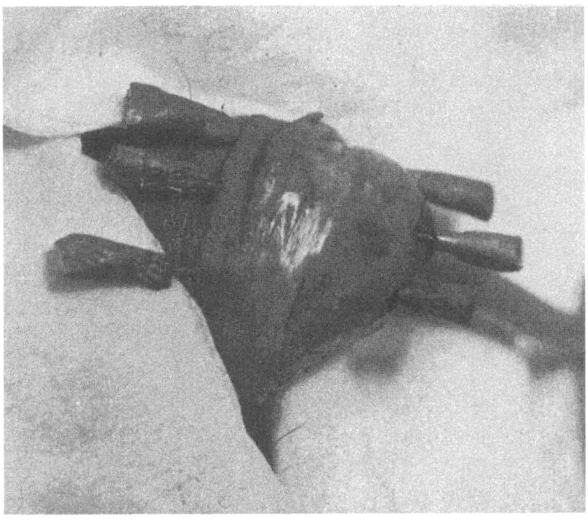

*Fig. 1. Implantation of $^{192}Ir$ by technique of intradermal wires. Circumferential, semicircular distribution of sources*

If the tumors were located circumferentially, $^{192}Ir$ was implanted in a semicircle, so that the urethra received a lower dose than the T-minimum dose.

The distribution of doses from three $^{192}Ir$ sources implanted in a semicircle in respect of circumferential penis invasion is illustrated by the isodose diagram, calculated by the technique of electronic calculations, in the Fortran language, according to Warsaw Institute program (1) (Fig. 2).

In this case the urethra received a dose lower by 60% than the T-minimum dose.

*Fig. 2. Distribution of doses from three sources implanted circumferentially in a semicircle, calculated by electronic technique*

## COMPARISON OF THERAPEUTIC RESULTS

The comparison of the results of $^{192}Ir$ and radium therapy at 3 years is shown in Table 2.

Table 2. Iridium and radium therapy results assessed at 3 years

| | $^{192}I$ No | % | $^{226}Ra$ No | % |
|---|---|---|---|---|
| Number of patients | 18 | 100 | 30 | 100 |
| Survival after 3 years | 16 | 89 | 25 | 83 |
| Mortality | | | | |
| Recurrence | 0 | 0 | 1 | 3 |
| Lymph node metastases | 2 | 11 | 2 | 7 |
| Other diseases | 0 | 0 | 2 | 7 |

The figures for the 3-year survival, depending on the local progression of the tumor, are shown in Table 3.

Table 3. Therapy results at 3 years depending on local progression of tumor

| | $^{192}Ir$ No of patients | Survived 3 years | $^{226}Ra$ No of patients | Survived 3 years |
|---|---|---|---|---|
| $T_1$ | 2 | 2 | 12 | 10 |
| $T_2$ | 6 | 6 | 10 | 9 |
| $T_3$ | 6 | 4 | 7 | 5 |
| Recurrence postoperation | 4 | 4 | 1 | 1 |
| Total | 18 | 16<br>89% | 25 | 30<br>83% |

In both compared groups, the percentage of patients who survived for 3 years is similar.

The patients who underwent radium therapy remained under observation for 5 or 10 years or even for longer periods of time. The rate of survival after longer observation decreases, due to natural mortality. During a 5-year observation period, 80% of the patients survived, and after 10 years 77% of the patients survived (5).

## COMPARISON OF FAILURE INCIDENCE, POSTTREATMENT COMPLICATIONS AND FINAL FUNCTIONAL EFFECTS

The incidence of local recurrences and postirradiation complications following $^{192}Ir$ and radium therapy is shown in Table 4.

Table 4. Comparison of incidence of local recurrences and posttreatment complications

| | $^{192}Ir$ No | % | $^{226}Ra$ No | % |
|---|---|---|---|---|
| Number of patients | 18 | 100 | 30 | 100 |
| Recurrence | | | | |
| Amputation | 1 | 5.5 | 2 | 7 |
| Local surgery | 1 | 5.5 | 0 | 0 |
| Postirradiation complications | | | | |
| None | 12 | 67 | 10 | 33 |
| Necrosis | 3 | 16.5 | 15 | 50 |
| Stricture | 0 | 0 | 2 | 7 |
| Amputation | 1 | 5.5 | 1 | 3 |

### Local Recurrence

After $^{192}Ir$ treatment, local recurrence was observed in one case, when the applied dose was too low (6000 rad). In this patient, a small recurrence seat was removed by surgery, without maiming. During a further 4-year observation, no recurrence of the disease was found. In the second case, the recurrence was probably due to high histologic malignancy of the tumor. This patient had two-thirds of his penis amputated.

After radium therapy, recurrences were observed also in two cases. In one case, the recurrence was caused by a very high degree of progression of the tumor. In the second case, the recurrence was probably due to an error in the therapeutic technique, i.e., inaccurate insertion of the mold. In both cases the patients underwent amputation.

## Early Radiation Reaction

Early radiation reaction in all cases was violent, with substantial pyorrhea and recurring swelling, which necessitated a repeated insertion of the catheter in three patients. The reaction lasted on the average for approximately 2 months.

## Radiation Necrosis

Analysis of Table 4 shows, that after $^{192}$Ir treatment the percentage of patients in whom no complications were observed was 2 times higher than after radium treatment, and the percentage of necrosis was 3 times lower. The higher incidence of necrosis after radium treatment was probably due to uneven distribution of the dose in irregularly shaped mold, adapted to the shape of the tumor. No relation was found between the amount of the total dose and the incidence of necrosis.

## Final Functional Effect

The final functional effect is a very important factor indicating the results of the therapy of patients with penis carcinoma, observed during a period of several years. In the classification of functional effects, three grades were adopted: very good condition, good condition, and bad condition. The results were evaluated as very good if the proper shape of the penis was preserved, miction was normal, and the organ could perform all functions (Fig. 3a,c). The results were evaluated as good if miction was normal but the organ showed disfiguring scars, which which nevertheless caused no discomform (Fig. 3b). The results were evaluated as bad, when the condition of the patient required amputation. The comparison of final functional effects after 3 years' observation is shown in Table 5.

Table 5. Comparison of final functional effects after 3-year observation

| | $^{192}$Ir No. | % | $^{226}$Ra No. | % |
|---|---|---|---|---|
| Survived 3 years | 16 | 100 | 25 | 100 |
| Functional effect: | | | | |
| Very good | 11 | 69 | 7 | 28 |
| Good | 3 | 19 | 15 | 60 |
| Amputation | 2 | 12 | 3 | 12 |
| Preserved organ (in relation to all patients) | 14/18 | 72 | 22/30 | 73 |

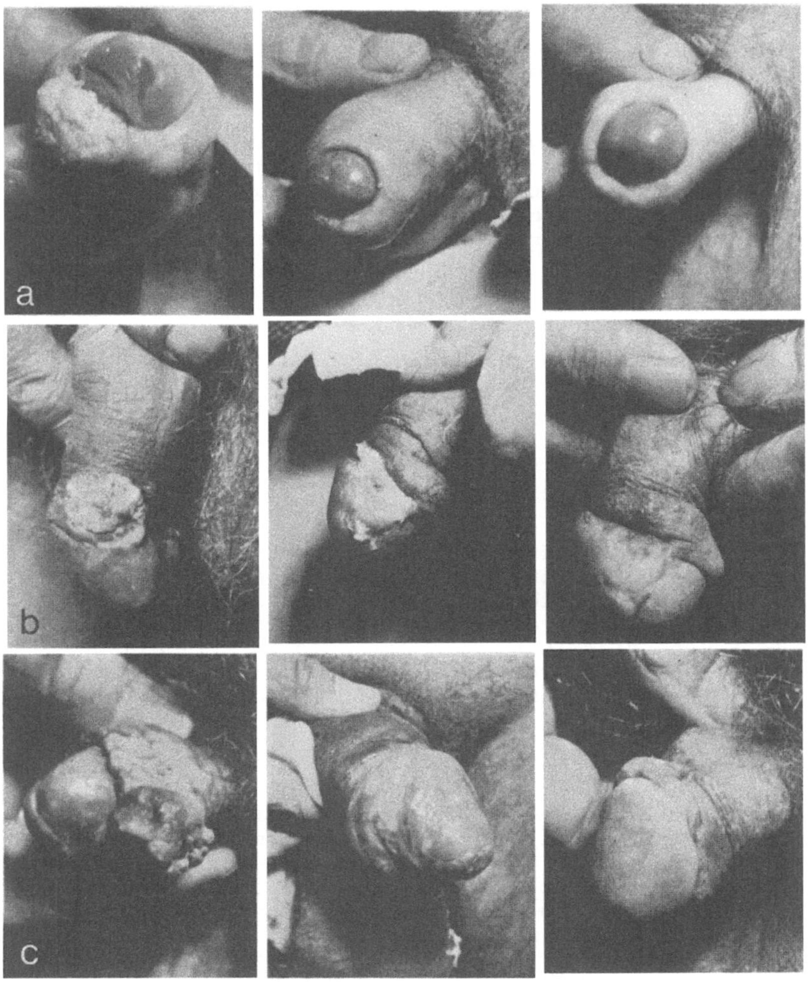


*Fig. 3a-c. Results of $^{192}Ir$ treatment: before (left); 6 weeks after (middle) and 6 months after treatment (right). (a) and (c) very good result; (b) good result*

DISCUSSION

The afterloading method for $^{192}Ir$ was introduced in the Institute of Oncology in Warsaw in order to obtain better therapeutic results and protect the personnel against radiation (3).

The results of iridium and radium therapy show that the results of the therapy assessed at 3 years are similar high (89% and 83%) for both groups of patients. The incidence of local recurrence (11% and 7%) of the tumor is also similar for both groups, bearing in mind that in patients cured with $^{192}Ir$ the growth process was more advanced.

Radiation necrosis occurs much more seldom after $^{192}Ir$ therapy, which is due to the afterloading technique that facilitates an accurate implantation of sources, and particularly their parallel location, thus avoiding overradiation of some areas. Thanks to proper implantation of sources, it was possible to avoid strictures of the urethra, described by JACKSON and DUCAN (6, 9).

In both compared groups of patients, a high percentage of patients with preserved organs (72% of the treated patients and 88% of the living patients) in comparison with results reported by other authors (6, 8 9, 11, 15, 16) was found, which is the main advantage of brachycurietherapy.

In evaluating the functional effects of treatment it should be emphasized that the percentage of very good functional effect was much higher for the group of patients treated with $^{192}Ir$ (69%) than in the group of patients treated with radium (28%). This difference is statistically significant. This fact is very important because half of the patients are under 50 years of age.

Research conducted in the Institute of Oncology showed that the application of afterloading technique for $^{192}Ir$ therapy lowered the radiation hazard to personnel during implantation approximately 50 times less than obtaining during application of radium in the form of a mold (4, 7).

## CONCLUSION

The use of brachycurietherapy for the treatment of patients with penis carcinoma is effective, due to a very high probability of the preservation of the organ.

Interstitial $^{192}Ir$ therapy by the afterloading method is more advantageous than radium therapy due to the higher chances of obtaining very good functional effects and lower hazard of after radiation complications, with equal chances of cure.

Moreover, the used of afterloading technique for $^{192}Ir$ therapy notably lessens the radiation hazard to the personnel as opposed to the application of radium.

## SUMMARY

The results of treatment of 30 patients with penis carcinoma cured with radium and 18 patients treated with $^{192}Ir$ were compared. In both groups of patients, cure assessed at 3 years was obtained for a similar percentage of patients (89% and 83%). After treatment with $^{192}Ir$, radiation necrosis was observed in 16%, and after treatment with radium in 50% of patients. In both groups a similar high percentage of patients (88%) with organs preserved after treatment was found. In the group of patients treated with $^{192}Ir$ the percentage of very good functional effects (69%) was much higher than in the group of patients treated with radium (28%).

## REFERENCES


1. Bulski, W., Majenka, I.: Use of electronic computers in the calculation of doses from the system of applicators of $^{192}Ir$ (in Ponish). Pol. Przegl. Radiol. 38, 71-77 (1974)
2. Classification of Malignant Tumours, TNM: Geneva: UICC 1968, rev. 1973
3. Dańczak, Z.: Early observations on therapeutic interstitial implantation of iridium-192. Radiol. biol. ther. 3, 305-309 (1971)
4. Dańczak, Z., Leszczyk, Cz.: Comparison of the results of radium treatment of cancer of the lower lip by the application of surface and interstitial methods (in Polish). Nowotwory 15, 257-263 (1972)
5. Dańczak, Z., Rajski, J.: Conservative radium treatment of cancer of the penis (in Polish). Nowotwory 22, 225-231 (1972)
6. Duncan, W., Jackson, S.M.: The treatment of early cancer of the penis with megavoltage X-rays. Clin. Radiol. 23, 246-248 (1972)
7. Dworakowski, M., Krystman-Mazgajska, E., Wysopolski, J.: Evaluation of the radiation exposure of the working staff during clinical application of iridium (in Polish). Nowotwory 25, 193-196 (1975)
8. Godan, F.: Erfahrung bei der Behandlung von Penismalignomen: Strahlentherapie 117, 432-443 (1962)
9. Jackson, S.M.: The treatment of carcinoma of the penis. Brit. J. Surg. 53, 33-35 (1966)
10. Koszarowski, T., Werner-Brzezińska, H., Nonnemacher, A.: Carcinoma vulvae et carcinoma penis. Nowotwory 16, 285-290 (1966)
11. Nevaishy, G.A., Deeley, T.J.: Radiotherapy in the treatment of carcinoma of the penis. Brit. J. Radiol. 41, 519-521 (1968)
12. Paterson, R.: The Treatment of Malignant Disease by Radiotherapy. London: Arnold, 1965
13. Pierquin, B.: Precis de Curiethérapie. Paris: Masson et Cie, 1964
14. Pierquin, B., Bunescu, N., Chassagne, D.: La radiothérapie des cancers de la verge par l'Iridium-192. J. Urol. Nephrol. 76, 1-8 (1970)
15. Veath, J.M., Green, J.P., Lowy, R.O.: Radiation therapy of carcinoma of the penis. Am. J. Roentgenol. 108, 130-135 (1970)
16. Woźniakowska, Z.: Radiation treatment of the primary focus of cancer of the penis (in Polish). Nowotwory 18, 365-370 (1967)

# Endocurietherapy of Penis Cancer

M. RAYNAL, D. CHASSAGNE, F. BAILLET, and B. PIERQUIN

Between 1966 and 1971, we applied endocurietherapy to 45 epitheliomas of the penis, first in our Institute Gustave Roussy, Villejuif, and then at the Hospital Henri Mondor, Créteil, using our special technique of afterloading with Iridium-192. These patients, whose lesions had received no previous treatment, were kept under observation for a minimum of 4 years.

## TECHNIQUES OF THERAPY

### 1. Primary Tumors

Our method utilizes hypodermic needles with mandrins of $^{192}Ir$ which are maintained in parallel position by plexiglass sheets. The particulars of the application techniques have been described previously (PIERQUIN et al., 1970) and need not be repeated; based upon recent experience it appears preferable to give some details of the conditions for implantation which assure an optimal target volume.

a) For small lesions with only minimal infiltration (less than 5 mm deep) we utilize a one-plane device observing two conditions (Fig. 1): The reference isodose (isodose 85%) must be strictly accounted for when it re-enters between the radioactive wire tips; therefore, the iridium wires must protrude considerably over the limits of the target volume (it may be useful to frame the lesion in its largest diameter) and the thickness of the target volume must be planned with great precision never to exceed 10 mm at the maximum.

b) For more extended lesions with infiltration we utilize a two-plane device shaped as a radioactive cage. A small cage of four lines (Fig. 2) will be sufficient to cover the whole glans, and adequate for treatment of lesions of less than 25 mm diameter. Here too, it is most important to observe with care the entering of the reference isodose, not only in the frontal plane where its flows through the radioactive lines but also in the frontal plane where it flows between the lines. We have always to keep in mind that endocurietherapy means treatment of a given volume; therefore the reference isodose must be controlled in all three dimensions in relation to the target volume. It is indispensable to have the radioactive lines sufficiently extended beyond the glans. According to our present experience, the maximal target volume must not exceed 40 mm in its maximum diameter which would correspond practically to a radioactive cage built of six radioactive lines. Clinically, this limit covers a marginal extension reaching the cavernous body (Fig. 3).

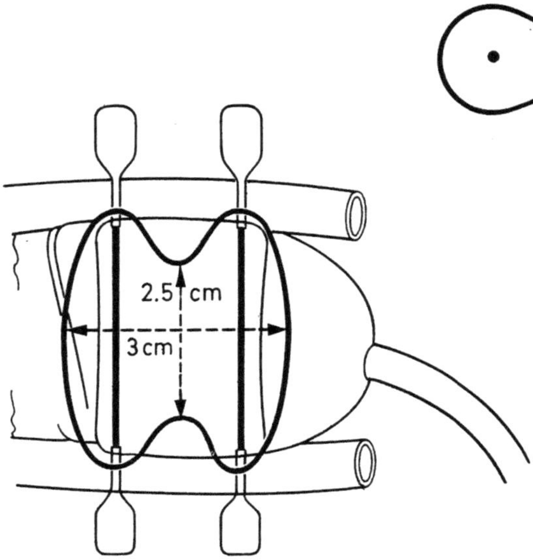


*Fig. 1. Superficial lesions, less than 1 cm thick. Single plane, 2 needles, spacing 1.8 cm. Reference isodose 85% DB, DB = 22. Length of needles = 4 cm, target volume = 7 cm³*

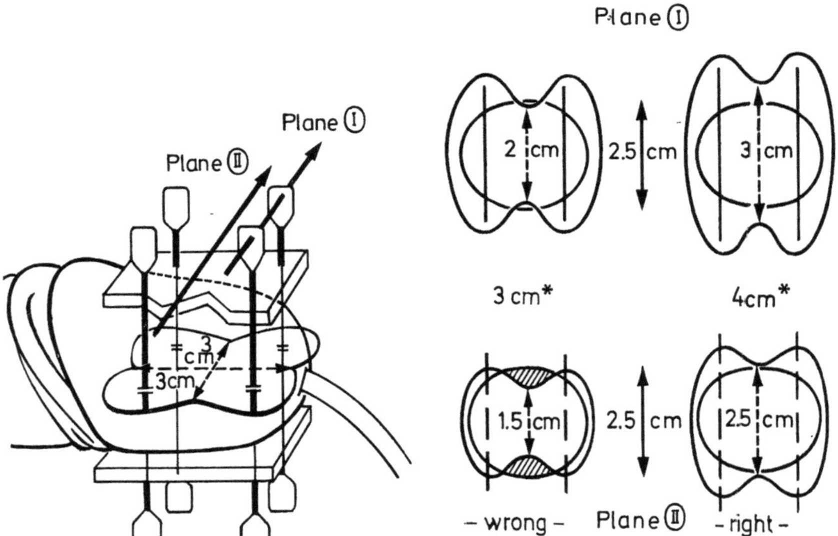


*Fig. 2. Infiltrating lesions, less than 2.5 cm long. Cage of 4 needles, spacing 1.8 cm. Reference isodose 85% DB, DB = 30. Length of needles = 4 cm, target volume = 20 cm³*

Therapeutic results are very satisfactory with the one-plane device for noninfiltrating lesions; with the two plane device, success is limited to cases of retractable sclerosis without major functional impairments (neither urinary nor sexual). In lesions that would require more than

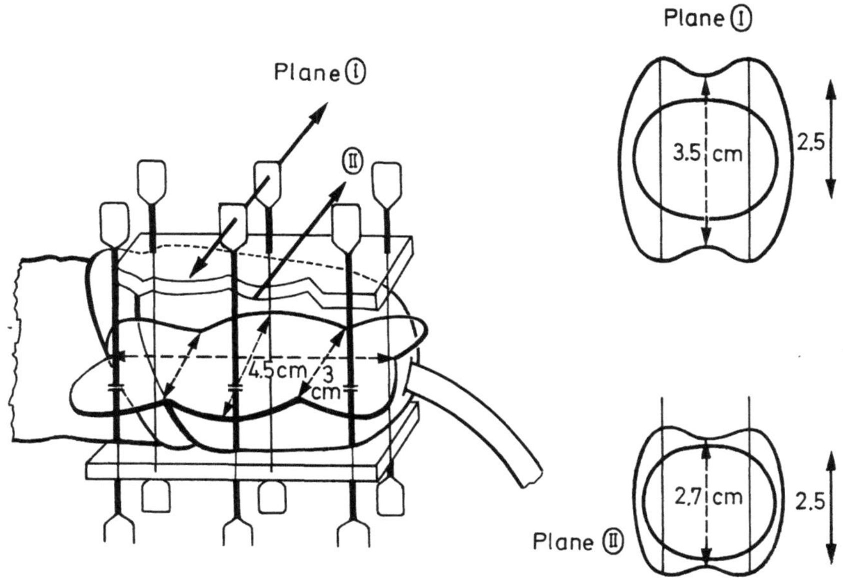


*Fig. 3. Infiltration lesions, less than 4 cm long. Cage of 6 needles, spacing 1.8 cm. Reference isodose 85% DB, DB = 35. Length of needles = 4 cm, target volume 35 $cm^3$*

six radioactive lines, the risks of protracted necrosis, associated with frequent recurrences, have convinced us that surgical amputation will be, from the start, preferable to this kind of radiotherapy.

The tumor dose was 6500-7000 rad upon reference isodose (85%) administered stepwise over 4-8 days.

2. Adenopathies (Lymphatic Involvement)

Until now we have refused or postponed treatment in all cases without clinical suspicion of lymphatic involvement (NO). In cases with lymphatic extensions (N1, N2, N3) we have mostly started by surgical exploration, uni- or bilateral with a limited curettage. In cases of N+, bilateral inguinal irradiation was subsequently administered to a dose of 5500 or 6000 rads (telecobalt or high voltage).

## RESULTS

Table 1 shows that of our 45 patients, 26 are still alive after 4 years with evidence of local healing, which means a total survival rate of 60%. A detailed survey of the results reveals three distinct groups with different prognoses:

1. Patients with noninfiltrating lesions of less than 30 mm maximum diameter (T1, T2). Their number was 14. The lesions remained limited to the glans and showed no lymphatic involvement at the beginning (NO). There were two local recurrences and two secondary adenopathies, but all these patients are still living after 4 years, with local healing in all 14 cases, and development of lymphatic extension in one.

Table 1. Carcinoma of the penis - Institut Gustave Roussy; Hôpital Henri Mondor. Results after 4 year follow-up

| T | cm Ø | no | N1, 2, 3 | Total |
|---|---|---|---|---|
| T1 - T2 | 3 | 14/14 | 0 | 14/14 |
| T3a | 4 | 9/17 | 2/7 | 11/24 |
| T3b-T4 | < 4 | 1/2 | 0/5 | 1/7 |
| Total | | 24/33 | 2/12 | 26/45 |

2. Patients with larger and infiltrating lesions of less than 40 mm maximum diameter (T3a). Their number was 24. Lesions of this kind can reach or even involve the cavernous body up to the balanoprepu- tial sulcus. Seven cases showed associated lymphatic involvement; 3 cases showed secondary adenopathies. Eleven of these patients are still living after 4 years. We found only 4 recurrences and 1 local necrosis eventually requiring an amputation.
3. Patients with infiltrating lesions over 40 mm maximum diameter (T3b and T4). Their number was 7. Five of them showed associated lymphatic involvement. There was 1 early death from aftereffects of radiotherapy; 4 patients had uncontrolled recurrences, 2 extensive necroses, and only 1 of them is still living after 4 years.

DISCUSSION

For all lesions under 40 mm the local results of endocurietherapy are most satisfactory. After careful dosimetric evaluation of the 6 recurrences among 38 cases we see that either an underestimation of the target volume relative to the tumor volume (marginal recurrence), or a faulty implantation (recurrence in situ) must have caused these inadequate results. With better technical skill such recurrences should become a rare exception. They were, however, eventually corrected by successful surgery. We have observed that the onset of recurrences is rather varying (between 1 and 4 years after treatment).

The quality of results is also satisfactory in these tumors locally curable by endocurietherapy. We found practically no embarrassing impairment after cures with not more than three radioactive lines. With four and more radioactive lines there may be delayed cicatrization and also, eventually, retractable sclerosis. The functions, however, are not very much impaired. The rare occurrence of urethral shrinking should be especially empharized. When more than six radioactive lines are required, we find as a rule, severe necrotic manifestations and mostly long and painful delays of cicatrization (1 or 2 years).

For tumors over 40 mm we agree that endocurietherapy is contraindicated, as well on account of necroses as of recurrences. Extensive surgical amputation appears to be the best solution for these cases from the start.

The problem of lymphatic involvement remains always difficult. Aware of the risk of major functional impairment after radiosurgery on the inguinocrural level, we hesitate before a decision in favor of a prophylactic treatment. On the other hand, the bad prognosis in manifest lymphatic involvement, would never indicate prolonged therapeutic with tumors under 40 mm, 12 have shown lymphatic involvement. Primary or secondary; 4 of these are under control for lymph nodes; the others have been up at distances.

Consequently we would recommend the following therapeutic guidelines (Table 2):

In tumors under 30 mm and without infiltration, the rareness of primary or secondary lymphatic involvement speaks in favor of therapeutic abstention when there is sufficient evidence of a NO, and on condition of careful and prolonged clinical surveillance.

In tumors between 30 and 40 mm with moderate infiltrations (this type is most frequent), surgical exploration with limited curettage imposes itself in all cases of even the slightest doubt, if necessary after pretreatment with antibiotics with respect to frequent superposed infections. Surgery will be followed by teleradiotherapy (5500 rad) if histologic examination has confirmed a N+. In cases of NO, prophylactic irradiation of the inguinocrural area to a dose of 5000 rad seems to involve the smallest risk.

In penis carcinoma the causes of death are rather difficult to arrange in a systematic classification. Among 19 of our patients who died or with whom we lost contact in the meantime, we found the following causes: 2 local and regional involvements, 6 metastases, 4 intervening affections, 4 deaths without precise diagnosis, 3 cases of lost contact.

Table 2. Carcinoma of the penis. Institut Gustave Roussy; Hôpital Henri Mondor. Proposed therapeutic schedule

| T | Therapy | NO | N1,2,3 |
|---|---|---|---|
| T1-T2 | $^{192}$Ir | Surveillance | Surgery, if N+: 5500 rad |
| T3a | $^{192}$Ir | 5000 rad | id. |
| T3b-T4 | Surgery | id. | id. |

## SUMMARY

Forty-five carcinomas of the penis have been treated with curietherapy using $^{192}$Ir to a dose of 6500 rad. With a minimum follow-up of 4 years, it appears that small lesions (less than 30 mm) have excellent local results (2 recurrences in 14 cases). With only a slight potential for lymphatic extension, these patients are alive without evidence of disease after 4 years. The lesions of moderate size (30-40 mm) have a poorer prognosis because of more frequent lymphatic extention and disseminated metastases; in contrast, the local results are still quite satisfactory (4 recurrences in 24 cases). The large lesions (more than 40 mm) recur or necrotize (5 recurrences and 2 necroses in 7 cases). In conclusion, curietherapy of epidermoid carcinomas of the penis is an excellent primary treatment for small or moderate lesions (T1, T2, and T3a) if one wishes to avoid surgical mutilation.

## REFERENCES

1. Pierquin, B., Bunescu, U., Chassagne, D., Jomain, J.: La radiothérapie des cancers de la verge par l'iridium-192. J. Urol. Néphrol. 76, 1-8 (1970)

# Chemotherapy of Penis Carcinoma

T. ICHIKAWA *

## INTRODUCTION

Chemotherapy of penis carcinoma is a milestone in the development of chemotherapy of solid tumors. The author was the first to test the effect of bleomycin in the treatment of this carcinoma and predicted bleomycin would be a specific drug against squamous cell carcinoma in general. The accuracy of this prediction has since been confirmed by many clinicians in various fields here and abroad and by animal experiments conducted by my coworkers and myself.

Bleomycin was discovered by H. UMEZAWA (28) in 1962 and reported on in 1965. At his request, we (6, 8) began its clinical trial in the treatment of urogenital malignancies in October 1965. During the first 2 months, a preliminary trial with bleomycin was made on several patients with carcinoma of the bladder and carcinoma of the prostate, one patient with carcinoma of the kidney and several cases with seminoma of the testicles. However, these treatments were not effective.

Subsequently , a patient with penis carcinoma responded dramatically to bleomycin; his tumor shrank by 50% after administration of 70 mg bleomycin given in three intravenous injections. This suggested a relationship between the effect of bleomycin and the properties of penis carcinoma. Histologically penis carcinoma is a squamous cell carcinoma and a special type of skin cancer. None of the carcinomas for which bleomycin had been used prior to penis carcinoma were squamous cell carcinomas and their primary sites of development were outside the skin (an ectodermal organ). These considerations prompted the following questions: Would not bleomycin be effective in all cases of squamous cell carcinoma, wherever the carcinoma might be? Were there any tumors of the brain - anectodermal organ - which would respond to bleomycin?

In order to prove that bleomycin is a specific drug against squamous cell carcinoma the author solicited the cooperation of clinicians in those fields of medicine where carcinoma of this kind is frequently encountered. At the same time the effect of bleomycin on squamous cell carcinoma chemically induced in animals was investigated.

---

* Emeritus Professor (Urology), The University of Tokyo. Honorary Director, National Medical Center Hospital. 1, Toyamacho, Shinjuku-ku, Tokyo 162, Japan.

## QUALITIES OF BLEOMYCIN

The following studies were performed (5, 7, 12, 29-32).

1. Physicochemistry: Bleomycin hydrochloride occurs as a water-soluble, basic, white powder. It can be fractionated chromatographically into fraction A ($A_{1-6}$, demethyl-$A_2$, $A_2'$-a, $A_2'$-b) and fraction B ($B_{1-6}$, $B_1'$). Bleomycin in present use chiefly comprises $A_2$ and $B_2$. It is a glycopeptide with a molecular weight of about 1400, consisting of carbon, hydrogen, nitrogen, oxygen, and sulfur.

2. Toxicity. In laboratory animals, bleomycin was shown to cause damage to the liver when given in high doses, although the damage is reversible. Chronic toxicity tests in most cases revealed changes of the skin and nails. Autopsy of animals dying before receiving heavy dosage demonstrated certain characteristic pulmonary changes but failed to reveal any significant toxic findings such as gastrointestinal ulceration or bleeding and impairment of hematopoietic organs.

3. Absorption, Distribution, Excretion, and Mode of Action. Bleomycin after being administered by intravenous, intramuscular, or intraarterial route, is distributed in the circulating blood and tissues, and is in most parts excreted in the urine.

Since the distribution of bleomycin in the tissues is important for the study of its mode of action, this was determined simultaneously with tritiated bleomycin by both radioactivity (total bleomycin: a) and antimicrobial activity (biologically active portion: b) in mice bearing squamous cell carcinoma or sarcoma induced experimentally with 20-methylcholanthrene solution. The b/a values are extremely important, for they indicate ratios of the biologically active portion to the total bleomycin distributed in tissues.

Table 1 shows that bleomycin was distributed in the squamous cell carcinoma much more widely than in sarcoma and was inactivated much less in the former than in the latter. This explains the exclusive antitumor effect of bleomycin in squamous cell carcinoma.

Table 1. Distribution of $^3$H-bleomycin in squamous cell carcinoma and sarcoma induced by 20-methylcholanthrene 1 h after s.c. injection

| Exp. | Carcinoma | | Sarcoma | |
|---|---|---|---|---|
| | Total BLM µg/g (a) | BLM by antibacterial activity µg/g (b) | Total BLM µg/g (a) | BLM by antibacterial activity µg/g (b) |
| 1 | 15.9 | 11.0 | 4.5 | 0.5 |
| 2 | 22.7 | 17.2 | 13.7 | 1.9 |
| 3 | 17.9 | 13.7 | 14.4 | 2.8 |

To mice bearing carcinoma: 65.1 mg/kg, 64.6 mg/kg, and 65.5 mg/kg were injected in Exp. 1, 2, 3.
To mice bearing sarcoma: 70.3 mg/kg, 70.6 mg/kg, and 62.7 mg/kg were injected in Exp. 1, 2, 3.
Radioactivity of $^3$H-bleomycin employed: 8.23 x $10^6$ dpm/mg in Exp. 1, 8.23 x $10^6$ dpm/mg in Exp. 2, 8.33 x $10^6$ dpm/mg in Exp. 3.

It was hypothesized that particular tissues show conspicuously higher antimicrobial activity levels than others due to differences in the content of enzyme inactivating bleomycin in the tissues. It was confirmed that such enzyme activity is abundant in sarcomas and scarce in squamous cell carcinoma (Fig. 1).

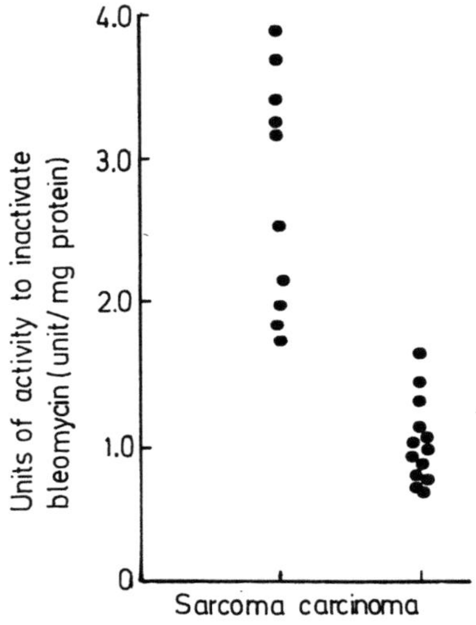


*Fig. 1. Activity of proteins obtained from squamous cell carcinoma and sarcoma induced by 20-methylcholanthrene in mice skin to inactivate bleomycin (1 unit inactivates 1.0 unit of bleomycin B in 1 min)*

4. Influence on Activity of Bone Marrow. Bleomycin does not result in lowered hematopoietic activity of bone marrow. According to SHIMADA (24), mitomycin C produced significant inhibition of total dehydrogenase of human bone marrow cells grown in vitro when added to the tissue culture medium at a concentration of 10 μg/ml, whereas no such inhibition was brought about by bleomycin, even at a concentration as high as 10 mg/ml.

5. Bleomycin and Immunosuppression. It has been observed by YAMAKI et al. (33), OHNO et al. (18) and MATHE et al. (16) that bleomycin does not interfere with immunologic reactions. This property sets also bleomycin apart from previously introduced antitumor drugs.

6. Effect of Bleomycin on Chemically Induced Malignancies. We (9, 10) attempted to confirm the specific effect of bleomycin on squamous cell carcinoma through the following experimentation.

a. Repeated cutaneous painting of mice with methylcholanthrene solution induces squamous cell carcinoma of skin. In our experiment parenteral administration of bleomycin significantly suppressed carcinogenesis.

b. Methylcholanthrene solution injected subcutaneously causes various kinds of sarcoma in mice. Parenteral tretament with bleomycin failed to inhibit sarcomatous development.

c. In rats supplied with N-diethylnitrosamine solution in place of fresh drinking water, esophageal carcinoma, hepatoma, and pulmonary metastasis of hepatoma normally develop. The development of esophageal carcinoma, which is a squamous cell carcinoma, can be effectively controlled with bleomycin. However, the medication has little effect on the development of hepatoma and its metastasis to the lung.

## DEVELOPMENT OF CLINICAL TRIALS

At the 5th International Congress of Chemotherapy held in Vienna in 1967 we (6) made a preliminary report on bleomycin therapy emphasizing the following two points:

1. Since bleomycin appears to be specific for squamous cell carcinoma an attempt should be made to treat all cases of squamous cell carcinoma with bleomycin, irrespective of site,

2. Since pulmonary fibrosis is the most serious of all side-effects of bleomycin appropiate precautions should be taken.

After this congress clinical trials of bleomycin spread to other hospitals and clinical fields of medicine so that enough data were made available to provide the content of a symposium at the 6th Annual Meeting of the Japan Society of Cancer Therapy held in Tokyo in 1968.

At this symposium my proposal to test bleomycin clinically was approved. Furthermore, it was recognized that bleomycin showed neither immunosuppression nor damage to hematopoietic organs. Several researchers (11, 26) reported on the combined effect of bleomycin with radiotherapy which resulted either in additive action in the intermittent combination treatment or in synergistic action in the simultaneous combination one. It is possible and recommended to combine surgery and bleomycin treatment; this is especially useful for the treatment of lymph node metastases. Combination treatment with bleomycin and other antitumor drugs is also available as has been done for malignant lymphoma (15) and some testicular carcinomas (14, 20, 23). The schemes of bleomycin therapy are listed in Table 2, its indications in Table 3.

Table 2. Scheme of bleomycin therapy

| | |
|---|---|
| I. | Treatment with bleomycin alone |
| II. | Intermittent combination treatment of bleomycin with radiotherapy and/or surgery |
| III. | Simultaneous combination treatment of bleomycin with radiotherapy and/or surgery |
| IV. | Combination treatment with bleomycin and other antitumor drugs |

Table 3. Indications for bleomycin therapy

| | |
|---|---|
| I. | Squamous cell carcinoma |
| II. | Some brain tumors |
| III. | Malignant lymphoma |
| IV. | Some testicular carcinomas |

I am of the opinion that the ideal antitumor drug should be capable of curing carcinoma with systemic administration and also should have such efficacy as to be comparable to streptomycin in the treatment of tuberculosis. In this meaning the specific effect of bleomycin is observed only in the treatment of squamous cell carcinoma; in three other indications bleomycin is not specific though it is important as one of the antitumor agents.

## METHOD OF ADMINISTRATION OF BLEOMYCIN

Bleomycin is usually injected. Only rarely it is applied externally with ointment, in solution with or without a gelatin sponge, powder, suppository, etc. An oil suspension is also available as a preparation having long-lasting action.

A single dose of bleomycin is usually 15 mg i.v. or i.m. administered 2 or 3 times a week. The total dosage in one series of treatment is usually 300 mg. If serious side-effects do not occur injections can be continued beyond 300 mg, but it is recommended that after this dosage the drug not be applied for 1-2 months.

The total dosage necessary for complete cure of squamous cell carcinoma seems to differ from case to case. In our experience it necessitates at least 300 mg administered gradually unless the lesion is small and of a well-differentiated type in the early stage. Thus, treatment with bleomycin alone may require long-term and large doses resulting in frequent occurrence of side-effects. Then, combination treatment of bleomycin with radiotherapy and/or surgery, particularly simultaneous combination treatment of bleomycin with radiotherapy and/or surgery, is recommended. Radiotherapy and/or surgery is known to produce good results in cases of squamous cell carcinoma.

Intermittent combination treatment with bleomycin and radiotherapy may be necessitated if bleomycin administration exceeds the standard dosage or causes severe side-effects. However, simultaneous combination treatment is becoming the standard method of bleomycin treatment because of the synergistic action of both agents reported on at the Tokyo symposium (11, 26). JØRGENSEN (13) presented similar experimental results at the 7th International Congress of Chemotherapy held in Prague in 1971. At the international symposium on "Bleomycin in the Treatment of Malignant Diseases" held in London in 1972, RYGÅRD et al. (21) and BERDAL et al. (2) strongly recommended combination therapy with bleomycin and radiotherapy.

In April 1975 at the symposium entitled "Chemotherapy of Cancer" held under the auspices of the 19th General Assembly of the Japanese Association of Medical Sciences, combination treatment was recommended for maxillary carcinoma by SUZUKI (27), for esophageal carcinoma by FUJIMAKI (4), for carcinoma of the uterine cervix by SAITO (22) and for penis carcinoma by ABE (1). At this symposium MATSUZAWA (17) gave as his opinion based upon his experience in the treatment of various kinds of lung cancer, that simultaneous combination treatment with bleomycin and radiotherapy may be effective against carcinomas other than squamous cell carcinoma.

## STATISTICAL OBSERVATIONS

The author has found himself compelled to shift from bleomycin to surgery and/or radiotherapy whenever the former failed to produce favorable progress. This is common clinical knowledge and a rule generally followed by the investigators in the 40 institutes whose data are shown in Table 4.

As shown in Table 4, treatment with bleomycin alone was performed in only 24 of 188 cases; the remaining patients received combination treatment of bleomycin with one or more antitumor agents, particularly surgery. This must be attributed to the small number of early cases and to the general reliance upon the long-standing therapeutic methods.

Table 4. Results of bleomycin and combined treatment of penis carcinoma at 40 institutes

| Treatment \ No. of patients | | Total | Alive | Dead |
|---|---|---|---|---|
| I. | B | 24 | 12 | 12 |
| II. | B and S | 92 | 74 | 18 |
| III. | B and R | 11 | 8 | 3 |
| IV. | B, R and S | 55 | 40 | 15 |
| V. | B, S and C | 1 | 0 | 1 |
| VI. | B, R, S and C | 5 | 1 | 4 |
| Total | | 188 | 135 | 53 |

B = bleomycin; R = radiotherapy; S = surgery; C = other cytostratics.

Next, the survival times and annual deaths in each group are shown in Table 5. Deaths occurred mostly within 1 year indicating a large number of the advanced cases. Therefore, if patients given bleomycin remain healthy for 1 year, they have a good chance of long survival.

Table 5. Survival times and annual deaths in groups shown in Table 4

| Groups | I | | II | | III | | IV | | V | | VI | | Total | |
|---|---|---|---|---|---|---|---|---|---|---|---|---|---|---|
| States / Follow-up time (year) | A | D | A | D | A | D | A | D | A | D | A | D | A | D |
| 0 - 1 | 1 | 8 | 19 | 14 | 4 | 3 | 18 | 14 | 0 | 0 | 0 | 4 | 42 | 43 |
| 1 - 2 | 5 | 4 | 11 | 4 | 1 | 0 | 7 | 0 | 0 | 1 | 0 | 0 | 24 | 9 |
| 2 - 3 | 0 | 0 | 17 | 0 | 1 | 0 | 5 | 1 | 0 | 0 | 0 | 0 | 23 | 1 |
| 3 - 4 | 3 | 0 | 19 | 0 | 2 | 0 | 3 | 0 | 0 | 0 | 0 | 0 | 27 | 0 |
| 4 - 5 | 3 | 0 | 8 | 0 | 0 | 0 | 6 | 0 | 0 | 0 | 1 | 0 | 18 | 0 |
| 5 - | 0 | 0 | 0 | 0 | 0 | 0 | 1 | 0 | 0 | 0 | 0 | 0 | 1 | 0 |
| | 12 | 12 | 74 | 18 | 8 | 3 | 40 | 15 | 0 | 1 | 1 | 4 | 135 | 53 |

A = Alive; D = Dead.

## CASE MATERIAL

Our own cases are tabulated in Table 6. Among 9 surviving cases, two surviving for over 7 years and one for over 5 years received bleomycin alone and another four cases received bleomycin and surgery; one of the remaining two patients received bleomycin, radiotherapy, and surgery, and the last patient is undergoing simultaneous combination treatment with bleomycin and radiotherapy.

Surgery for penis carcinoma usually means amputation of the penis, but among our own cases only one underwent amputation and another four received excision of the tumor or excision and plastic surgery to retain the original form and function of the penis.

Table 6. Author's own case material

| Prognosis | Alive 9 | Dead 9 |
|---|---|---|
| Follow-up time (year) | (Treatment) | (Cause of death) |
| 0 - 1 | 1<br>(receiving simultaneous combination treatment with bleomycin and radiotherapy) | 7<br>3 (metastases)<br>1 (stomach cancer)<br>1 (cardiac failure)<br>1 (pneumonia)<br>1 (pulmonary fibrosis) |
| 1 - 2 | 0 | 0 |
| 2 - 3 | 0 | 1<br>(cardiac failure) |
| 3 - 4 | 1[b]<br>(bleomycin 1240 mg, i.v. $^{60}Co$: 2000 rad and ampuattion of penis during 1 year and 7 months) | 0 |
| 4 - 5 | 0 | 0 |
| 5 - 6 | 4<br>1[a](bleomycin 300 mg, i.v. during 4 months)<br>1 (bleomycin 300 mg, i.v. and excision during 6 months)<br>1 (bleomycin 120 mg, i.v., 25.5 mg, local and excision during 2 years)<br>1 (bleomycin 870 mg, i.v. excision and plastic surgery during 11 months) | 1<br>(cardiac failure) |
| 6 - 7 | 1<br>(bleomycin 220 mg, i.v. and excision during 8 months) | 0 |
| 7 - 8 | 2<br>1[a](bleomycin 255 mg, i.m. during 3 months)<br>1[a](bleomycin 1010 mg, i.v. during 1 year and 2 months) | 0 |

[a] Cases treated with bleomycin alone.

[b] Case having amputation of penis.

Typical cases are as follows. Case 1, 53 years old (Figs. 2 and 3). The patient was given 1010 mg bleomycin i.v. between December 1966 and February 1968, divided in four series of treatment, each varying dosage and length of intermission period. For 7 years and 8 months he has been free of relapse and quite healthy without additional treatment. The skin of his palms is slightly thickened as evidence of the chronic toxicity of the drug, but it does not disturb his daily life.

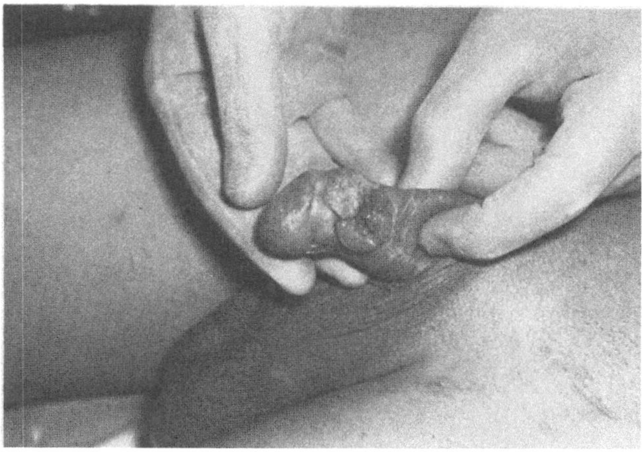

*Fig. 2. Case 1. See text*

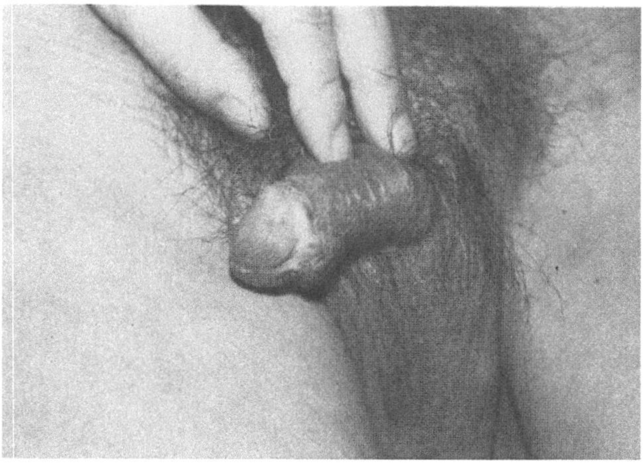

*Fig. 3. Case 1. See text*

Case 2, 58 years old (Figs. 4 and 5). The patient received 255 mg bleomycin i.m. between November 1967 and February 1968 in the outpatient department. This patient has been also free of relapse for 7 years and 8 months without additional treatment. He has no side-effects.

Case 3, 58 years old (Figs. 6-9). This patient received 870 mg bleomycin between March and October 1969; resection of the shrunken tumor was performed in November and a plastic operation with scrotal skin in January 1970. The patient has been healthy for 5 years and 9 months.

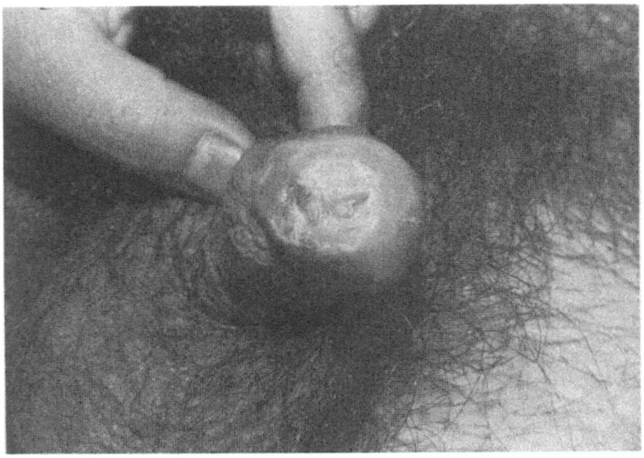

*Fig. 4. Case 2. See text*

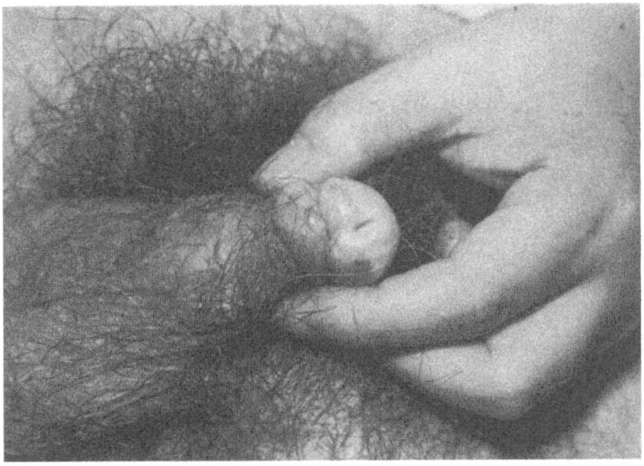

*Fig. 5. Case 2. See text*

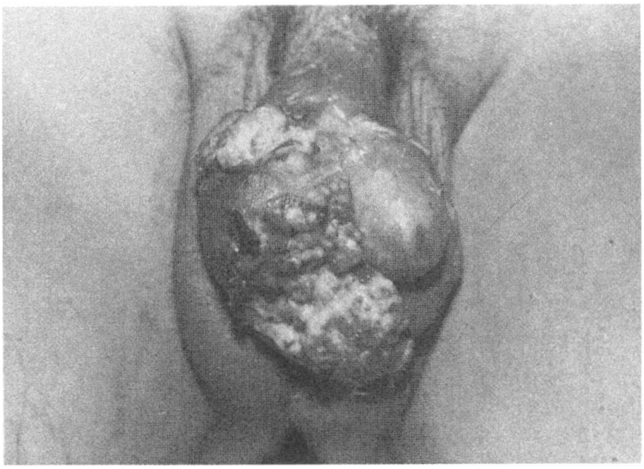

*Fig. 6. Case 3. See text*

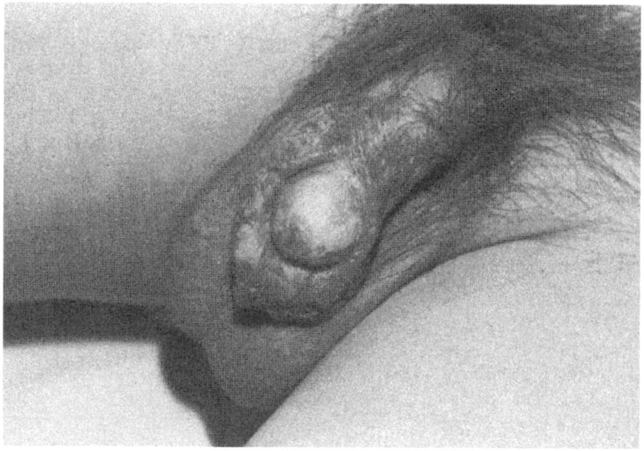

*Fig. 7.*
*Case 3. See text*

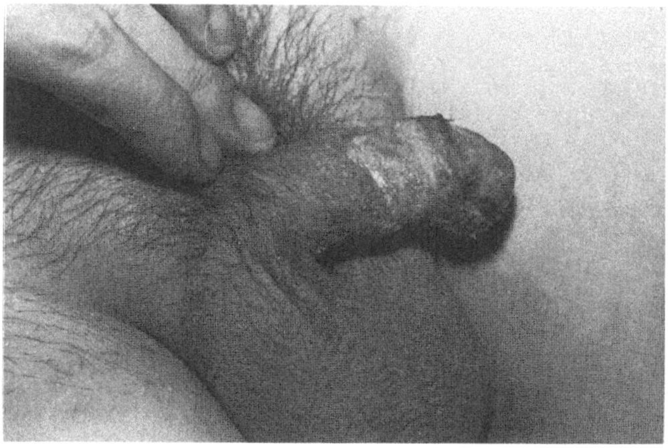

*Fig. 8.*
*Case 3. See text*

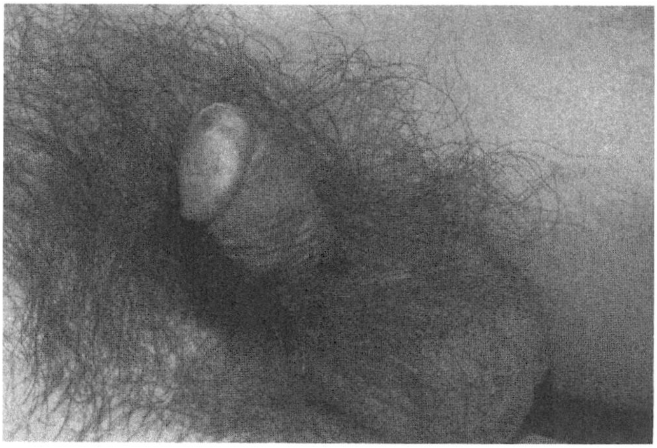

*Fig. 9.*
*Case 3. See text*

After I confirmed complete cure of penile cancer treated with bleomycin alone I switched to simultaneous combination treatment with bleomycin and radiotherapy, but since not enough time has elapsed to demonstrate the superiority of the latter, the cases of ABE et al. (1) will be cited here (Table 7). ABE et al. have confirmed that simultaneous combination treatment can bring about complete cure of penis carcinoma with smaller doses of both agents and more quickly than by treatment with bleomycin alone.

Table 7. Combined treatment of penile cancer (squamous cell carcinoma)[a]

| No. | Age | Grade of Differentiation | TNM | Treatment | | | Prognosis (inguired in March 1974) | Side-effects |
|---|---|---|---|---|---|---|---|---|
| | | | | Bleomycin | Radiotherapy | Length of time | | |
| 1 | 59 | well differentiated | $T_2N_0$ | i.v. 2/w<br>20 mg x 1<br>30 mg x 9<br>Total:<br>290 mg | (4 Mev betatron) daily used<br>200 r. x 28<br>300 r. x 1<br>100 r. x 1<br>Total: 6000 r./40 days | 1 month and 8 days | Excellent after 5 y. and 10 m. | - |
| 2 | 46 | do. | $T_3N_1$ | i.v. 2/w<br>30 mg x 10<br>Total:<br>300 mg | (6 Mev betatron) daily used<br>200 r. x 29<br>Total: 5800 r./39 days<br>(Dissection of inguinal lymph nodes) | 1 month and 9 days | Excellent after 4 y. and 9 m. | - |
| 3 | 67 | moderately differentiated | $T_3N_0$ | i.v. 2/w<br>15 mg x 10<br>Total:<br>150 mg | (15 Mev betatron) daily used<br>200 r. x 25<br>Total: 5000 r./30 days | 1 month | Excellent after 4 y. and 1 m. | - |
| 4 | 40 | well differentiated | $T_2N_0$ | i.v. 2/w<br>15 mg x 10<br>Total:<br>150 mg | (4 Mev betatron) daily used<br>200 r. x 22<br>Total: 4400 r./39 days | 1 month and 8 days | Excellent after 1 y. and 10 m. | - |
| 5 | 36 | do. | $T_3N_0$ | i.v. 2/w<br>15 mg x 10<br>Total:<br>150 mg | (12 Mev betatron) 2/w used<br>500 r. x 10<br>Total: 5000 r./33 days | 1 month and 3 days | Excellent after 7 m. | - |

[a] From ABE (1).

## SIDE-EFFECTS

The clinical toxicity of bleomycin may be divided into acute and subacute or chronic reactions; the former include mostly systemic side-effects and the latter consist of local toxicity in the majority of cases.

BLUM et al. (3) summarized the common manifestations of bleomycin toxicity in four groups (Table 8).

### 1. Acute Toxicity

The symptoms of acute toxicity, such as pyrexia, loss of appetite, nausea, vomiting, headache, fatigue, are liable to occur early - even on the first injection - when the usual single dose of 15 mg is given 2 or 3 times a week. If so, the dosage has to be reduced to less than 5 mg; sometimes antipyretics and/or antihistamines are applied to suppress the symptoms. Most symptoms resemble those occurring on intravenous injection and on other drugs. Shock may occur. Pyrexia has a characteristic pattern; it begins commonly several hours after intravenous injection of bleomycin and disappears after about 7-8 h. Sometimes it is accompanied by local pain at the lesion similar to Herxheimer's reaction in the treatment of syphilis. According to MATHE (16) the incidence of hyperpyrexia due to bleomycin is much less with intramuscular than with intravenous administration. BLUM et al. (3) collected four cases of fulminant reactions of unknown cause and which progressed to death. We experienced one case of severe shocklike toxicity which fortunately recovered.

Table 8. Common manifestations of bleomycin toxicity

| | U.S. 808 | Japan 540 | E.O.R.T.C. 237 | Scandinavia 154 |
|---|---|---|---|---|
| Mucositis | 22% | Stomatitis 4% | 20% | 38% |
| Alopecia | 13% | 29% (27.7%)[a] | 20% | 41% |
| Pigmentation | 8% | 20% (18.3%)[a] | - | 16% |
| Pyrexia | 26% | 36% (31.6%)[a] | 50% (IV) 15% (IM) | 20% |
| Anorexia | 17% | 32% (29.9%)[a] | - | - |
| Vomiting | 14% | 42% (9.8%)[a] | 5% | - |
| Nausea | 10% | (9.8%)[a] | | 15% |
| Pulmonary toxicity | 10% | 9% (Pneumonitis) 4.2%[a] (Fibrosis 3.4%)[a] | 3% | 12% |

[a] Author's case material.

## 2. Subacute or Chronic Toxicity

The symptoms of subacute or chronic toxicity, which tended to occur after a fairly large total dose was reached, were alopecia, swelling and thickening of fingers and toes, pigmentation of skin, sclerosis and obstruction of veins, pneumonitis, and pulmonary fibrosis.

Table 9 shows the correlation between dose and the actual number of patients having skin symptoms among our 455 cases, but not the incidence of such symptoms. Skin symptoms appeared most frequently as a side-effect of chronic toxicity, but the symptoms disappeared slowly if the drug was withdrawn.

Table 9. Correlation between dose and skin symptoms

| Dose (mg) / Symptoms | 0 ∿ 100 | 101 ∿ 200 | 201 ∿ 300 | 301 ∿ 400 | 401 ∿ 500 | 501 ∿ 600 | 601 ∿ 700 | 701 ∿ 800 | 801 ∿ 900 | 901 ∿ 1000 | >1000 | Unknown |
|---|---|---|---|---|---|---|---|---|---|---|---|---|
| Alopecia | 7 | 48 | 46 | 6 | 5 | 2 | 0 | 1 | 0 | 0 | 0 | 15 |
| Change of finger and hand | 7 | 46 | 52 | 3 | 3 | 3 | 1 | 1 | 0 | 0 | 0 | 9 |
| Change of toe and foot | 6 | 36 | 45 | 3 | 3 | 2 | 1 | 1 | 0 | 0 | 0 | 10 |
| Pigmentation | 7 | 32 | 30 | 3 | 7 | 0 | 1 | 0 | 0 | 0 | 0 | 6 |
| Change of nail | 7 | 46 | 49 | 6 | 2 | 1 | 2 | 0 | 0 | 0 | 0 | 7 |

Pneumonitis and pulmonary fibrosis, particularly the latter, is the most dangerous side-effect of bleomycin. Patients usually have slight dyspnea and fever. Examination discloses leukocytosis and abnormal conditions in the chest. According to OKA (19) pulmonary complications are liable to occur in cases having pulmonary dysfunction. Therefore, bleomycin must be administered very carefully in the elderly and in those cases with lung cancer. OKA reported that such complications can be prevented by monitoring of (1) vital capacity (%VC), (2) arterial oxygen tension ($PaO_2$), (3) direct reaction of bleomycin injection, e.g., fever, anorexia, etc., and (4) diffusing capacity ($D_{LCO}$).

The facts mentioned above agree with the results of our basic study which showed that the distribution of bleomycin after repeated administration was such that its content was high in both skin and lung.

BLUM et al. (3) found the greatest incidence of pulmonary toxicity after administration of 450-550 mg; the number of our cases having side-effects was greatest after about 300 mg of bleomycin (Table 10). In our material there were 20 cases of pneumonitis and 16 of pulmonary fibrosis among 455 patients treated with bleomycin injection and 6 of the 36 cases were fatal. We have treated 13 cases with local application of bleomycin with no correlation to pulmonary complications. In the USA 43 patients were at risk of pulmonary toxicity due to bleomycin administration; 7 deaths occurred (Table 10). It has been found in both countries that the danger to life increases with the increase of dose and age of patient.

The pulmonary toxicity of antitumor drugs seems to have been first noted with the clinical use of bleomycin. However, this side-effect has been observed upon administration of other antitumor drugs, too, although its incidence is not as great as with bleomycin, according SHIMOSATO

Table 10. Pulmonary toxicity after bleomycin administration

| Japan | | | U.S.A. | | |
|---|---|---|---|---|---|
| Dose (mg) | Number of patients | Death | Dose (mg) | Number of patients | Death |
| 0- 50 | 0 | 0 | 0- 49 | 2 | 0 |
| 51- 100 | 1 | | 50-149 | 5 | 0 |
| 101- 150 | 3 | | 150-249 | 10 | 1 |
| 151- 200 | 3 | | | | |
| 201- 250 | 2 | | | | |
| 251- 300 | 11 | 3 | 250-349 | 11 | 2 |
| 301- 350 | 2 | | | | |
| 351- 400 | 3 | | 350-449 | 5 | 0 |
| 401- 500 | 1 | | 450-549 | 5 | 1 |
| 501- 600 | 3 | | >550 | 5 | 3 |
| 601- 800 | 4 | 1 | | | |
| 801- 900 | 2 | 1 | | | |
| 901-1000 | 0 | 1 | | | |
| >1000 | 1 | | | | |
| | 36 | 6 | | 43 | 7 |

et al. (25). According to these authors bleomycin was often only the trigger of pulmonary toxicity which was initiated by another drug, e.g., by mitomycin C.

The above-described chronic side-effects, particularly those of pulmonary complications, will in the future be greatly reduced with the popularization of simultaneous combination treatment with bleomycin and radiotherapy. The total dosage of bleomycin utilized in this treatment is so lowered that pulmonary toxicity barely occurs.

## DISCUSSION

My associates and I have recognized bleomycin to be an excellent drug for treating carcinoma of the penis, although it has no effect against carcinoma of the prostate (adenocarcinoma), carcinoma of the bladder (transitional cell carcinoma), carcinoma of the kidney or seminoma of the testicles. These facts indicate that bleomycin has a specific effect on squamous cell carcinoma although treatment must be applied gradually unless the lesion is small and well differentiated. In such cases several courses must be repeated, resulting in an increased total dosage of bleomycin.

In 1967, the author proposed that bleomycin should be investigated in various clinical fields regardless of its specificity; at the same time attention was called to its dangerous side-effect pulmonary fibrosis. IGARASHI (11) reported on the superiority of simultaneous combination treatment of bleomycin and radiotherapy after he observed for 1 year an old female patient with relapsed mandibular carcinoma to be quite healthy; this patient has been given 300 mg of bleomycin and 4000 rad ($^{60}Co$) during 5 weeks. This clinical experience was confirmed by JØRGENSEN with animal experiments in 1971 (13). Thereafter, several reports on the superiority of this combination treatment appeared here and abroad.

## CONCLUSION

1. Bleomycin can completely cure squamous cell carcinoma when the case is of a well-differentiated type in the early stage and bleomycin is given as the first treatment.

2. Combination treatment, particularly simulzaneous combination of bleomycin with radiotherapy, is superior to treatment with bleomycin alone because it is also effective for the not well-differentiated type of this carcinoma, can shorten the term of treatment, and reduce the total dosage of both agents, resulting in disminishing their undue side-effects. Furthermore, it can not only simplify the operative technique but can also make surgery unnecessary in the early stage and increase operability in the advanced stage.

3. Of the undue side-effects, one that endangers the life of the patient is pulmonary fibrosis, and it is necessary to monitor pulmonary function not only during the administration of bleomycin but also for some time after it. This is particularly important for patients having pulmonary dysfunction, and in simultaneous combination treatment of carcinoma of both lung and esophagus.

4. The important problem for the future is to establish the most effective schedule of simultaneous combination treatment with bleomycin and radiotherapy against squamous cell carcinoma and to investigate whether carcinomas other than squamous cell carcinoma respond to bleomycin or not when it is used immediately after the radiotherapy.

5. We confirmed that the antitumor drug could be effective for the tumor, having a close relationship with the tissues where the drug was distributed in high concentration and inactivated not strongly.

## REFERENCES


1. Abe, N.: Simultaneous combination treatment with bleomycin and radiotherapy for the penile cancer (personal communication)
2. Berdal, P., Ekroll, T., Iversen, O.H., Weyde, R.: Bleomycin and radiotherapy in the treatment of squamous cell carcinoma of the head and neck - A clinical and histological study. In: Proc. Internat. Symp. Bleomycin in the Treatment of Malignant Diseases, London, November, 1972. Dorking, Surrey, England: Bartholomew Press. pp. 53-61
3. Blum, R.H., Carter, S.K., Agre, K.: A clinical review of bleomycin - A new antineoplastic agent. Cancer (Philad.) 31, 903-924 (1973)
4. Fujimaki, M.: Chemotherapy of esophageal carcinoma; particularly, on the combination with bleomycin and radiotherapy (in Japanese). In: Proc. 19th Gen. Ass. Jap. Assoc. Med. Sci. 1975, pp. 230-231
5. Fujita, H., Kimura, K.: Blood level, tissue distribution, excretion and inactivation of bleomycin. In: Progress in Antimicrobial and Anticancer Chemotherapy. Proc. 6th Internat. Congr. Chemotherapy. Tokyo: University of Tokyo Press, 1970, Vol. II, p. 309

6. Ichikawa, T., Matsumoto, K., Umezawa, H.: Clinical study of a new antitumor antibiotic bleomycin (preliminary report). Proc. 5th Internat. Congr. Chemother. A IV-4/34, 507-516 (1967)
7. Ichikawa, T., Matsuda, A., Yamamoto, K., Tsubosaki, M., Kaihara, T., Sakamoto, K., Umezawa, H.: Biological studies on bleomycin A. J. Antibiot. Ser. A. (Tokyo) 149-155 (1967)
8. Ichikawa, T., Nakano, I., Hirokawa, I.: Bleomycin treatment of the tumors of penis and scrotum. J. Urol. (Baltimore) 102, 699-707 (1969)
9. Ichikawa, T., Ohashi, S., Takeuchi, T., Hori, S.: Influence of bleomycin against esophageal carcinoma induced chemically in rats. In: Proc. 29th Ann. Meet. Jap. Cancer Ass. 1970, p. 251
10. Ichikawa, T., Umezawa, H., Ohashi, S., Takeuchi, T., Ishizuka, M., Hori, H.: Animal experiments confirming the specific effect on bleomycin against squamous cell carcinoma. Progr. antimicrob. and anticancer Chemother. 2, 315-316 (1970)
11. Igarashi, S.: Discussion on bleomycin treatment in oral surgery, (in Japanese). In: Proc. Symp. New Antitumor Antibiotic Bleomycin. 6th Ann. Meet. Jap. Soc. Cancer Ther. Tokyo, 1968, pp. 124-129
12. Ishizuka, M., Takayama, H., Takeuchi, T., Umezawa, H.: Activity and toxicity of bleomycin. J. Antibiot. Ser. A. (Tokyo) 20, 15-24 (1967)
13. Jørgensen, S.J.: a) Dose schedule in bleomycin treatment. Europ. J. Cancer 8, 93-97 (1972); b) Time-dose relationship in combined bleomycin treatment and radiotherapy. Europ. J. Cancer 8, 531-534 (1972)
14. Kawai, T., Nakao, H., Okano, S., Tsuya, A.: On the treatment of embryonal carcinoma of testicles. Abstr. of the 11th Congr. Jap. Soc. Cancer Ther. 1973, p. 183
15. Kimura, K., Sakai, Y., Konda, C., Shimoyama, M., Kitahara, T., Mikuni, M.: Chemotherapy of malignant lymphoma with special reference to the effects of sequential therapy with bleomycin and vinca alkaloids. In: Advances in Antimicrobial and Antineoplastic Chemotherapy. Proc. 7th Internat. Congr. Chemother., Prague, 1971. Munich-Berlin-Vienna: Urban & Schwarzenberg, 1972, Vol. II, pp. 667-671
16. Mathé, G.: Study of clinical efficacy of bleomycin in human cancer. Brit. med. J. 13, 643-645 (1970)
17. Matsuzawa, T.: Personal communication
18. Ohno, R., Nishihara, H., Kawashima, K., Uetani, T., Hirano, M., Miura, M., Yamada, K.: Lack of immunosuppressive effect of bleomycin on the primary response of mice to sheep red blood cells. Gann 62, 207 (1971)
19. Oka, S.: Treatment of lung cancer with bleomycin (in Japansese). Proc. 19th Gen. Ass. Jap. Assoc. Med. Sci. 1975, pp. 232-233
20. Rathert, P.: Bleomycin beim metastasierenden Teratocarcinom des Hodens. Verh. dtsch. Ges. Urol. 187-188 (1972)
21. Rygård, J., Hansen, H.S.: Bleomycin and radiotherapy as primary treatment for head and neck tumors. In: Proc. Internat. Symp. Bleomycin in the Tretament of Malignant Diseases, London, November 1972. Dorking, Surrey, England: Bartholomew Press pp. 39-52
22. Saito, M.: Chemotherapy of carcinoma of the uterine cervix; particularly, on the combined treatment with bleomycin and radiotherapy (in Japanese). In: Proc. 19th Gen. Ass Jap. Assoc. Med. Sci. 1975, pp. 231-232
23. Samuels, M.L.: Bleomycin in the therapy of testicualr tumors. In: Proc. New Drug Seminar on Bleomycin. NIH, Feb. 15, 1974, pp. 124-150
24. Shimada, M.: Sensitivity of bone marrow from a tumor-bearing human host to bleomycin. Progr. Antimicrob. Anticancer Chemother. 2, 715 (1970)

25. Shimosato, Y., Baba, K., Watanabe, S.: Pulmonary lesions produced by antitumor drugs - Studies on autopsy cases (in Japanese). Gann No Rinsho 17, 21-34 (1971)
26. Soda, T., Matsumura, Y., Takesue, M.: Effect of bleomycin on the carcinoma of larynx and maxilla (in Japanese). In: Proc. New Antitumor Antibiotic Bleomycin. 6th Ann. Meet. Jap. Soc. Cancer Ther. Tokyo, 1968, pp. 124-129
27. Suzuki, Y.: Chemotherapy of carcinoma of the head and neck (in Japanese). In: Proc. 19th Gen. Ass. Jap. Assoc. Med. Sci. 1975, pp. 227-229
28. Umezawa, H.: Bleomycin and other antitumor antibiotics of high molecular weight. Antimicrobial Agents and Chemotherapy 1079-1085 (1965)
29. Umezawa, H.: Natural and artificial bleomycins: chemical and antitumor activities. Pure appl. Chem. 28, 665-680 (1971)
30. Umezawa, H., Ishizuka, M., Hori, S., Chimura, H., Takeuchi, T.: The distribution of $^{3}$H-bleomycin in mouse tissue. J. Antibiot. Ser. A. (Tokyo) 21, 638-642 (1968)
31. Umezawa, H., Maeda, K., Takeuchi, T., Okami, Y.: New antibiotics, bleomycin A and B. J. Antibiot. Ser. A. (Tokyo) 19, 200-209 (1966)
32. Umezawa, H., Suhara, Y., Takita, T., Maeda, K.: Purification of bleomycin. J. Antibiot. Ser. A. (Tokyo) 19, 210-215 (1966)
33. Yamaki, H., Tanaka, N., Umezawa, H.: Effects of several tumor-inhibitory antibiotics on immunological responses. J. Antibiot. 22, 315-321 (1969)

# III. Carcinoma of the Seminal Vesicles

## Diagnosis and Treatment of Primary Malignant Tumors of the Seminal Vesicles

J. BOREAU

All papers on primary malignant tumors of the seminal vesicles start with this sentence: "Malignant tumors of the seminal vesicles are rare". But papers on this disease are becoming more and more numerous! It would, moreover, be surprising if the seminal vesicles were the only organ which did not undergo malignant degeneration. It is difficult to say what is the true frequency of these tumors for two reasons:

The first is that they are not sought carefully enough. The published cases concern, mostly, very extensive lesions which cannot possibly be missed. Nevertheless, one usually has to wait for the autopsy for full assessment. There are surely earlier forms which one must learn to detect.

The second reason is that it is difficult to say, clinically, whether the tumor is primary or not. Similarly, in the cases published in the literature, it is not always easy to separate truly primary malignant lesions of the seminal vesicles, i.e., those derived from the vesicular tissues from vesicular lesions due to spread from carcinomas of neighboring organs. These include, first, the prostate, then the bladder, then embryonal tumors developing in the retrovesical region, and finally, and much more rarely, rectal or sigmoidal carcinomas which only spread to the genital and urinary tracts at a late stage of the disease.

One may consider that, if only forty authentic cases of these primary tumors of the seminal vesicles have been reported, this is because medical attention has not been sufficiently attracted to the pathology of these organs.

In fact, few clinical signs orient one straightaway toward a vesicular lesion. Lesions of the intrapelvic seminal system may give rise to abdominal, pelvic, lumbar, or perineal pain and only inguinal lesions give rise to more suggestive symptoms.

Involvement of the seminal vesicles may be responsible for any genital or urinary symptom, e.g., cystitis, dysurea, burning pain on micturition, partial or total retention of urine, hematuria, or, also, hemospermia and ejaculation disorders. Rectal tenesmus, associated with symptoms of epididymitis or orchitis, may also be seen. None of these symptoms are pathognomic.

The main clinical investigation is rectal palpation of the prostate, which is already insufficient to determine prostatic involvement and - unless carried out under general anesthesia - one cannot detect lesions of the seminal vesicles unless they are already of large volume.

Urethroscopy and cystoscopy are more useful. These examinations may reveal abnormalities, deformities of the posterior urethra in the area of the veru montanum, of the ejaculatory ducts, or changes in the appearance and orientation of the trigone, which are indicative of a lesion of the seminal vesicles.

A transurethral needle biopsy is not easy to carry out. A transrectal is dangerous, and a transperineal or transvesical (during cystostomy) may pass to one side of the degenerative focus. Certain authors have, however, used them successfully.

Laboratory examinations are not of great use. The most useful are, in certain cases, sperm analysis and urocytography. Cellular changes noted or the appearance of abnormal cells, may suggest a lesion of the secretory cells.

The best information at present is given, by radiology. Urethrography and cystography may be carried out routinely. One should expose the films at different stages of filling, with multiple views and tomography. Thus one may note abnormal appearances, such as irregularity of one border, amputation or haziness of part of the film, various filling defects or deformities which are nevertheless constant.

Urography and retrograde ureteropyelography give further information on the state of the terminal ureter and possible effects on the kidney. The latter may be observed in cases where the original lesion has already compressed the terminal part of the ureter, i.e., at an advanced stage of the disease.

The best way to observe the seminal vesicles is to opacify them. This is almost always possible using deferentovesiculography. In view of the simplicity, perfect innocuousness, and efficacy of this procedure it is surprising that it is not used routinely when there is serious doubt concerning the possibility of disease of the ampullae or the seminal vesicles.

Vasopuncture of the vas deferens is easy to carry out and injection of contrast medium into its lumen gives images which usually permit to make the diagnosis, or at least, are highly suggestive.

It is obviously ideal to have available a powerful, modern radiological apparatus with which one can follow progression of the contrast medium under fluoroscopy, using an image amplifier or television. One may use a rapid selector, with a mobile grill, to take numerous films with short periods of exposure. But the simplest apparatus is quite able to give perfectly suitable films for everyday practice.

The injection of a dose of 2.5 cc is necessary and sufficient to obtain satisfactory X-ray appearances. If any excess fluid passes into the bladder and masks the area to be examined, a bladder washout is sufficient to get rid of it.

We must emphasize the fact that deferentovesiculography is the basic examination. It should be carried out early when there is the slightest doubt. Its role is not to detect relapses, as suggested by some authors, but to give the best early diagnostic information.

Vesiculodeferentography should always be carried out on both sides. One vas deferens may be obstructed by the tumor, or by previous disease, but such obstruction is rarely bilateral. The image obtained on the permeable side is usually characteristic, either of bilateral involvement or of the effects of a lesion on the opposite side. This may then give rise to topographic changes by displacement, compression, or deformity, which is common, or by invasion, which is more rare.

Malignant disease of the seminal vesicles, rather than the ampullae, usually gives rise to amputations, filling defects, irregular spasm, but also rigidity and imperfect borders. There may be associated changes in the axis or orientation which are not noted in other diseases. In fact, all types of ampullary or vesicular images may be seen in malignant tumors of the seminal vesicles but none truly resemble common lesions of infection or congenital abnormalities. There is always an appearance of disorder or chaos, which is characteristic. One should note that a stretching out and rise in the curve of the vas deferens is rather suggestive.

To analyze all these changes, as in examination of the ejaculatory ducts, which may be distended or compressed, it is also essential to carry out several views.

In cases of impermeability of both vasa deferentia, one may attempt catheterization of the ejaculatory ducts at the level of the veru montanum, but this maneuver is always technically difficult, and sometimes anatomically impossible.

Xeroradiography gives rise to images which have the same appearance. They permit a slightly different analysis of the parietal images.

Attempts at echotomography, investigation by ultrasound of this type of lesion, are not yet sufficiently numerous for us to have a definite opinion of their value.

Angiography is, however, now well known. Several observations have confirmed the undoubted value of this examination. Selective arteriography of the internal iliac artery permits to one examine the pelvis. One may see an increase in the size and number of the arterial branches. One may note changes in their course. There may also exist around the tumor, patches of contrast medium, and arteriovenous fistulas have also been noted at this level.

It is very important when there are abnormal genital or urinary signs, to obtain a rapid etiologic diagnosis if there is may possibility of a vesicular lesion, for it seems that adenocarcinomas of the seminal vesicles, which are the commonest primary tumors, remain for a long time included within dense fibrous tissue and only spread later. The ideal would be to treat the seminal lesion before urinary spread. It should be possible to do this with the means now at our disposal.

*Surgical treatment* has obvious indications. It should be considered at practically all stages of the development of the tumor. At an early stage, to carry out removal of a lesion which seems to remain, for long time, locally malignant, and later, to remove a primary focus and relieve compression or spread to genital or urinary organs.

The seminal vesicles may be approached by numerous routes, which are as follows.

## A. Anterior Routes

1. The supra-pubic route is subumbilical or subserous laparotomy. One has to pass around the lateral and posterior walls of the bladder and this requires blunt dissection during which it is difficult to avoid opening the bladder. One should distinguish this complication from

2. The transvesical route where the bladder is opened deliberately through the anterior wall, in order to seek the seminal vesicles by means of a T-shaped incision of the posterior wall. The vertical part of the T passes on the midline between the two ureteral orifices. The horizontal part, which is 2-3 cm long, passes immediately behind the ureteral orifice.

3. The inguinal route is a paramedian laparotomy which passes down to the root of the scrotum. The vas deferens may then be used to guide one toward the posterior surface of the bladder, after ligature of the epigastric artery. In my opinion, it is much simpler to dissect out the ureter first, and follow the latter, for the technique adopted for the remainder of the operation depends more on the state of the ureter than on that of the vas deferens. This route can only be used if one wishes to operate on one side only, for two identical inguinal incisions are very mutilating.

B. Posterior Routes

These have been very successful for they give much better exposure of the lesions, which can thus be treated under direct vision. They permit treatment of both seminal vesicles through a single incision. Four posterior routes have been described:

1. The sacral route by resection of the coccyx and the left half of the sacrum. This has been practically abandoned in the treatment of carcinoma of the rectum, owing to the considerable damage caused and I consider that it should also be abandoned in surgery of the seminal vesicles.

2. The parasacral route leaves the bone intact but requires division of the gluteus maximus, the sacrosciatic ligament, the upper part of the levator ani, and the ischiococcygeal muscle before one can mobilize the rectum downward. This series of movements is also very traumatic.

3. The coccyperineal route permits one, by disarticulation of the coccyx, to avoid muscular damage, but there is very narrow access to the vesicles.

4. The anococcygeal route passes through a median vertical incision behind the anus to the base of the coccyx, resection of which permits displacement of the rectum. In its lower part, the incision extends into the perineum.

C. Inferior Routes

1. The perineal route. This is the classical route for perineal prostatectomy. Through a preanal incision, concave backward, from one ischial tuberosity to the other, one may approach the anterior part of the perineum. The essential stage of the dissection is the identification and careful division of the rectourethral raphe. But cleavage, which should lead well above the upper border of the prostate, sometimes raises insoluble problems.

2. The ischiorectal route partly avoids these difficulties. The incision passes through the left lateral border of the anus to reach the fourth part of the sacrum. One is then higher up in the pelvis but, finally, this technique includes the disadvantages of the posterior routes and those of the perineal route.

In fact, all these methods have the same disadvantage, i.e., the possibility of operating only on the seminal vesicles. They can only be considered if one is certain that the lesion is strictly limited to the spermatic reservoirs, which is very difficult to say definitely.

We now know that spread to the ejaculatory ducts and the prostate is common. In certain cases it may even occur early. We know that adhesions occur more rapidly forward, toward the bladder, than backward toward the rectum.

A study of all these cases shows that the most frequent complications include compression of the lower part of the ureter with its effect on the upper urinary tract. Thus, apart from very limited lesions, which are not easy to diagnose, it is necessary during operation (1) to verify the state of the bladder, and treat it, if necessary, (2) to operate, if necessary, on the prostate, and (3) to relieve low ureteral stenosis.

It thus seems that <u>the anterior transvesical route</u> alone permits one to solve all these problems. However, with an open bladder, the precise nature of the operation depends on what one finds.

Except in cases seen very early, where removal of the vas deferens, ampulla and vesicle on one side only may be indicated, I believe that prostatectomy and vesiculectomy, removing one or two vesicles, is the safest operation. It includes total removal of the lesion and prevention of spread to the prostate, which is, moreover, rarely completely unaffected.

Our attitude toward the ureter depends on its state. If it is normal and has not been damaged during dissection, it may then be left intact. If it is simply compressed by the mass of the seminal vesicle, removal of the latter may permit the ureter to return to normal. If a tumor has spread into it, it must be sacrificed in order to obtain complete removal of the tumor. One may then carry out reimplantation of the ureter into the bladder by one of the classical techniques.

Invasion of the lower part of the ureter is often associated with vesical spread. It is rare for partial cystectomy to be possible in view of the number of sutures which must then be made in the bladder.

If the vesicular lesions are bilateral, like those of the ureters, if the area of the trigone or the ureteral orifices are invaded, the treatment of choice is total cystectomy with prostatectomy.

Our attitude toward the ureter depends not only on the lesions noted but also the age and general condition of the patient. One may carry out either intestinal implantation of the urinary tract or double cutaneous ureterostomy.

If the tumor spreads into the rectum or sigmoid, which seems to occur at a later stage, one cannot simply operate on the seminal vesicles; bypass operations are necessary. These depend on the nature and site of the obstruction, before starting palliative treatment.

<u>Lymph node involvement</u> along the iliac chain of lymph nodes detected, if necessary, by lymphography, may require lymphadenectomy or removal of pelvic connective tissue. These complementary operations cannot be considered during the same stage as the treatment of the primary lesion. Removal of lymph nodes, if necessary, will be carried out later.

*Treatment by radiotherapy* is of undoubted value. In view of the difficulty of surgery on these organs deeply situated in the pelvis, it is obvious that treatment by radiotherapy, without surgery, would be ideal if one could make the diagnosis before the onset of signs of mechanical and organic invasion of the urinary tract.

Radiotherapy can always be used, even before surgical operation and it can also be undertaken as complementary treatment of the pelvic focus or of the chain of lymph nodes. One may consider treatment by high-energy radiotherapy, e.g., cobalt, radioisotope teletherapy, betatron or linear accelerator. The conditions for detection, centering, and dose measurement are the same as for the prostate. One may advise a fairly large target-volume initial dose of about 4500 rad (Dose applied by a "volume-technic" or in only one A axis). One may complete this by a direct high-energy electron beam by the perineal route with a dose of about 2500 rad (20-25 MeV at a distance of about 7-8 cm) which represents a total of 7000 rad. This seems to us sufficient. On relapses, this is the only possible therapeutic weapon available.

As far as metastases are concerned, their treatment depends both on their site and on their nature, but radiotherapy is often used to attempt to halt their development.

Certain authors emphasize the importance of the association of hormones with other forms of treatment. Estrogens, in particular, seem to have improved a few cases and diethylstilbestrol is quoted sometimes as having a beneficial effect.

In fact, it is difficult to say whether primary tumors of the seminal vesicles are more sensitive than others to this type of drug. Hormone therapy seems to act mainly on seminal tumors with marked prostatic involvement and it is more on the prostate than on the vesicular lesion that these drugs act.

Finally, one should attempt *chemotherapy* although the rules are still not yet fully drawn up. I do not think that one can avoid using this treatment, which seems to give very favorable results.

As in any malignant disease, the prognosis of primary tumors of the seminal vesicles depends on early diagnosis, which itself is necessary for rapidly bringing into play appropriate treatment. At present, among the means available, it seems that vesiculography is the simplest and best method of diagnosis.

## SUMMARY

The author, after suggesting that malignant tumors of the seminal vesicles are not as rare as usually believed, considers the best method of early diagnosis to be deferentovesiculography carried out in all suspected cases. Surgery of these tumors includes vesiculectomy by the transvesical route which permits simultaneous treatment of vesicular, ureteral. vesical, and prostatic lesions. A place of choice is reserved for high-energy radiotherapy.

# *IV. Epididymal Tumors*

## Tumors of the Epididymis

E. ELSÄSSER

Tumors of the epididymis, both primary and secondary - whether benign or malignant - are rare phenomena. I myself have hitherto encountered only five benign tumors of the epididymis and discovered, in my predecessor's records, a single malignant tumor, a leiomyosarcoma of the spermatic cord. How frequent or rare are extratesticular tumors really?

At the Urologic University Clinic in Munich over a 10-year period only five tumors of the epididymis - four adenomatoid tumors and a benign cystic lymphangioma - were observed in addition to 108 testicular tumors (10). Of the 1039 intrascrotal tumors systematically recorded in Great Britain by the Testicular Tumor Panel and Registry in the years 1958-1963 there are only 44 tumors of the epididymis and spermatic cord compared with 995 testicular tumors (5, 7, 16). In both cases the percentage is not quite 5%. Since in the testis itself tumors not originating from the germinal epithelium also represent about 5% of testicular tumors, one gains the impression that the elements of the spermatic duct system, whether inside the testis or outside it in the epididymis and spermatic cord, exhibit the same slight tendency toward tumorous growth, being only 1/20 of that of the germinal epithelium. If, as extensive statistics show, 20-25 out of a million males are afflicted annually with a testicular tumor (7), the chances are that only one of them is suffering from an extratesticular tumor.

As the aforementioned 44 extratesticular tumors in Great Britain were recorded within a certain time and population, they also provide a representative cross section of the relative frequency of the various extratesticular tumors (Table 1).

The adenomatoid tumor, a peculiar benign tumor of still disputed histogenesis that is typical for the genital regions in both sexes, is featured 11 times, i.e., in a quarter of the cases. Rhabdomyosarcoma and embryonic sarcoma, the sarcomas of children and juveniles, make up a second quarter with, again, 11 cases, the remaining sarcomas - fibro-, leiomyo-, lipo-, and undifferentiated sarcomas, the sarcomas of adults and the aged - constitute a third quarter also with 11 cases; the remaining quarter is distributed over benign tumors of connective tissue, 1 metastatic tumor, 2 miscellaneous tumors, and 3 cases of uncertain diagnosis.

It is striking that in these rather extensive records there are no epithelial tumors. It is therefore appropriate to recall briefly the development of these organs. The origin of the gonads already becomes visible in very young embryos on the medial side of the mesonephric plica as a thickening of the mesothelium on the dorsal circumference of the coelom on both sides of the mesenteric radix (Fig. 1). From the endoderm the primordial germ cells traverse the mesentery into this region, where they induce the formation of testicles or ovaries.

Table 1

| Relative frequency of testicular and extratesticular tumors | | | | |
|---|---|---|---|---|
| | Urologische Universitätsklinik München 1960-1970 | | Testicular tumor Panel & Registry Great Britain 1958-1963 | |
| Testicular tumors | 108 | 95.58% | 995 | 95.77% |
| Extratesticular tumors | 5 | 4.42% | 44 | 4.23% |
| Total number of cases | 113 | 100% | 1039 | 100% |
| **Relative frequency of different types of paratesticular tumors** | | | | |
| Adenomatoid | 4 | 80% | 11 | 25% |
| Rhabdomyosarcoma and embryonic sarcoma | - | - | 11 | 25% |
| Leiomyosarcoma | - | - | 5 | |
| Fibrosarcoma | - | - | 3 | 25% |
| Liposarcoma | - | - | 2 | |
| Undifferentiated sarcoma | - | - | 1 | |
| Benign mesenchymal tumors | 1 | 20% | 5 | |
| Miscellaneous tumors | - | - | 2 | 25% |
| Metastases | - | - | 1 | |
| Tumors of uncertain diagnosis | - | - | 3 | |
| Total number of cases | 5 | 100 | 44 | 100% |

The mesenchyma below the thickening of the mesothelium condenses to form the so-called mesenchymal nucleus and the primitive sex cords, from which the testicular tubules and the rete testis emerge.

The primordial germ cells are admitted to these tubules and are later differentiated to stem spermatogonia, which give rise to the germinal epithelium. The ductuli efferentes originate from the distal residue of the mesonephric tubules, which are already connected with the wolffian duct, the subsequent ductus epididymis. Both the wolffian duct and the mesonephric tubules as well as the müllerian duct and the glomeruli and tubular apparatus of the metanephros originate from the mesothelium of the coelom, which was displaced or had advanced far down.

Of the fully developed organs only the testis contains true epithelium in the form of germinal epithelium, which is derived from embryonic covering cells, the primordial germ cells from the endoderm. The elements of the testicular tubules themselves, the Sertoli cells and epithelia of the rete testis, originate from the embryonic mesenchyme.

The epithelia of Bowman's capsule and of the tubular apparatus of the remaining kidney as well as the ductuli efferentes of the globus major of the epididymis are descendants of meso- and metanephrogenic tissue. It should be particularly noted that the ductuli efferentes of the globus major represent structures analogous to the distal tubules of the remaining kidney; descendants of the wolffian duct are in the urinary tract the collecting ducts of the kidney, the renal pelvis,

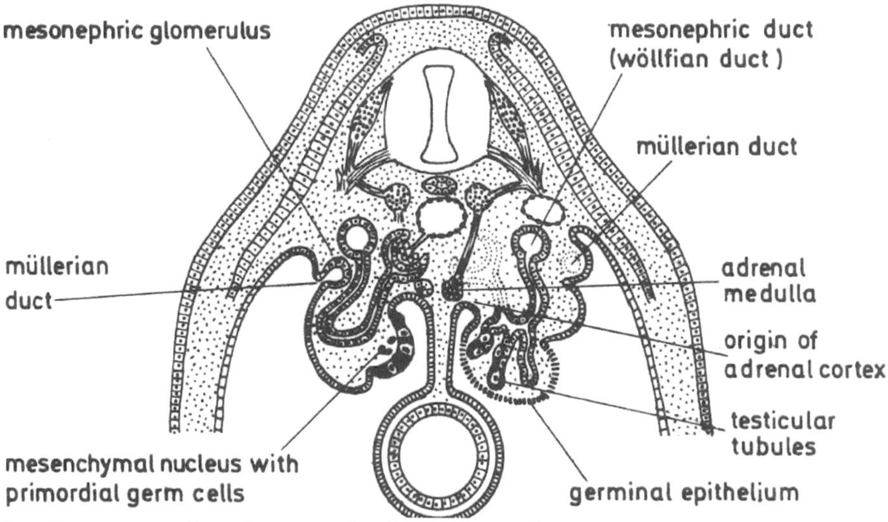


*Fig. 1. Development of male gonad. Cross section through a human embryo of about 5 mm. The left side shows the younger, the right side the elder stage. From HEINKE and DOEPFMER (17)*

the ureter, the trigone of the bladder and the dorsal part of the urethra down to the veru montanum and in the genital tract the ductus epididymis, ductus deferens, the seminal vesicles, and the ductuli ejaculatorii.

It is easy to imagine that in the case of tumorous growth, which is always accompanied by a certain loss of differentiation , the epithelia of all these ducts remember their mesodermal origin and more or less lose their epithelial character again.

What kind of tumors occur in the epididymis and spermatic cord? Table 2 is based on a compilation of CZVALINGA and GÖTZ (8). In addition to four cases of their own, these authors were able to collect as many as 547 cases from the world literature and I have, as was possible, supplemented them with further reports, without wishing to lay claim to completeness.

There are epithelial tumors that also occur in the epididymis, even though only in small numbers. The most frequent tumor of the epididymis is without doubt the so-called adenomatoid tumor, which is reported in 355 cases. The purely descriptive term adenomatoid tumor, chosen by GOLDEN and ASH (15), shows that the histogenesis of these tumors is still controversial. The mesothelium, endothelium, residues of the wolffian or müllerian duct and the mesonephric ducts, etc., have been considered initial tissue (2, 4, 5, 8, 10, 14, 18, 19, 23, 24). The histologic appearance of adenomatoid tumors is characterized by the simultaneous occurrence of stroma and adenomatoid cells, which traverse the tumor in the form of solid threads, but which may also enclose tubes or reticularly connected cavities, as can be observed in one of our cases (Fig. 2). The stroma between the cavities may have a varying content of reticular or fibrous connective tissue, smooth muscle cells, capillaries, and lymphocytic infiltrates. The adenomatoid cells range from cubic to flat and are frequently vacuolated. Since in individual cases the different components of the tumor may predominate or diminish, the histologic appearance may vary appreciably. Accordingly, the tumor

Table 2. Tumors of epididymis, spermatic cord, and appendages

| Benign tumors | | Malignant tumors | |
|---|---|---|---|
| Epithelial | | Epithelial | |
| Papillary cystadenoma (4, 6, 8, 23) | 40 | Carcinomas (4, 8, 12, 25) | 20 |
| Papilloma in spermatocele (23) | 2 | Seminoma (8) | 11 |
| Adenoma of adrenal gland cortex (8) | 1 | Carcinoid (8) | 1 |
| Mesenchymal | | Mesenchymal | |
| Adenomatoid tumor (2,4,8,10,14,16,18,24) | 355 | Malignant adenomatoid tumor (8, 12) | 12 |
| Leiomyoma (8, 16) | 34 | Rhabdomyosarcoma and embryonic sarcoma (8,13,16,26) | 39 |
| Fibroma (8, 9) | 22 | Undifferentiated sarcoma (8, 16) | 8 |
| Lipoma (8, 18) | 4 | Leiomyosarcoma (8, 16) | 12 |
| Neurofibroma (8) | 2 | Fibrosarcoma (8, 16) | 11 |
| Angioma (8) | 15 | Liposarcoma (21, 23) | 2 |
| Lmyphangioma (10) | 1 | Chondrosarcoma (8) | 1 |
| Miscellaneous tumors | | Angiosarcoma (8) | 1 |
| Melanotic hamartoma (8, 23, 30) | 8 | Malignant schwannoma (4, 8) | 2 |
| Dermoid cysts (8, 23) | 4 | Melanosarcoma (8) | 2 |
| Teratoma adultum (8) | 5 | Malignant mesothelioma (11) | 1 |
| Cholesteatoma (8) | 6 | Myxosarcoma (1) | 1 |
| Brenner tumor (23) | 1 | Miscellaneous tumors | |
| | | Embryonic teratosarcoma (8) | 9 |
| | | Malignant lymphoma (3, 4, 8, 20) (sarcoidosis, reticuloendotheliosarcoma, lymphosarcoma, lymphatic leukemia) | 15 |
| | | Metastatic tumors (4, 8, 28) (carcinoma of the prostate, carcinoma of the stomach, renal carcinoma, carcinoma of the sigmoid colon, argentaffin carcinoma of the ileum) | 17 |

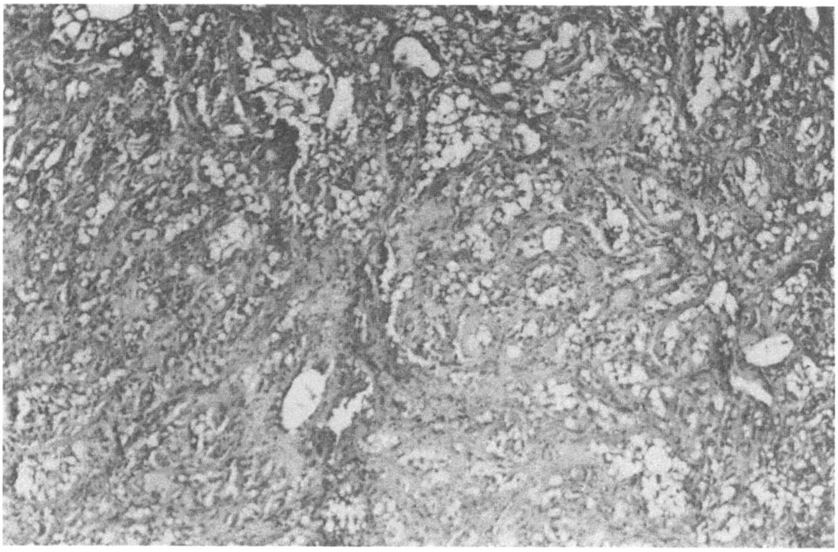

*Fig. 2. Histologic appearance of an adenomatoid tumor situated in globus minor of epididymis of a 36-year-old man.* x *40*

has already been classified as adenofibroma, adenofibromyoma, angiomatoid tumor, lymphadenoma, mesothelioma, to name just a few examples. Most authors seem to consider the mesothelial genesis of the tumor to be the most likely (2, 4, 10, 14, 23), particularly since it is supported by histochemical investigations (4). Although MOSTOFI and PRICE 1973 also assume a mesothelial genesis of the tumor (23), these authors nevertheless prefer to draw a distinction between it and the "true mesotheliomata." They would possibly designate one of our adenomatoid tumors (Fig. 3) as a true mesothelioma.

Adenomatoid tumors grow slowly, seldom attain more than the size of a pea or cherry, cause little pain to the sufferer and, in the male, have a close affinity with the epididymis, usually in the globus minor and rarely in the region of the globus major, and are not necessarily connected to the duct sytem of the epididymis. In one case we were able to separate two cherry-sized adenomatoid tumors from the globus minor without injuring the duct system, while two others could only be removed with the epididymis. Adenomatoid tumors often seem - as in one of our cases - to occur as an incidental finding in cases of severe inflammation of the epididymis calling for semicastration, which thus demonstrates their close relation to reactive mesothelial proliferation (23).

It seems to me that the adenomatoid tumor reveals the pluripotential of the mesothelium of the urogenital region, which in the course of its development has to form both epithelium-lined ducts and their coating of muscular and connective tissue. As a urologist I have encountered, particularly in experimental urologic surgery, similar formations in the course of regeneration processes in the spermatic and urinary tracts.

Other benign tumors of connective tissue are described (Table 2), the most frequent of which are leiomyomas, which are found in a ratio of 1 : 10 with adenomatoid tumors, and which have already been regarded

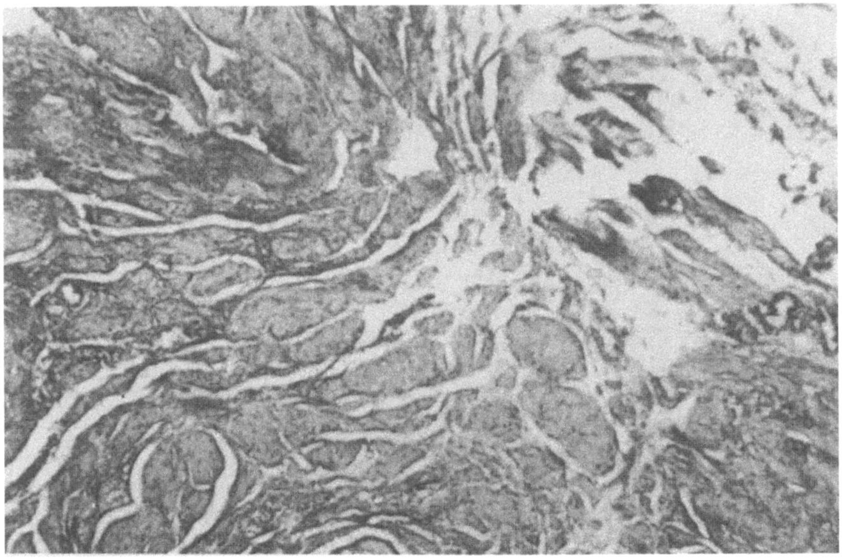

*Fig. 3. Adenomatoid tumor found in epididymis of a 43-year-old man resembling tumors classified by MOSTOFI and PRICE (23) as true mesothelioma.* x *40*

as adenomatoid tumors with a unilateral development. Fibromas, including a giant fibroma weighing 2 kg, lipomas - mostly of the spermatic cord - neurofibromas, angiomas, and lymphangiomas occur.

There is only one tumor of the epididymis which has preserved a purely epithelial character: the papillary cystadenoma of the globus major, which develops inside the duct system of the ductuli efferentes. As I myself have not experienced such a case, I am obliged to MOSTOFI and PRICE (23) for Figures 4 and 5. The serous content of these cystic tumors can, as in a case of CHAN et al. (6), also fill the duct system of the epididymis and the rete testis. This tumor often occurs bilaterally and is then apparently a partial manifestation of Hippel-Lindau's disease which, as is known, is accompanied by angiomatous, gliomatous, or cystic tumors in the cerebellum, on the retina, and in the pancreas.

The isolated and unilateral papillary cystadenomas of the epididymis have therefore adready been regarded as a forme fruste of Hippel-Lindau's disease. Particularly interesting are two cases of papillary cystadenoma, one of which developed simultaneously with a tumor of the epididymis, the other 8 years later with a renal carcinoma. Morphologically, too, there seem to be similarities between parts from a papillary cystadenoma (Fig. 5) and some renal carcinomas, which point to the already mentioned analogy between ductuli efferentes and the distal tubule apparatus of the kidney.

It is a case of BROTH et al. (4) where there was coincidence of epithelial cystadenoma of the epididymis and carcinoma of the prostate in an 81-year old man.

Similar mural papillomas have also been found in spermatic cysts (23).

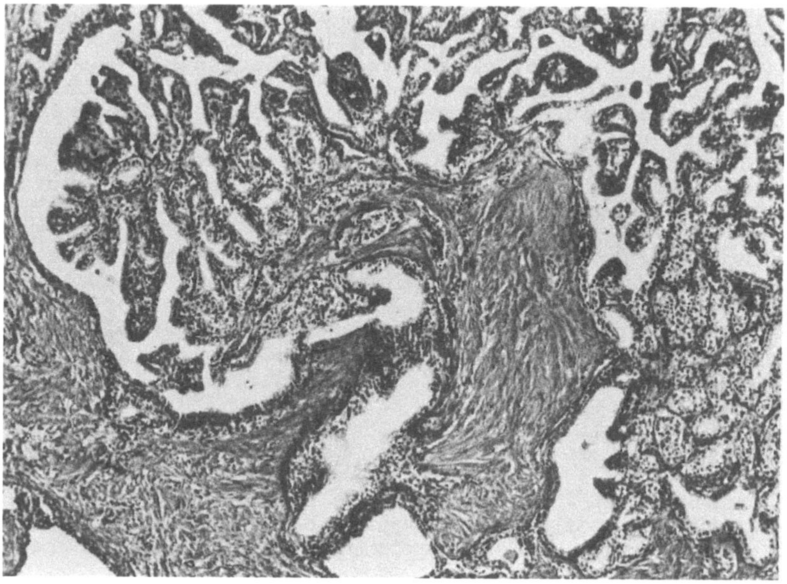

*Fig. 4. Cystadenoma of epididymis. Ectatic efferent ducts and microcystic spaces are seen; the latter are nearly filled with multiple complex papillary processes covered by clear cells. Stroma is fibrous with focal hyalinization. x 80 (From MOSTOFI and PRICE (23))*

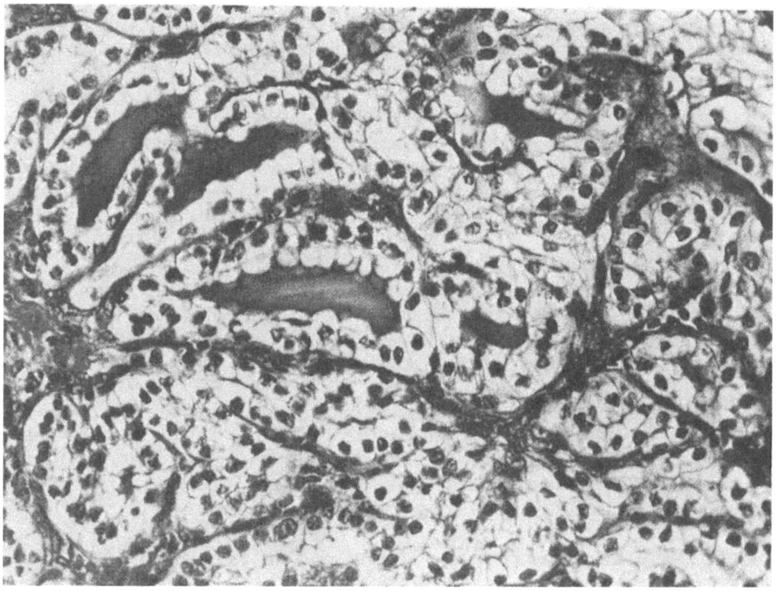

*Fig. 5. Cystadenoma of epididymis, same case as Figure 4. Papillary processes are covered and glandlike spaces are lined by cuboidal to columnar epithelial cells with clear or vacuolated cytoplasm. Spaces between papillae and lumens of glandlike structures are filled with a deeply eosinophilic homogeneous material resembling colloid. x 300 (From MOSTOFI and PRICE (23))*

It is true that malignant epithelial tumors, or carcinomas of the epididymis have also been described (see Table 2). Most of this work, however, is contained in not readily accessible reports from before the Second World War. More recently, just a few individual reports have appeared, at least one of which seems not to rule out that metastasis of an unknown primary tumor was present (25). It is known in any case that particularly carcinoma of the prostate and stomach and also occasionally renal carcinoma and intestinal tumors can metastasize into the epididymis (see Table 2).

Seminomas of the epididymis are also described (Table 2). They would have to be derived from displaced elements of the germinal epithelium. One must always, however, reckon with the possibility that malignant lymphomas, which not infrequently afflict the epididymis and testicular region mostly together, have been misdiagnosed as seminomas since histologic differential diagnosis is apparently difficult, as is stressed in the relevant reports (3, 22). Particularly when the malignant lymphoma is primarily manifested in the epididymis, there is the likelihood of the misdiagnosis "seminoma."

As mentioned at the outset, it is necessary in the case of malignant mesenchymal tumors to distinguish between the sarcomas of juveniles, on the one hand, and the sarcomas of adults and the aged, on the other.

The first group comprises the extremely malignant rhabdomyosarcomas and embryonic sarcomas, which apparently have a special affinity with the urogenital tract and occur not only in the spermatic cord and epididymis but also in the prostate, bladder, uterus, and vagina as well as in the pelvic connective tissue of children and juveniles. An important point is WILLIS's (28) observation that the majority of rhabdomyosarcomas in juveniles occur outside the striated voluntary musculature. He concludes from this, that the usual source of rhabdomyosarcomas is the embryonic mesenchyma.

Malignant adenomatoid tumors, where described, also seem to be a disease of juveniles (8, 12). Whether, however, there is a group of tumors that are rightly designated as malignant adenomatoid tumors is a question for pathologists to answer. Their malignancy or their character as an adenomatoid tumor has already been doubted (12, 18, 23).

The other sarcomas of various differentiation which occur in adults and the aged are not distinguished by their behavior from sarcomas located elsewhere. Like the sarcomas of juveniles, they, too, originate more frequently from the spermatic cord than from the epididymis and can - as in our case (Fig. 6) - undergo very rapid development.

The 76-year-old leiomyosarcoma patient from my predecessor's records observed an increase in size of the content of the right scrotal cavity over a 6-month period. With inguinal semicastration it was no longer possible to remove the tumor totally. Within 2 months the patient died of cachexia and general metastasization.

Miscellaneous tumors also occur both in benign and malignant forms: Whereas the melanotic hamartoma - also called retinal anlage tumor - has been found in the epididymis itself (8, 23, 29), dermoid cysts and both benign and malignant teratomas predominate in the spermatic cord (8, 23).

On the diagnosis of these tumors, which are readily accessible to palpation, not much need be said: Every tumorous alteration of the scrotal

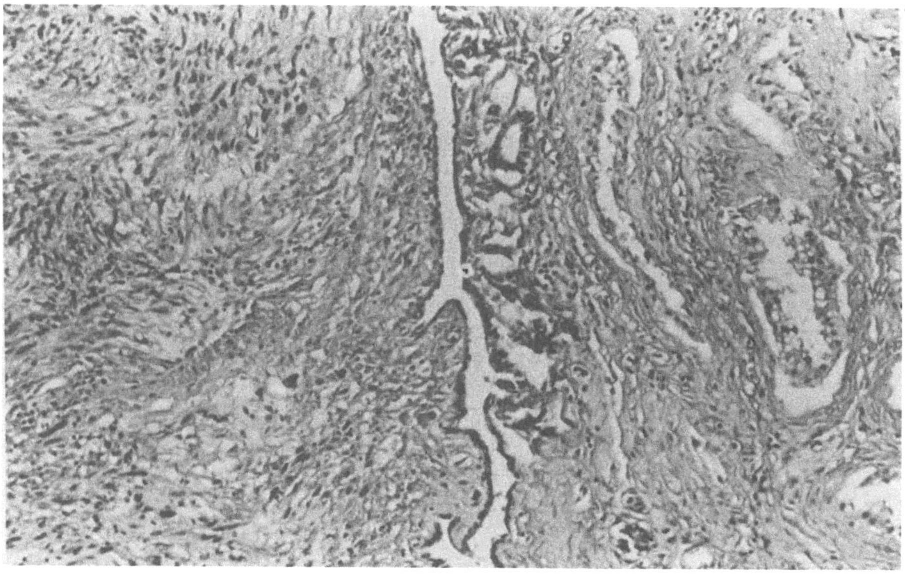

*Fig. 6. Leiomyosarcoma of spermatic cord in a 76-year-old man, already involving epididymis and testis*

content must be regarded as potentially malignant and should thus be histologically clarified.

Hydroceles, which hamper exact palpation, should not be punctured, but always operated on, it being then possible to assess the scrotal content. Symptomatic hydroceles are described in about 10% of benign tumors and more frequently in the case of malignant tumors. Serious difficulties may be present in the differential diagnosis between a rapidly growing malignoma of the epididymis and a subacute epididymitis.
In adults the relative painlessness of the swelling should always lead one to suspect a tumor, while in children, before puberty, one should primarily assume a tumor.

For the prognosis of extratesticular malignomas it is difficult to gain a reliable picture from the literature because the reported observation periods are too short as a rule and data on the stage of the disease at the start of treatment are mostly lacking. The high malignancy of these tumors is revealed in the report of the Testicular Tumor Panel and Registry in Great Britain: of 11 patients with rhabdomyosarcomas and 11 with other sarcomas, 8 and 5 respectively died within 2 years. Only liposarcoma of the spermatic cord seems to be relatively benign. In 1970 BANOWSKY and SCHULTZ found among 101 case histories in the literature on extratesticular sarcomas only 73 with follow-up (1). Of these 73 only a third survived without signs in the reported observation periods of various durations. Two-thirds of this patients have either died or developed metastases. In origin the metastasization was purely lymphatic in 53% of these cases, both lymphatic and, probably secondarily, hematogenous in 37%, and primarily hematogenous in only 10%. Malignomas of the epididymis, like testicular tumors, can apparently develop retroperitoneal metastases along the lymphatic ducts of the vasa spermatica. The closer, however, they are situated to the spermatic cord, the more they affect the lymphatic nodes of the iliac region, in keeping with the course of the vasa diferentia, and particularly the inguinal lymphatic nodes, in keeping with the spread of the vasa cremasterica.

It is thererore not surprising that therapeutic success such as reported by GHAVIMI et al. (13) has only been achieved since the introduction of radical surgery with inguinal semicastration and both retroperitoneal and, primarily, inguinal lymphadenectomy. GHAVIMI et al. first performed such radical operations on 11 children with extratesticular rhabdomyosarcomas, in some cases even removing the affected half of the scrotum, and then subjected all patients to a course of intermittent treatment repeated in cycles for periods of up to 2 years with four different cytostatics: dactinomycin, adriamycin, vincristine, and cyclophosphamide (Fig. 7). Six of these children, five of whom were in stage IA and one in stage IB at the start of treatment, survived between 2 and 10 years without signs. A seventh child, already affected in the para-aortal lymphatic nodes, i.e., in stage III, was treated 28 months without signs by applying additional local and para-aortal radiation therapy (4000 rad). Only three children with primary stages III and IV died early in spite of this intensive treatment.

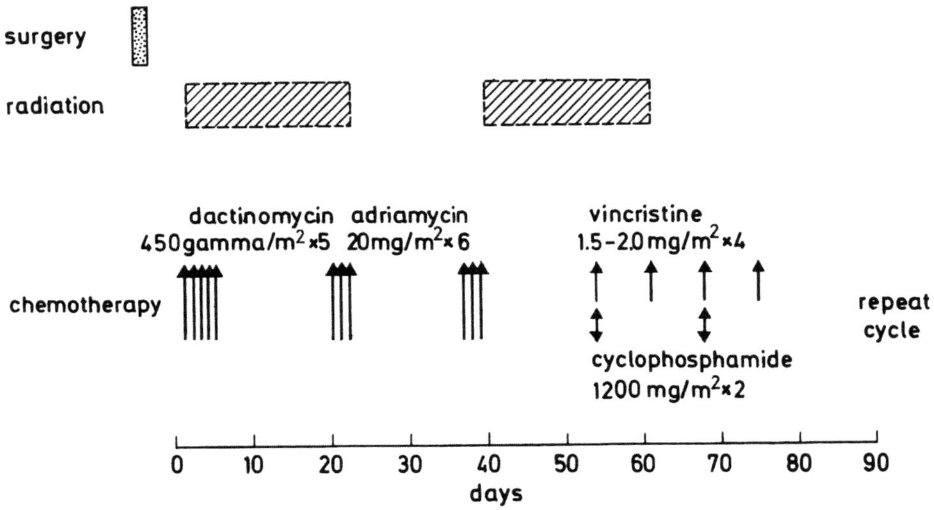


*Fig. 7. Multidisciplinary protocol for treatment of embryonal rhabdomyosarcoma. From GHAVIMI et al. (13)*

I am not prepared to state that this elaborate therapy or components of it were decisive for the favorable outcome. Since cases of survival including long-term survival, have been reported repeatedly, also in accounts of less recent origin, it seems to me that the most essential factor is early diagnosis and removal of the malignoma in a still favorable stage. The conclusion to be drawn by the clinician is therefore to regard every intrascotal swelling as potentially malignant and to explore it surgically once too often rather than one time too few.

Biopsy, of course, may only be performed when facilities for immediate histologic examination are available, and only on the basis of an inguinal incision, so that inguinal semicastration with inguinal lymphadenectomy can, if necessary, be performed immediately. As with testicular tumors, lymphography followed by retroperitoneal lymphadenectomy should, as a rule, be performed. If histologic examination reveals an epithelial tumor further investigations must be done. These include, in cases of papillary cystadenoma, checks for other manifestations of Hippel-Lindau's disease, and in cases of carcinoma of the epididymis, checks for a possible, hitherto unknown primary tumor of the prostate, intestinal tract, or kidney.

Whether one should, in principle, then continue treatment, either chemotherapeutically or radiotherapeutically, or do so only when there is evidence of metastasis, is a question that remain open.

## SUMMARY

Tumors of the epididymis, both primary and secondary, whether benign or malignant are very rare. The elements of the spermatic duct system, whether inside the testis or outside it in the epididymis and spermatic cord, exhibit only 1/20th of that of the germinal epithelium. In accordance with the mesodermal, or mesothelial origin of the whole spermatic duct system, tumors of the epididymis and spermatic cord are - with few exceptions - mesenchymal tumors, the most frequent of these being the so-called adenomatoid tumor, a benign slowly growing tumor. With regard to the relative frequency of the various extratesticular tumors, a British panel has shown that one quarter of its cases are adenomatoid tumors, a second quarter sarcomas of children and juveniles (rhabdomyosarcomas and embryonic sarcomas), a third quarter sarcomas of adults and the aged, while the last quarter includes simple benign mesenchymal tumors, mixed tumors, metastatic tumors, and others. There is only one extremely rare epithelial tumor of the epididymis, the papillary cystadenoma, which seems to be a partial manifestation or forme fruste of Hippel-Lindau's disease. So far only 40 cases have been described in the world literature.

Therapy of intrascrotal but extratesticular tumors always ought to be surgical: If the tumor proves to be benign, simple excision suffices. In cases of malignancy, immediate inguinal lymphadenectomy and - as with testicular tumors - lymphography followed by retroperitoneal lymphadenectomy. Whether one should, in principle, then continue treatment either chemotherapeutically or radiotherapeutically, or do so only when there is evidence of metastasis, is a question which still remains open.

## ACKNOWLEDGMENTS

The author wishes to thank Prof. Dr. med. E. LANGER, chief pathologist, Städtisches Krankenhaus München-Schwabing for the histologic examination and the microphotographs of the tumors shown in Figures 2 and 3, and also Prof. Dr. F. OCCHIONERO, Munich pathologist, for the histologic examination and the microphotograph of the leiomyosarcoma shown in Figure 6.

REFERENCES


1. Banowsky, L.H., Schultz, G.N.: Sarcoma of the spermatic cord and tunics: review of the literature case report and idscussion of the role of retroperitoneal lymph node dissection. J. Urol. (Baltimore) 103, 628-631 (1970)
2. Bibus, B., Zeitlhofer, J.: Tumorartige Bildungen und Tumoren im Bereiche des Nebenhodens und des Samenstranges. Z. Urol. 62, 529-534 (1969)
3. Bichler, K.H., Büscher, K.H., Tauber, R., Naber, K.: Lymphoreticuläre Sarkome des Hodens und Nebenhodens. Akt. Urol. 5, 221-228 (1974)
4. Broth, G., Bullock, W.K., Morrow, J.: Epididymal tumors: 1. Report of 15 new cases including review of literature. 2. Histochemical study of the so-called adenomatoid tumor. J. Urol. (Baltimore) 100, 530-536 (1968)
5. Brown, N.J.: Miscellaneous tumors of mainly epithelial type. Brit. J. Urol. 36, 70-77 (1964)
6. Chan, Y.H., Schinella, R.A., Draper, J.W.: Papillary clear cell cystadenoma of the epididymis. J. Urol. (Baltimore) 100, 661-665 (1968)
7. Collins, D.H., Pugh, R.C.: Classification and frequency of testicular tumors. Brit. J. Urol. Suppl. June 1964, 36, 1-11 (1964)
8. Czvalinga, I., Götz, F.: Über die Geschwülste des Nebenhodens. Z. Urol. 65, 175-186 (1972)
9. Dandia, S.D., OJha, D.G.: Giant fibroma of the epididymis: a case report. J. Urol. (Baltimore) 96, 941-943 (1966)
10. Elsässer, E., Carl, P.: Primäre Tumoren des Nebenhodens. Münch. med. Wschr. 20, 978-981 (1972)
11. Fishelovitch, J., Meiraz, D., Keinan, Z., Green, I.: Malignant mesothelioma of the testicular tunica vaginalis. Brit. J. Urol. 47, 208 (1975)
12. Fisher, E.R., Klieger, H.: Epididymal carcinoma (malignant adenomatoid tumor , mesonephric mesodermal carcinoma of epididymis). J. Urol. (Baltimore) 95, 568-572 (1966)
13. Ghavimi, F., Exelby, P.R., D'Angio, G.J., Whitmore, W.F., Jr., Lieberman, P.H., Lewis, J.L., Jr., Mike, V., Murphy, M.L.: Combination therapy of urogenital embryonal rhabdomyosarcoma in children. Cancer (Philad.) 32, 1178-1185 (1973)
14. Glantz, M.G.: Adenomatoid tumor of the epididymis: a review of 5 new cases including a case report associated with hydrocele. J. Urol. (Baltimore) 95, 227-233 (1966)
15. Golden, A., Ash, J.E.: Adenomatoid tumors of genital tract. Amer. J. Path. 21, 63-79 (1945)
16. Gowing, N.F.C., Morgan, A.D.: Paratesticular tumors of connective tissue and muscle. In: The Pathology of Testicular Tumors. Edinburgh and London: Livingstone, 1964. Brit. J. Urol. Suppl. 36, 78-84 (1964)
17. Heinke, E., Doepfmer, R.: In: Handbuch der Haut- und Geschlechtskrankheiten, Suppl. VI/3, Schuermann, H., Doepfmer, R. (eds.). Berlin-Göttingen-Heidelberg: Springer-Verlag 1960, p. 32
18. Jablokow, V.R., Jagatic, J., Rubnitz, M.E.: Adenomatoid tumors of the genital tract: Report of 12 cases and review of the literature. J. Urol. (Baltimore) 95, 573-576 (1966)
19. Longo, V.J., McDonald, J.R., Thompson, G.J.: Primary neoplasms of the epididymis. J. Amer. med. Ass. 147, 937-941 (1951)
20. McGowan, A.J., Jr., Smith, E.H.: Urological implications of sarcoidosis. J. Urol. (Baltimore) 97, 1090-1093 (1967)
21. MacKenzie, I., Roberts, G.H.: Liposarcoma of paratesticular origin: a case report. Brit. J. Urol. 46, 467-470 (1974)

22. Mostofi, F.K.: Testicular tumors. Epidemiologic etiologic and pathologic features. Cancer (Philad.) 32, 1186-1201 (1973)
23. Mostofi, F.K., Price, E.B., Jr.: Tumor of the male genital system. In: Atlas of Tumor Pathology. Washington, D.C.: Armed Forces Inst. Path. 1973, Fasc-7, Series 2, pp. 143-175
24. Pap, S.: Über den adenomatösen Tumor des Nebenhodens. Z. Urol. 61, 393-395 (1968)
25. Reichel, O.: Maligne Neubildungen des Nebenhodens. Z. Urol. 61, 869-871 (1968)
26. Satter, E.J., Heidner, F.C., Wear, J.B.: Primary sarcoma of the spermatic cord and epididymis. J. Urol. (Baltimore) 82, 148-152 (1959)
27. Wachtel, T.L., Mehan, D.J.: Metastatic tumors of the epididymis. J. Urol. (Baltimore) 103, 624-627 (1970)
28. Willis, R.A.: Pathology of tumors. Cited in Gowing,N.F.C., Morgan, A.D.
29. Zone, R.M.: Retinal anlage tumor of the epididymis: a case report. J. Urol. (Baltimore) 103, 106-107 (1970)

## *V. Testicular Tumors*

# Epidemiology and Pathology of Tumors of Human Testis

F. K. MOSTOFI

The incidence of testicular tumors in Germany is unknown. In the USA it is 3.1 per 100,000 (3) and 2.5 in Ontario (11). In the USA 0.64% of all male cancer deaths are attributed to testicular tumors. In England the corresponding figures are 0.52%. In both USA and Canada testicular tumors account for 11-13% of all cancer deaths in the age group 15-34 years. In the age group of 20-34 years old, testicular tumors constitute the most frequent malignant tumor following leukemia, Hodgkin's and melanomas.

HOWDEN in Auckland (9), GRUMET and McMAHAN in the USA (8), and CLEMENSEN in Denmark (4) have observed a doubling of the mortality rate from testicular tumors from the period 1943-1947 to 1958-1962.

## Geographic and Racial Distribution

Testicular tumors are rare in Asia (1, 2, 20), in Finland (22), in New Zealand (9), in Africa (5, 6, 10, 19, 23), and in American blacks.

It is of interest to note that the frequency of testicular tumors varies with age: they are common in infants and children, the highest peak incidence is in age group 18-40, and a third peak occurs in men over 50 years of age. The histologic types vary with age (14).

## Pathology

To understand the pathology of testicular tumors it is essential to remember that there are five components in the testis. The most important of these is the germ cell which is located in seminiferous tubules and presents a variety of histologic appearances depending on the stage of its maturation. The germ cell is supported by two cell types - the sustentacular cells of Sertoli and the interstitial cells of Leydig. These we have designated as the specialized gonadal stromal cells. The excretory ductal system serves to transport the spermatozoa out of the testis. These elements are supported by a fibrovascular stroma and the entire organs is covered by a fibromuscular capsule.

Germ cells constitute the largest cell population and their tumors comprise over 90% of primary testicular tumors. Next in frequency are the tumors of specialized gonadal stroma which constitute 4-6% of testis tumors. Tumors of the excretory ductal system - the collecting tubules, rete, epididymis, and spermatic cord - constitute a very small proportion as do also tumors of fibrovascular connective tissue and the capsule. As in other organs the testis is subject to invasion by metastatic tumors. These are also very rare except in older patients in whom they constitute a relatively large proportion of tumors.

## Classification of Testicular Tumors

The classification herein reported is essentially the proposed World Health Organization's international histologic classification of testis tumors:

### HISTOLOGIC CLASSIFICATION OF TESTIS TUMORS

I. Germ cell tumors

- A. Tumors of one histologic type
  1. Seminoma
  2. Spermatocytic seminoma
  3. Embryonal carcinoma
  4. Yolk sac tumor, embryonal carcinoma - infantile type
  5. Polyembryoma
  6. Choriocarcinoma
  7. Teratoma
     - a) mature
     - b) immature
     - c) with malignant transformation (other than 1-6)
- B. Tumors of more than one histologic type
  1. Embryonal carcinoma + teratoma (teratocarcinoma)
  2. Choriocarcinoma and any other type (specify types)
  3. Other combinations (specify)

II. Sex cord/stromal tumors

1. Leydig cell tumors
2. Sertoli cell tumors
3. Granulosa cell tumors
4. Mixed forms (specify)
5. Incompletely differentiated forms

III. Tumors and tumorlike conditions containing both germ cell and sex cord/stromal elements

- A. Gonadoblastoma
- B. Others

IV. Miscellaneous tumors

- A. Carcinoids
- B. Others

V. Lymphoid and hematopoietic tumors

VI. Secondary tumors

VII. Tumors of collecting ducts, rete, epididymis, spermatic cord, capsule, supporting structures, and appendices

VIII. Unclassified tumors

IX. Tumorlike conditions

The various categories in the classification have been discussed in detail elsewhere (15, 16). For this presentation only category I will be considered in detail. The others are mentioned for the purpose of completeness.

## I. GERM CELL TUMORS

The classification and postorchiectomy management of all testicular tumors, more particularly germ cell tumors, are based entirely on their pathomorphology. A clear understanding of various categories and their relationships is essential to the proper management of these tumors.

To understand the pathomorphology and pathophysiology of germ cell tumors it is essential to realize that in its natural habitat the cell of origin, i.e., the germ cell, is a dynamic constantly changing cell. Under certain environmental conditions, e.g., penetration into an ovum, it may develop into normal or abnormal embryonic and extra embryonic tissue. Such capability is reflected in neoplasms of this cell resulting in a diversity of histologic patterns ranging fron single cell tumor to complex neoplasms.

About 60% of these tumors consist of one cell type; 40% of more than one cell type. This phenomenon is observed not only in the primary tumor but in the metastases as well. In the majority of instances the histology of metastases is the same as that of the primary; however, in many instances the metastases are either of different cell type or show multiple elements that may not be visible in the primary.

The histologic types to be described each have different clinical behavior, survival, and mortality rates. We have shown that 90% of deaths from testes tumors occur in the first 2 years and almost all deaths in 5 years. NEFZGER and MOSTOFI (17) demonstrated in a 17-year follow-up of 834 patients with testicular tumors that only 2 patients died of metastases after 6 years. We observed that 81% of patients who lived for 2 years were alive after 15 years. We have, however, seen patients with seminoma present with metastases 10 or 20 years later. Such cases should always raise the possibility of a second primary testicular tumor.

### A. Germ Cell Tumors of One Histological Type

1. Seminoma. Seminoma constitutes about 40% of germ cell tumors of testis and is the most common tumor found in cryptorchid testes. The testis is usually enlarged and may attain a very large size but it may be normal or even smaller. The enlargement is usually diffuse but may be nodular. Tunical vessels are usually dilated, the tunica may be smooth and glistening or rough, dull, fibrous, or thick. The cut surfaces show a homogeneous lobulated grayish-white and glistening tissue. The consistency is usually soft but may be hard, depending on the amount of fibrous tissue. Areas of hemorrhage and necrosis are rare. The tumor is not encapsulated from the surrounding testicular parenchyma. In a few cases the tumor may be found to extend beyond the capsule, usually through the sites of entry of blood vessels. Extension to the hilus, the rete testes, epididymis, and the spermatic cord occur and affect the prognosis.

Histologically, the typical seminoma is composed of uniform cells supported by a delicate connective tissue stroma (Fig. 1). The cells are large, round, or polyhedral. The nucleus is centrally placed, large, spherical, and has an irregular nuclear membrane, distinct and granular chromatin distribution, and one or two large basophilic nucleoli. The cytoplasm is clear or granular and contains varying amounts of glycogen and rarely lipid material. The cells have a distinct border forming a cobblestone or mosaic arrangement. Mitoses and giant cells are rare.

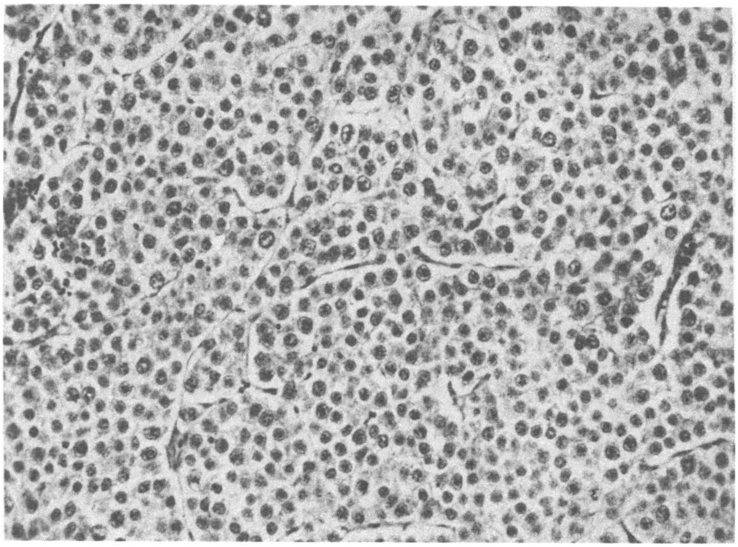

*Fig. 1. Seminoma. Tumor is made up of uniform cells supported by a delicate stroma. AFIP Neg. 75-14722* x *190*

The cells occur in lobules, rows, or cords but may be intratubular or diffusely infiltrating the parenchyma.

The stroma consists of delicate fibrovascular tissue which divides the tumor cells into lobules of varying sizes (Fig. 2). Varying amounts of lymphocytic infiltration and granulomatous reaction are seen in every case but in about 20% these are quite marked, and are indicative of immune response. Stromal hyalinization is seen occasionally.

Most seminomas present a fairly uniform cell population. In about 10%, however, variations in size, shape, and staining of the cells are seen. In a number of these there is a definite increase in mitotic activity. This may be focal or diffuse. We have felt that since variation in size, shape, and staining of cells is so often a function of fixation and processing and are subjective, the most reliable criterion for anaplasia and increased aggressiveness is the increased mitotic activity - an average of 3 mitoses in 10 high power fields (Fig. 3). We have shown that the majority of seminomas that metastasize have increased mitotic activity in their primary and MAIER et al. (12) have shown that anaplastic seminomas have a higher mortality than typical seminomas.

Seminomas tend to spread most frequently through the lymphatics. The route and frequent sites of metastases have been described elsewhere. Suffice it to say that in 65% of metastasizing seminomas the metastases consist of seminomas, 26% embryonal carcinomas, and in 4% as teratomas. We have seen three instances of tumors that were pure seminomas in the primary metastasize as choriocarcinomas.

The significance of these observations is that if a patient with seminoma does not respond to radiation it is probably due to the fact that the metastases are something else. While most of metastases occur in the first 2 years and almost all within 5 years, we have seen instances of delayed metastases occurring 10-20 years later.

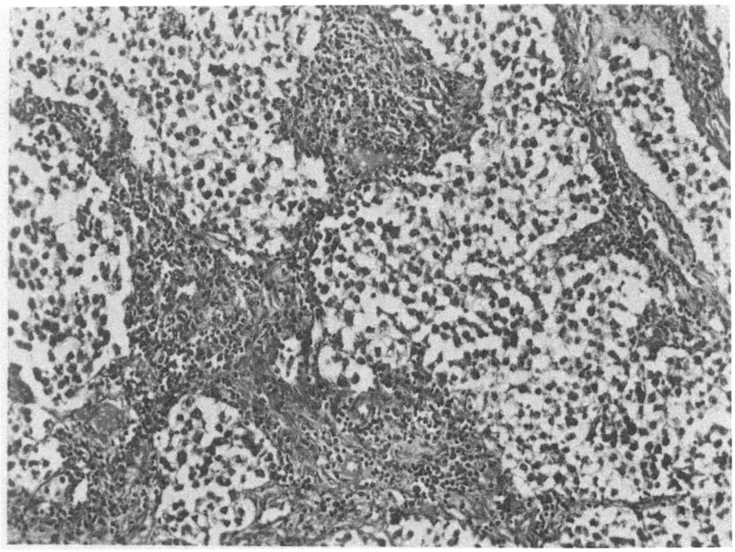

*Fig. 2. Seminoma. Seminoma cells are vacuolated. They occur in lobules separated by fibrous tissue showing granulomatous reaction and lymphoid infiltration. AFIP Neg. 75-14331* x *130*

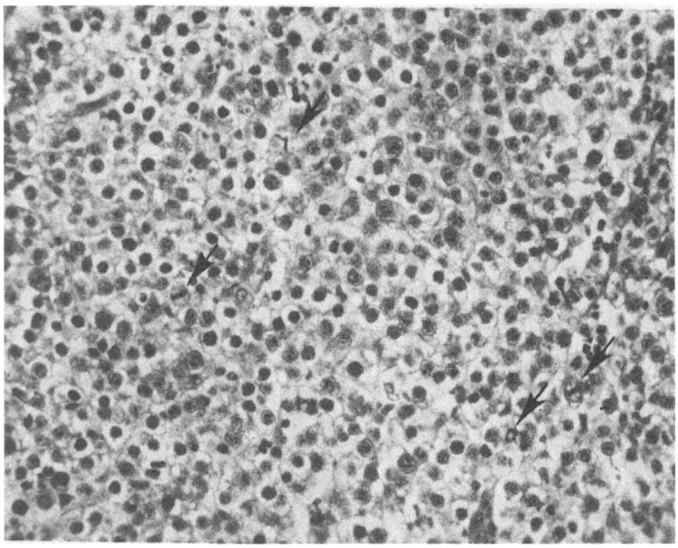

*Fig. 3. Anaplastic seminoma. Several mitotic figures are present. AFIP Neg. 75-12559* x *200*

2. Spermatocytic Seminoma. Described first by MASSON in 1946 (13), this tumor is grossly and microscopically different from seminoma. Its frequency varies with the age of the patient population, being more frequent in older age patients. It grows slowly and it less symptomatic. Grossly, it is yellowish in color, soft, and slightly mucoid, and it has cystic areas.

Histologically, the tumor shows three cell types (Fig. 4); the majority of the cell population, however, consists of medium-sized cells with a round nucleus and considerable amount of eosinophilic cytoplasm. The second cell type is a small, lymphocyte-like cell with a round basophilic glassy nucleus surrounded by a distinct rim of eosinphilic cytoplasm. The cells are reminiscent of secondary spermatocytes. The third cell type consists of huge mono- or multinucleated giant cells with round or oval nuclei surrounded by a considerable amount of eosinophilic cytoplasm. The nuclei in the intermediate and the giant cells have characteristic spireme or filamentous arrangement of chromatin resembling the meiotic phase of normal primary spermatocytes (Fig. 5). Moderate numbers of mitotic figures are present and some are abnormal. The cytoplasm is devoid of glycogen so that PAS stains are negative.

The tumor cells occur in sheets with large and small lakes containing an eosinophilic precipitate and cell debris. The stroma is scant and there is no lymphocytic or granulomatous reaction.

The histology suggests a high degree of radiosensitivity.

Spermatic seminoma would seem to have a good prognosis as very few deaths have been reported (15).

3. Embryonal Carcinoma (Figs. 6-9). Embryonal carcinoma is usually the smallest of testis tumors. It constitutes about 20% of germ cell tumors. The cut surfaces show a variegated appearance with granular or smooth grayish-white soft tissue. Hemorrhage and necrosis are frequent. The tumor is not encapsulated.

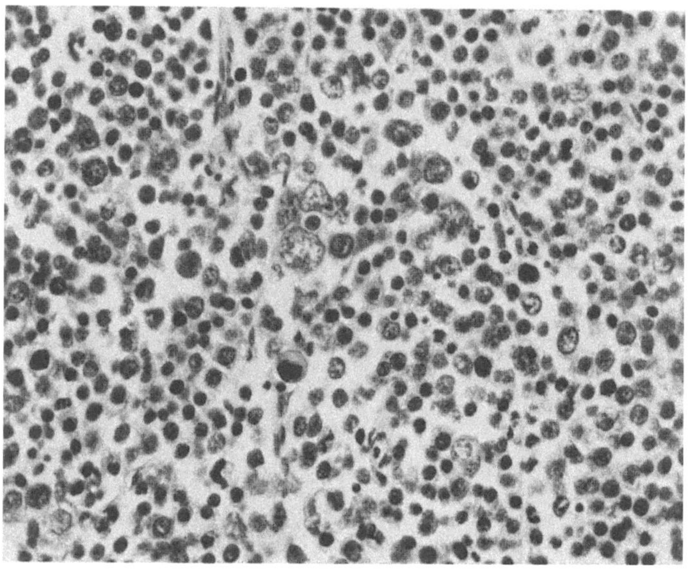

*Fig. 4. Spermatocytic seminoma. Tumor shows three cell types: large mononuclear cells, intermediate-sized cells, and small lymphocyte-like cells. Note absence of lymphocytic or granulomatous reaction. AFIP Neg. 73-7374 x 350*

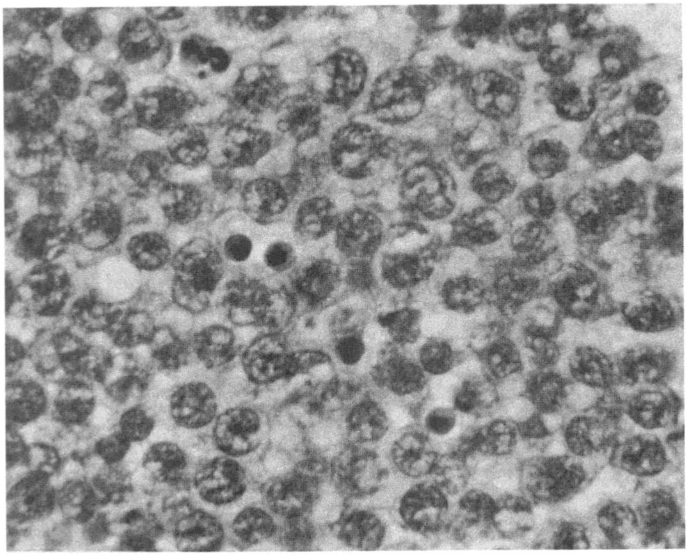

*Fig. 5. Spermatocytic seminoma. Another case showing spireme arrangement of nuclei. Note frequent mitotic figures. AFIP Neg. 73-6023* x *625*

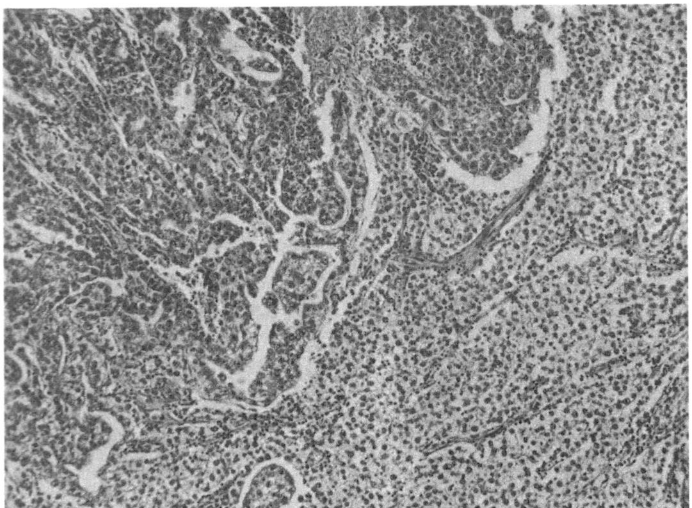

*Fig. 6. Embryonal carcinoma and seminoma.Right portion of field shows seminoma with fairly uniformly sized and staining cells occurring in lobules. Left portion shows papillary carcinoma. AFIP Neg. 73-5153* x *90*

Microscopically, the cells have an embryonic malignant epithelial appearance, The size, shape, and arrangement of cells vary considerably. The cells may be cuboidal, flattened, or columnar. The cytoplasm is usually homogeneously amphophilic or vacuolated. The cell borders are usually indistinct. The nuclei are irregularly round or oval with an irregular, coarse nuclear vacuolization. Mononuclear and multinucleated giant cells are frequent, as are mitotic figures.

The most frequent pattern of growth is the acinar; less frequently tubular, papillary or reticular arrangements may be seen. The acini, tubules, or papillary structures may be small or large. Occasionally the tumor may consist, in part or toto, of solid sheets resembling seminoma. However, the cells are distinctly epithelial, they are usually larger, display more variation in size, shape, and staining, the cell borders are usually absent, lymphocytic and granulomatous reactions are infrequent, and the lobular pattern of seminoma is absent.

In a number of embryonal carcinomas syncytiotrophoblastic cells may be seen.

A number of investigators have considered embryonal carcinomas as the primitive tumor of a totipotential cell which has the capability of going into somatic or trophoblastic differentiation. That there is a totipotential cell in germ cell malignancy which has the capability of developing into teratoma or carcinoma is further supported by the classic work of STEVENS (21), and PIERCE and DIXON (18).

In man, however, no evidence has been presented to date to show that once an embryonal carcinoma has developed it retains any other capability but that of unlimited growth.

A majority of embryonal carcinomas metastasize as embryonal carcinoma, a few metastases show foci of teratoma and/or choriocarcinoma. The preaortic and iliac lymph nodes are most frequently involved, followed by the lungs, liver, pleura, bone, and gastrointestinal tract.

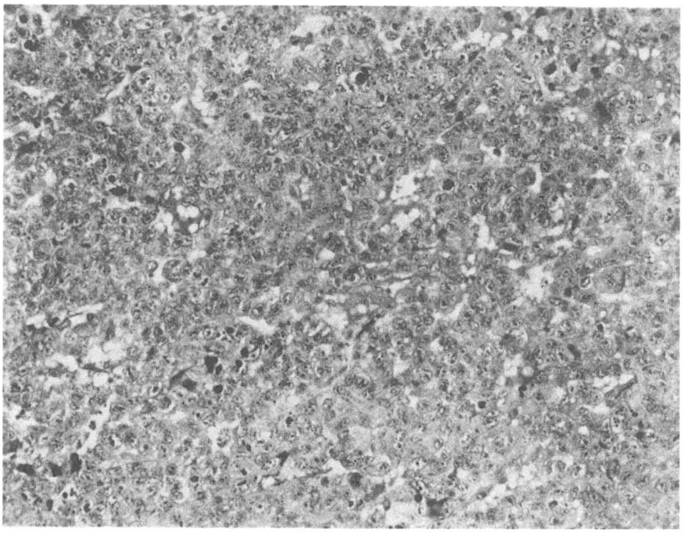

*Fig. 7. Embryonal carcinoma - solid pattern. Cells vary considerably in size and staining qualities. In contrast to Fig. 1 cell borders are not apparent and there is a suggestion of glandular pattern. AFIP Neg. 75-14902 x 130*

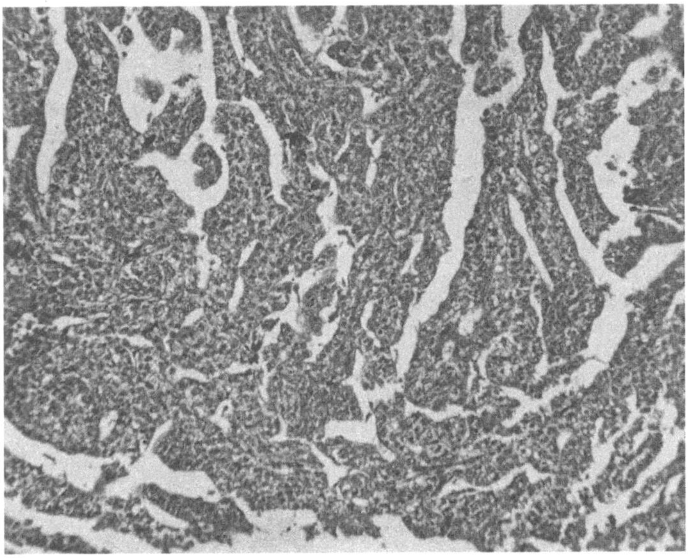

*Fig. 8. Embryonal carcinoma. Tumor shows papillary and glandular patterns. AFIP Neg. 73-8966* x *115*

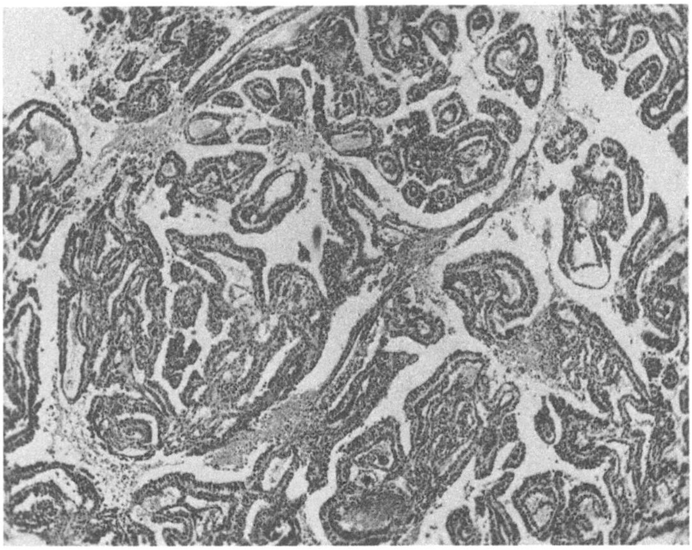

*Fig. 9. Embryonal carcinoma. Tumor shows a papillary pattern with double layer of cells. AFIP Neg. 71-10291* x *50*

4. Polyembryoma. Constituting a very small percentage of testis tumors this neoplasm has no gross characteristics. To be designated as such microscopically, the tumor must consist entirely or predominantly of embryoid bodies: a disc of single or multilayered undifferentiated cells, a cavity resembling amniotic cavity, and a tubular form resembling entoderm, and surrounded by loose mesenchyme in which a few

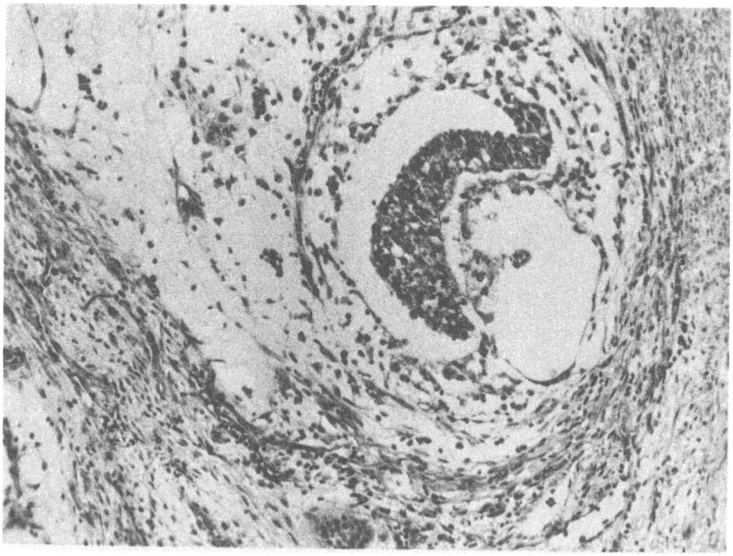

*Fig. 10. Embryonal body with a distinct cell disc and two cystic structures contained in a myxomatous stroma. AFIP Neg. 75-12733 x 150*

syncytio- and rarely cytotrophoblastic cells may be present (Fig. 10). These resemble embryos of 1-2 weeks gestation. Not all of these show the characteristic features we have described but many variations occur and the reader is referred to the classic work of EVANS (7).

What would develop if such an embryoid body of a testicular tumor were to be transplanted or allowed to grow is not known. In mice, STEVENS has demonstrated that when a highly pleomorphic murine testicular tumor is transplanted into the peritoneal cavity, thousands of embryoid bodies are produced (21). When these are transplanted subcutaneously in the same strain of mice, fully differentiated teratomas and teratocarcinomas developed. When the embryonal bodies were retransplanted intraperitoneally they developed into a anaplastic carcinoma. While pure polyembryomas are extremely rare, many embryonal carcinomas and teratocarcinomas contain enbryoid bodies.

5. Yolk Sac Tumor, Infantile Embryonal Carcinoma (Endodermal Sinus Tumor). This tumor occurs rarely in adults but is the most common testicular tumor of infancy and childhood. It presents a homogeneous grayish-white, lobulated, resilient, fatty, and mucinous appearance.

Microscopically, the tumor has a characteristic pattern: anastomosing glandular and ductal structures lined by low columnar, cuboidal, or flattened endothelial-like cells (Fig. 11). Solid sheets or papillary projections (Schiller-Duval bodies) may be seen which have misled to diagnosis of mesonephroma. The nuclei are usually large and irregularly shaped and have a variable chromatin distribution and one or two nucleoli. Sometimes the nuclei are closely parked suggesting syncytial cells. They are usually round or oval but sometimes elongated and spindle-shaped. The cytoplasm is usually vacuolated and the vacuoles may coalesce. The cytoplasm contains glycogen and lipid material.

The reticular pattern with large and small vacuoles, the anastomosing glands alternating with papillary structures and solid areas are the

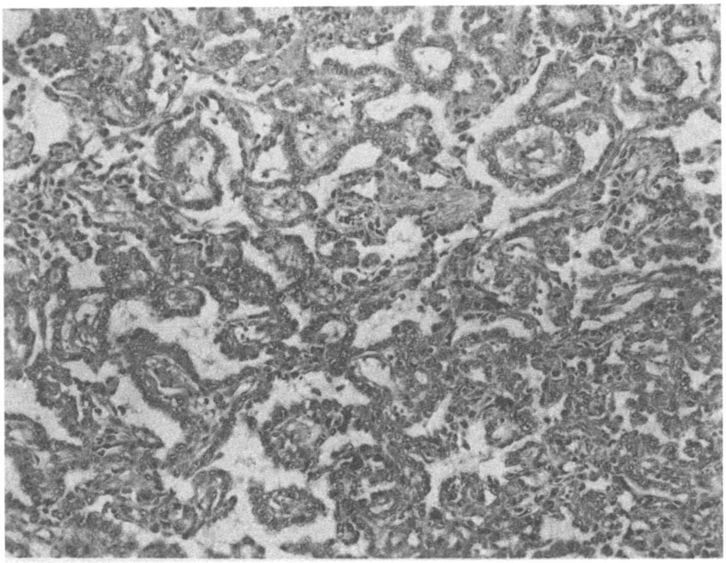

*Fig. 11. Embryonal carcinoma - infantile type. Tumor consists of anastomosing glandular structures lined by cuboidal epithelium. Note many Schiller-Duval bodies. AFIP Neg. 75-14903* x *100*

characteristic features of the tumor. In many of these tumors careful examination shows some teratoid structures - mucous glands, nests of cartilage, and squamous cysts. Metastases always show the carcinomatous components and the distribution is both by lymphatics and vascular channels.

6. Choriocarcinoma. In its pure form choriocarcinoma is extremely rare. We found 18 in the first 6000 testicular tumors in the American Testicular Tumor Registry. In most cases the patients present with symptoms referable to metastasis, which, on histologic examination, reveals the existence of choriocarcinoma. The patients have gynecomastia and marked elevation of chorionic gonadotropins.

Grossly, the testis is usually normal or small, but may be enlarged because of hemorrhage which is an invariable accompaniment of the tumor. The surface shows a hemorrhagic mass with some grayish-white tissue at the periphery.

Microscopically, for the diagnosis of choriocarcinoma we maintain that two distinct cell components must be clearly indentified: syncytiotrophoblasts and cytotrophoblasts (Fig. 12). Typically, the former is large, multinucleated, with many hyperchromatic irregular nuclei in a cytoplasm that is either eosoniphilic or amphophilic and has many vacuoles of varying sizes. These appear empty but may contain red cells. Others may be spindle-shaped resembling those of older placentas. Cytotrophoblasts are uniform, small, and closely parked. They have a clear cytoplasm, distinct cell border, and a single, uniform moderately sized vesicular nucleus. Syncytiotrophoblasts form the advancing edge of the tumor but no true villi are seen.

In our experience pure choriocarcinoma of the testis invariably metastasizes as choriocarcinoma and terminates fatally within 9 months. Metastases are via the bloodstream.

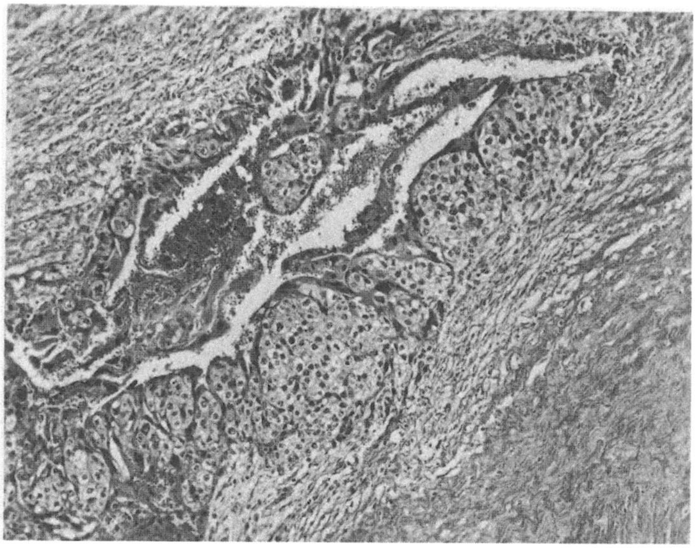

*Fig. 12. Choriocarcinoma. Tumor consists of two cell types: syncytiotrophoblasts and cytotrophoblasts. AFIP Neg. 75-10564* x *120*

While pure choriocarcinoma is extremely rare, choriocarcinomatous areas and more frequently syncytiotrophoblasts are not infrequently found in association with embryonal carcinoma, teratoma, or seminoma. We have seen several hundred such cases. It has been customary to designate a tumor by its most malignant component; however, in testicular tumors we reserve the term choriocarcinoma for those of the pure variety, i.e., where no other testicular tumor is found. When choriocarcinomatous foci are found in combination with other histologic types, they are classified in accordance with the components that are present, e.g., embryonal carcinoma and choriocarcinoma.

7. Teratoma (Fig. 13). Teratoma is defined as a complex tumor showing recognizable elements of more than one germ layer (ectoderm, mesoderm, and endoderm) in various stages of maturation often arranged in such a manner as to suggest abortive organ formation. These tumors constitute less than 10% of germ cell tumors.

The testis is usually enlarged. The tunica is irregularly distorted and nodular. The tumor cuts with varying degrees of resistance and the cut surface reveals cysts of various sizes filled with clear, gelatinous, or mucinous substances. Varying amounts of solid tissue are present in between. Cartilage and bone are not infrequent.

Microscopically, teratoma is applied to tumors that show elements derivable from more than one of three germ layers: ectoderm, represented by squamous epithelium with or without keratinization and nerve tissue; endoderm, represented by gastrointestinal and respiratory tissue and mucous glands, and mesodern, represented by bone, cartilage, and muscle. However, when multiple tissues representing only one germ layer are present, e.g., squamous cysts and brain tissue, such a tumor is regarded as teratoma. Also, when a single type of differentiated tissue, e.g., cartilage or squamous cyst or mucous gland is seen in association with seminoma or embryonal carcinoma, such areas are regarded as teratoma. Teratomas are further histologically classified as immature or

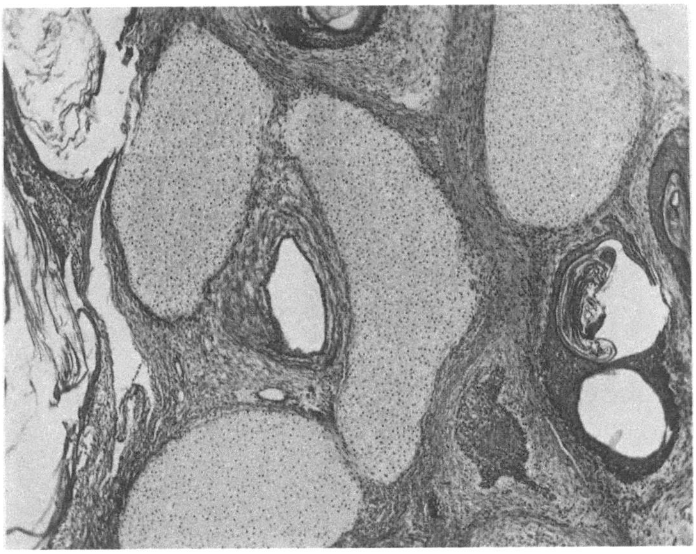

*Fig. 13. Mature teratoma. Tumor is made up of many nests of cartilage, squamous casts, and glandular structures. AFIP Neg. 75-10363* x 50

mature. By immature teratoma we mean teratomas which consist of primitive neuroectoderm, endoderm, or mesoderm. The distinguishing feature is that although the cells are primitive, an embryonic structure is identifiable.

Mature teratoma is characterized by the presence of recognizable tissue: cartilage, bone, mucous glands, squamous, transitional, cuboidal or columnar epithelial cells, smooth or skeletal muscle, and/or abortive organ formation - gastrointestinal, respiratory tissue, eye, pancreas, liver, choroid plexus, brain, and bone marrow. Most teratomas are entirely mature and pure immature teratomas are extremely rare as there are usually some nature elements in all immature teratomas.

Although no malignant areas may be found in a mature teratoma, testicular teratomas should never be diagnosed as benign since they are potentially malignant and capable of invasion of lymphatics and local extension.

Rarely a teratoma, mature or immature, may show malignant areas not identifiable as embryonal carcinoma, seminoma, or choriocarcinoma. Such areas can be recognized as undifferentiated or differentiated sarcomas, adenocarcinoma, or squamous carcinomas. These are designated as teratoma with malignant areas.

Teratomas metastasize via lymphatics and the earliest and most frequent sites of metastases are the preaortic and iliac lymph nodes, liver, lungs, bones, pleura, and intestines. Most teratomas metastasize as teratoma or embryonal carcinoma, a few as choriocarcinoma.

Dermoid cyst is quite common in the ovary but rather rare in the testis. We have seen 15 such cases. The distinguishing feature is a cyst of keratinized stratified squamous epithelium with skin appendages: hair, sebaceous and keratohyaline material, teeth, and pancreas. We have not seen metastases from any pure dermoid cysts.

Two lesions of the testis are generally regarded as one-sided developments of teratoma but, if seen by themselves, they should not be designated as such.

1. Epidermal cyst. Epidermal cysts contain keratohyaline material and are lined by stratified squamous epithelium but they contain no skin appendages. At times the wall may be ruptured with extrusion of contents and foreign body and lipogranulomatous reaction. Price has shown that tumors that consisted entirely of an epidermal cyst without any other elements or any scars, showed no metastases.

2. Carcinoid. Carcinoids of the testis may be primary or secondary. They may occur in a teratoma or no teratomatous structures may be identified. They may be functional or nonfunctional - the majority are nonfunctional. They should be regarded as potentially malignant

## B. Germ Cell Tumors Showing More Than One Histological Pattern

Forty percent of germ cell tumors show more than one of the basic histologic patterns and the most common of these is embryonal carcinoma and teratoma (24%), teratoma, embryonal carcinoma, and seminoma (6.4%). Other combinations are less frequent. When encountered the components should be listed in the diagnosis.

Teratocarcinoma has come to be applied to tumors of testis that consist of embryonal carcinoma and teratoma (Figs. 14 and 15). Grossly, these tumors show features of teratoma - cysts, cartilage and bone, and solid areas. They are usually the largest of testis tumors and replace the parenchyma. Microscopically, the tumor consists of varying proportions of definite embryonal carcinoma and teratoma.

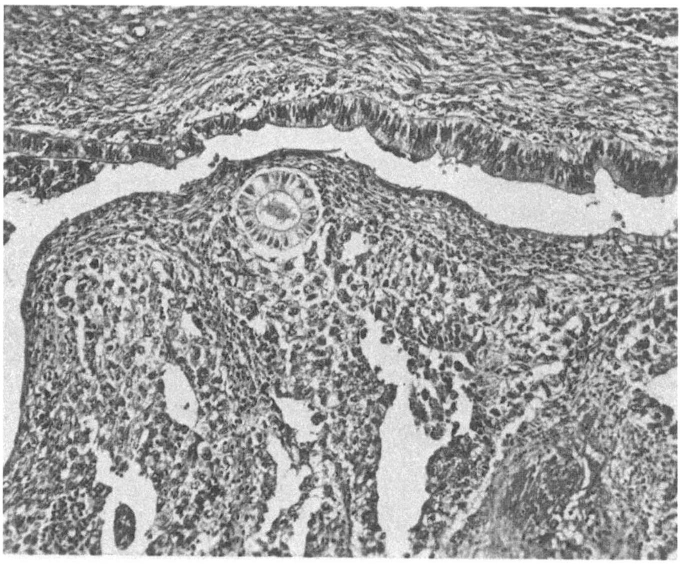

*Fig. 14. Teratocarcinoma. Tumor shows a mucous gland, a structure lined by tall columnar epithelium (teratoma), and there is also an embryonal carcinoma. AFIP 74-5834 x 130*

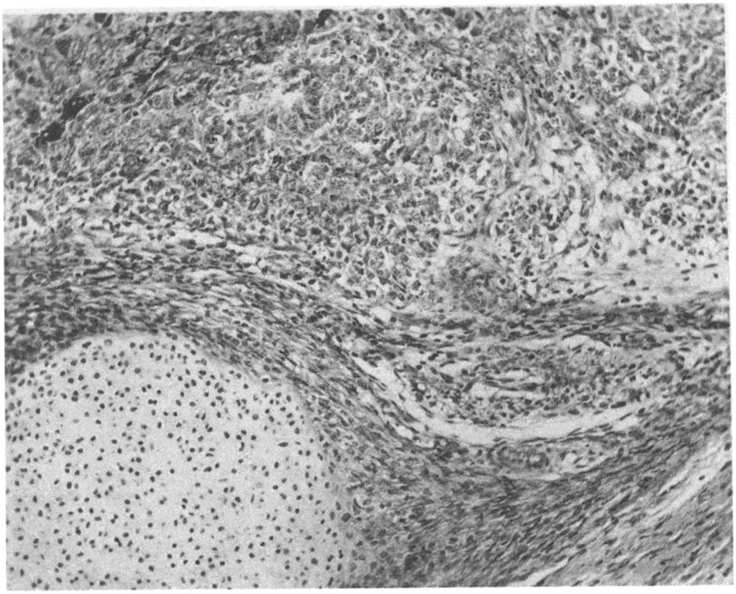

*Fig. 15. Teratocarcinoma. Tumor shows both embryonal carcinoma and a nest of cartilage (teratomatous components). AFIP Neg. 75-10364* x *115*

These tumors metastasize mostly as embryonal carcinoma but teratoma and choriocarcinoma may also be seen in the metastases. The routes of metastases are via the lymphatics and the bloodstream, and the sites of metastases are similar to those of embryonal carcinoma.

### C. The Nature of Metastases in Germ Cell Tumors

As mentioned earlier, in most germ cell tumors the metastases are similar to the primary, but it is not uncommon for a tumor of a single cell pattern to show either a mixture of cell patterns or a totally different cytology, e.g., a seminoma may show teratoma, embryonal carcinoma, or choriocarcinoma in the metastases. Three possible explanations have been offered for this phenomenon: (1) a small focus may have been missed in the primary; (2) the primitive totipotential malignant germ cell may have developed into one type in the testis and the same or one or more of the other types in the metastases, and (3) the environment may have affected the histology of the tumor. The last two theories could also explain the phenomenon that a tumor which is histologically entirely benign should metastasize or that the metastases of an embryonal carcinoma or teratocarcinoma may consist of histologically benign-appearing teratomatous tissue.

## II. SEX CORD STROMAL TUMORS

About 6% of our testicular tumors consist of Leydig cells, Sertoli cells, granulosa or theca cell-like tumors, or mixtures of these. The frequency with which combinations of these tumors occur led the author to postulate a common cell origin - the specialized gonadal stroma - for these tumors.

1. Leydig Cell tumors. Grossly, the testis may be diffusely enlarged or may show one or more nodules. In 5-9% the tumors are bilateral and these should arouse the suspicion of adrenogenital syndrome. The size may vary from 1-10 cm or more. The cut surfaces are usually homogeneously yellow to mahogany brown and bulging. There may be areas of hyalinization and calcification.

Microscopically, several cell types have been described. The most frequent cell is medium-sized, hexagonal with indistinct borders, with an eosinophilic or vacuolated cytoplasm surrounding a regular round or oval nucleus. The nuclei are vesicular, the chromatin is delicate, and there is a small basophilic nucleolus. Large cells, and binucleated or multinucleated cells are occasionally seen and should not lead to the diagnosis of malignancy. The cells usually have an endocrine pattern of vascularity. They occur in cords, fascicles, islands, and nests. The stroma is usually delicate but may be hyalinized and even calcified.

Leydig cells contain varying amounts of lipofuscin pigment and lipid material. The characteristic features of Leydig cells is Reinke's crystal which is cigar-shaped cytoplasmic inclusion of varying size. Unfortunately, it is seen only in about 40% of Leydig cells tumors.

The tumor may consist of large cells, finely and coarsely vacuolated, small hyperchromatic cells, or elongated spindle cells. The tumor is usually encapsulated but it may merge with the surrounding parenchyma.

Many Leydig cell tumors begin as hyperplasia, and at times it is difficult to distinguish between hyperplasia and tumor, especially in patients with the adrenogenital syndrome. Hyperplasia is usually diffuse and not focal, the hyperplastic cells fill and distend prexisting intertubular spaces without destroying or displacing tubules. If there is a distinct mass of Leydig cells without any entrapped seminiferous tubules and if there is compression at the periphery it is probably a tumor. At times the advancing edge of the tumor may have the appearance of hyperplasia with tumor cells in between seminiferous tubules.

About 90% of Leydig cell tumors are benign. Unfortunately, histologically it is often difficult to distinguish between a benign and a malignant tumor. Some tumors that present a uniform cellular population may be malignant as manifested by metastases, while tumors that show variations in size, shape, and staining of cells, double and multinucleated cells suggesting malignancy, may behave as benign. We have found the following criteria of value in differentiating between benign and malignant tumors: invasion of rete, the adnexae or vascular or lymphatic spaces, and/or increased mitotic activity. The most reliable criterion is development of metastases.

It should be emphasized that the diagnosis of malignancy should be made with great restraint. Glandular and acinar structures should be looked for, and a secondary carcinoma should be ruled out before a diagnosis of malignant Leydig cell tumor is made. Metastases are usually late in development (4-5 years) although we have seen it appear within 1 year.

2. Sertoli Cell, Granulosa Cell and Theca Cell Tumors. Sertoli cell, granulosa cell, and theca cell tumors and admixtures may be discussed together because, clinically, it is impossible to distinguish them from each other. Most of them have no endocrine manifestations but about 30% show gynecomastia irrespective of the specific histology.

Grossly, the tumors vary from 1 to 10 cm in diameter. They are usually solitary, lobulated, well-circumcribed, grayish-yellow to yellow, and usually homogeneous. Occasional cysts may be found but hemorrhage and necrosis are rare.

Microscopically, the tumors may consist of Sertoli cells, granulosa cells, or a mixture of these or be incompletely differentiated. The epithelium of Sertoli cell tumors may vary from hexagonal to tall columnar. The nuclei are large, round, or oval with a vesicular chro chromatin distribution and one small distinct basophilic nucleolus. The cytoplasm may be scantor abundant, vacuolated, eosinophilic, or basophilic. Many contain lipid material. Mitoses and giant cells are rare. The cells usually form tubules or rows and columns. In granulosa cell tumors the cells are smaller, more cuboidal, and have a follicular arrangement resembling graafian follicles.

In some cases either alone or in admixture with the other two, the cells are large, and have a ground-glass eosinophilic cytoplasm suggesting Leydig or Lutein cells; however, the cells form distinct tubules or are intermingled with spindle-shaped stromal cells. In group 5 tumors consist of spindle-shaped cells with eosinophilic or vacuolated cytoplasm and an elongated nucleus. The cells usually occur in bands in between Sertoli-lined tubules but rarely may be the sole component. Macrophages and lipid-loaded epithelial cells are not unusual.

It should be emphasized that tubules of Sertoli cells or immature tubules often encountered in cryptorchid testis should not be labeled Sertoli cell adenoma or tumor unless there is distinct capsule.

The majority of tumors of this group are benign; about 10% are malignant. The criteria for malignancy are the same as those for Leydig cells. Most of those that metastasize do so within a year.

## III. TUMORS WITH BOTH GERM CELL AND GONADAL STROMAL ELEMENTS

We have recognized two categories of these - the extremely rare instances in which there are two separate tumors: a germ cell neoplasm, e.g., seminoma, and a gonadal stromal tumor, e.g., Sertoli; and the more frequent but still quite rare instances where the two are intermingled.

Scully has designated this group as gonadoblastomas. The tumors are almost entirely in individuals with dysgenetic gonads and abnormal secondary sex organs.

Grossly, the tumor varies from 1 or 2 to 30 cm but the majority are less than 10 cm in diameter. The color and consistency depend on the relative proportions of germ cell or gonadal stromal elements; if the former predominates, they are grayish; if the latter, yellow or brown. The tumors may be soft and fleshy or hard. Calcific foci are frequent.

Microscopically, the tumor shows actively proliferating neoplastic germ cells - seminoma or embryonal carcinoma intermingled with Sertoli-granulosa, Leydig, or Theca cells. Of the germ cell elements, seminoma is the most frequent and occasionally this may be so prominent as to mask the gonadal stromal elements. It is the germ cell element that usually metastasizes.

## IV. MISCELLANEOUS TUMORS

### A. Carcinoids

This group may be a part of a teratoma or it may be secondary, in which event it should be so designated. If it is neither of these it should be listed in this category.

## V. LYMPHOID AND HEMATOPOIETIC TUMORS

### A. Malignant Lymphoma

Although the tumor may occur at any age, it is most often seen in older age patients. Not infrequently it is bilateral.

Grossly, the testes are usually diffusely enlarged. The cut surfaces are grayish-white, bulging, granular, solid with areas of necrosis and hemorrhage.

Microscopically, the tumors are usually very cellular and the infiltration is in the interstitium. It is often confused with seminoma and embryonal carcinoma. The cytology of the tumor varies greatly depending on the specific type of lymphoma and whether it is mixed or pure. Generally speaking, lymphoma cells are smaller, not as distinctly outlined as seminoma or embryonal carcinoma cells; they have scant cytoplasm, the nuclear chromatin distribution is different. The seminiferous tubules are separated from each other; they may be compressed and eventually infiltrated from outside.

In our experience most of these patients develop evidence of generalized lymphoma within 2 years.

## VI. SECONDARY TUMORS

Metastatic tumors are occasionally encountered in the testis. These are usually autopsy findings but rarely they may be clinical. The most frequent primary sites are lungs and prostate. The tumor is interstitial and there is invariably a considerable amount of vascular invasion.

## VII. TUMORS OF COLLECTING DUCTS, RETE, EPIDIDYMIS, SPERMATIC CORD, CAPSULE, SUPPORTING STRUCTURES AND APPENDICES

### A. Benign

1. The most common of these are adenomatoid tumors. They are usually small but may reach 5 cm or more in diameter. They are hard, well-encapsulated, and usually attached to the tunica. They cut with the consistency of fibrous tissue revealing a grayish-tan or white surfaces.

Microscopically, the tumors consist of epithelial-like cells and fibrous stroma with or without smooth muscle and lymphocytic infiltration. The histology varies a great deal. The epithelial cells are usually arranged in solid strands, cords or interlacing pseudotubular structures or dilated spaces. The cells may be cuboidal, low columnar or flattened and endothelial-like, or they may be vacuolated. The nuclei are round or oval, vesicular or hyperchromatic. The stroma varies from dense collagenized to loose connective tissue. Varying amounts of lymphocytic infiltration are seen and some of the tumors contain smooth muscle fibers.

2. Papillary cystadenoma of epididymis is rare and is usually associated with von Hipple-Lindau's disease.

3. Mesenchymal tumors are rare.

B. Malignant Tumors

1. Carcinoma. This is extremely rare and is usually secondary.

2. Rhabdomyosarcomas are the most frequent tumors of the spermatic cord. They occur most often in the first 3 decades and in all races.

Grossly, the tumor may range from 1 to 2 cm. It is circumscibed but not encapsulated. The cut surface is tan or grayish-white and fibrous.

Microscopically, the tumors may range from undifferentiated mesenchymal through the myxomatous stage to spindle cell, alveolar, or pleomorphic patterns.

Other types of sarcomas may occur but they are all rare.

## CONCLUSION

The question may well be asked as to why we should have a new classification. There would be no need for any effort in this respect if there was a reasonable international agreement on classification of testis tumors. Unfortunately, this situation does not exist, even among English-speaking people. There is a French classification, a Russian classification, a Scandinavian classification, and a British classification plus an American classification. Of these, the American classification is the most commonly used.

In developing an international histologic classification of these tumors the World Health Organization convened a meeting of a number of pathologists who have made major constributions to the pathology of these tumors: Prof. TEILUM (Denmark), Prof. CABANNE (France), Dr. PUGH (U.K.), Prof. HEDINGER (Switzerland), Prof. GANINA (USSR), Prof. RAPAPORT (Argentina), Dr. McMOVERN (Australia), and Dr. MOSTOFI (USA), who served as Chairman. In addition to these, Prof. SEROV (USSR) and Dr. SCULLY (USA) represented the Ovarian Panel; Prof. WILLIAMS (U.K.), the Endocrine Panel. Before the meeting a small panel had formulated recommendations relative to the basis of the classification and the panel modified this as a tentative WHO classifictaion.

In accordance with WHO policy, which requires that these classifications be based on histology of the tumor, the proposed WHO classification is essentially the Scandinavian and American classifications with certain modifications.

An internationally agreed upon histologic classification is absolutely essential, otherwise it is impossible to compare the epidemiologic, survival, and mortality data, or the results of therapy.

REFERENCES


1. Ahluwalia, H.S., Duguid, J.B.: Malignant tumors in Malaya. Brit. J. Cancer 20, 12-15 (1966)
2. Akasaka, H., Imamura, K., Lijima, H., Nakanishi, K., Maruyama, Y., Suga, T., Kondo, I., Kai, Y.: Report on 14 cases of testicular tumors, with special reference to the statistical study on malignant tumors of the testis. Jap. J. Urol. 56, 597-615 (1965)
3. Clarke, B.G.: The relative frequency and age incidence of principal urological diseases. J. Urol (Baltimore) 98, 701-705 (1967)
4. Clemensen, J.A.: Doubling of morbility from testis carcinoma in Copenhagen, 1943-1962. Acta path. microbiol. scand. 72, 348-349 (1968)
5. Davies, J.N., Owor, R.: The diagnosis of primary carcinoma of the liver; an assessment of the reliability of clinical diagnosis in Uganda Africans. E. Afr. med. J. 37, 249-254 (1970)
6. Edington, G.M., MacLean, C.M.: A cancer rate survey in Ibadan, Western Nigeria, 1960-1963. Brit. J. Cancer 19, 470-481 (1965)
7. Evans, R.W.: Developmental stages of embryo-like bodies in teratoma testis. J. clin. Path. 10, 31-39 (1957)
8. Grumet, R.F., MacMahon, B.: Trends in mortality from neoplasms of the testis. Cancer (Philad.) 11, 790-797 (1958)
9. Howden, P.F.: Carcinoma of the testicle. N. Z. med. J. 67, 215-217 (1968)
10. Hutt, M.S., Burkitt, D.: Geographical distribution of cancer in East Africa. A new clinicopathological approach. Brit. med. J. 5464, 719-722 (1965)
11. MacKay, E.N., Sellers, A.H.: A statistical review of malignant testicular tumours based on the experience of the Ontario Cancer Foundation Clinics, 1938-1961. Canad. med. Ass. J. 94, 889 (1966)
12. Maier, J.G., Sulak, M.H., Mittenmeyer, B.T.: Seminoma of the testis: Analysis of treatment success and failure. Amer. J. Roentgenol. 102, 596-602 (1968)
13. Masson, P.: Etude sur le sêminome. Rev. canad. Biol. 5, 361-387 (1946)
14. Mostofi, F.K.: Testicular tumors. Epidemiologic, etiologic, and pathologic features. Cancer (Philad.) 32, 1186-1201 (1973)
15. Mostofi, F.K., Price, E.B.: Tumors of the male genital system. AFIP Fascicle 8 (1973)
16. Mostofi, F.K., Sobin, L.H.: Histological typing of testicular tumors. Wld. Hth. Org. 1977
17. Nefzger, M.D., Mostofi, F.K.: Survival after surgery for germinal malignancies of the testis. II. Effects of surgery and radiation therapy . Cancer (Philad.) 30, 1233-1240 (1972)
18. Pierce, G.B., Dixon, F.J., Jr.: Testicular teratomas. I. Demonstration of teratogenesis by metamorphosis of multipotential cells. Cancer (Philad.) 12, 573-583 (1959)
19. Prates, M.D., Torres, F.O.: A cancer survey in Lourenco Marques, Portuguese East Africa. J. nat. Cancer Inst. 35, 729-757 (1965)
20. Reddy, D.B., Ranganayakamma, I.: Review of 56 cases of testicular tumours. Indian. J. Cancer 3, 255-271 (1966)
21. Stevens, L.C.: Embryonic potency of embryoid bodies derived from a transplantable testicular teratoma of the mouse. Develop. Biol. 2, 285-297 (1960)
22. Teppo, L.: The histopathological classification of testicular tumors and its clinical implications. Duodecim 83, 1261-1274 (1967)
23. Williams, E.H.: A local registry in a mission hospital in Uganda. E. Afr. med. J. 43, 200-207 (1966)

# The Endocrinology of Testicular Tumors

P. C. WALSH

Feminization and precocious pubertal development are manifestations of hormone production by both benign and malignant testicular tumors. The pathophysiologic mechanisms underlying these clinical syndromes vary not only with the cell type of the tumor but also with the age of the host. Recent refinements in the ability to measure both steroidal and polypeptide hormones have provided both a new insight into these mechanisms and also useful parameters for monitoring therapy in these disorders.

## BACKGROUND

The endocrine manifestations of testicular tumors can be produced by one of three mechanisms: (1) direct synthesis of androgens or estrogens by the tumors; (2) synthesis of gonadotropins that stimulate secondary secretion of androgens or estrogens; or (3) alteration of the peripheral metabolism of androgens. Before discussing these mechanisms further, it is important to review briefly some normal physiology. It is well known that the testis is the major site of testosterone secretion in the male and that the synthesis of testosterone by the Leydig cell is under the regulation of luteinizing hormone (LH). Plasma testosterone levels, which are low in childhood, rise during puberty over an extended period of time to reach the normal adult male level. This increase in plasma testosterone correlates well with increasing LH levels during puberty. In adulthood, testosterone production rates are 7 mg/day and plasma levels are approximately 500 ng/100 ml.

In contrast to testosterone, which is secreted mainly by the testes, estrogen in the normal man arises principally from aromatization of plasma androstenedione and testosterone at some peripheral sites (14). The average daily production of estradiol in men is 45 µg/day, of which approximately 15 µg arises from testosterone, 20 µg arises from androstenedione, and 10 µg is directly secreted by the testes. Consequently, it can be concluded that peripheral formation of estradiol from circulating precursors accounts for at least three-fourths of estradiol production and the remainder arises from direct testicular secretion.

Although the testis is a normal site for androgen and estrogen production, it does not normally secrete gonadotropins or other polypeptide hormones. However, all cells of an organism contain genetic material coded with the same information. Presumably much of this information is repressed as differentiation proceeds and special cell functions are derived. However, with the development of neoplasia derepression may occur and result in the elaboration of new polypeptides.

Presumably, the synthesis of a polypeptide chain requires only a single alteration in cellular genetic material. This is the explanation for the production of ectopic gonadotropin by malignant testicular tumors. It is of interest, that in addition to gonadotropin production, many of these tumors perform a number of the same biochemical functions as normal placental tissues. The placenta has many important endocrinologic functions: (1) production of human chorionic gonadotropin (HCG); (2) secretion of human chorionic somatomammotropin (HCS), prolactin-like substance (18); and (3) transformation of dehydroepiandrosterone sulfate (an inactive androgen made by the fetal adrenal) to estradiol (16). The production of these polypeptide hormones by testicular tumors, coupled with their ability to alter the peripheral metabolism of androgens, results in several mechanisms that give rise to the endocrinologic manifestations of these tumors.

Based on this general discussion, we will now turn to the specific mechanism underlying the production of either feminization or precocious puberty by testicular neoplasms.

## STEROID-SECRETING TUMORS

Leydig cell tumors are the most common nongerminal tumors of the testis in both adults and children. Although in all prepubertal patients isosexual precocity is the primary clinical presenting symptom, in the majority of adults these tumors are usually without clinical manifestation. However, approximately 20-25% of adult patients do develop gynecomastia (6). These tumors are always benign in prepubertal children but approximately 10% of adult patients with Leydig cell tumors develop metastases.

It has been well demonstrated that Leydig cell tumors produce androgens and this provided a ready explanation for the development of isosexual precocity in prepubertal patients. Likewise, in adults who are full-masculinized, it is understandable why only a small proportion of patients develop symptoms. In the adult patients who develop gynecomastia, there is recent excellent documentation of increased estradiol production. Three independent studies have demonstrated high spermatic venous estradiol levels from the side of the tumor and in one patient estradiol levels were elevated 35 times that in the nontumorous side (6, 10, 13).

Sertoli cell tumors are extremely rare testicular neoplasms that are histopathologically distinct from Leydig cell tumors. However, their biochemical and biological characteristics are similar to the findings in feminizing intersital cell tumors and gynecomastia occurs in approximately 30% of patients (15). Because these tumors are rare, there is little information about their endocrinology. Available hormonal studies have reported increased gonadotropins, estrogens, androgens, and normal levels in individual cases. However, from studies performed in dogs, a species in which nongerminal tumors are quite common, these tumors appear to have all of the enzymatic capabilities of normal Leydig cells (12).

## GONADOTROPIN-SECRETING TUMORS

It is well known that choriocarcinoma of the testis, as well as some malignant testicular teratomas, secrete chorionic gonadotropin. Until recently, the laboratory determination of chorionic gonadotropin depended upon relatively intensitive urinary tests or upon a radioimmunoassay for pituitary luteinizing hormone (LH) which nonspecifically cross-reacts with HCG. However, recently a sensitive specific radioimmunoassay for HCG has been developed which makes it possible to identify specifically tumor gonadotropin.

Four polypeptide hormones (LH, FSH, TSH, and HCG) are composed of two polypeptide chains, designated α or β. Within the same species, although the α subunits of these hormones are identical in all respects, the β subunits have distinct immunologic differences and confer biological specificity to the hormone. Because the β subunits of LH and HCG differ in only 26-29 terminal amino acids, radioimmunoassays for LH consistently cross-react with HCG. However, with the recent elucidation of gonadotropin structure it has become possible to separate the α and β subunits of HCG and to develop an assay specific for HCG-β that does not cross-react with LH (1).

With the development of this specific assay, it is now recognized that many tumors are capable of producing HCG in minute amounts. Using the older assay methods, it was estimated that only 7-13% of seminomas and 11-30% of embryonal carcinomas produced chorionic gonadotropin (4, 7). However, these studies generally utilized urinary pregnancy tests that are only designed to respond to more than 500-1000 IU of chorionic gonadotropin per liter of urine. Because the excretion of LH in normal men usually ranges between 1 and 20 IU per 24 h, it can be seen that a great range of abnormal gonadotropin could exist and not be detected by the standard pregnancy tests. Recently, utilizing the specific HCG-β assay, BRAUNSTEIN et al. (1) have reported that 37.5% of seminomas and 56% of embryonal carcinomas produce gonadotropin. Not only is this assay sensitive, it is also specific. Because HCG-β is never produced in normal men its presence in the serum is an absolute marker of tumor activity. Consequently, one can assume with certainty that the presence of chorionic gonadotropin in the blood of a man implies the presence of an associated neoplasm.

Utilizing this assay to study a group of 53 patients with malignant testicular tumors, COCHRAN et al. (3) have made some interesting observations. They found that 11 of 15 men with detectable HCG-β in the serum had negative urinary tests for gonadotropin; thus reliance on a urinary screening test to detect chorionic gonadotropin would have given a false negative result in 80% of patients with a positive serum level. Second, they found that after unilateral orchiectomy elevations of serum LH werecommon, presumably due to a compensatory response at the hypothalamic pituitary axis to correct for the loss of Leydig cells. Consequently, if serum LH were used as the sole index of HCG production, half of the patients following orchiectomy would have a false positive elevation. However, only those patients with residual tumor have elevated HCG-β levels. Third, although elevated FSH levels were frequently present following unilateral orchiectomy, serum FSH levels were suppressed in those patients with elevated levels of HCG-β. This suppression of serum FSH correlated well with elevated levels of plasma estradiol. Finally, in all patients in this study, there was an excellent correlation between HCG-β levels and response to therapy, suggesting that this test should be useful in selecting patients for adjunctive irradiation or chemotherapy and in assessing the results of such treatment. However, some other investigators utilizing assays for alpha fetoprotein, placental alkaline phosphatase, and human placental lactogen (HPL) have occasionally found tumors producing more than one of these markers. Previous work indicates that these proteins are not produced under coordinate control and that in tumors producing more than one markers a fall in the level of one polypeptide may not necessarily reflect the overall tumor activity (2). Consequently, in evaluating the response to therapy in patients with testicular malignancies, one should use many tumor markers as possible.

## MECHANISMS RESPONSIBLE FOR THE DEVELOPMENT OF GYNECOMASTIA

Although it is well known that gynecomastia develops in patients with benign and malignant testicular tumors, the mechanism by which this occurs was not well understood until recently. However, several studies have provided insight into the etiology of gynecomastia and have helped to explain the breast enlargement that occurs in men with testicular tumors.

The breast is a target organ for this action of both androgen and estrogen. In normal men, the breast fails to enlarge because there is a quantitative predominance of androgen production over estrogen secretion. However, when the normal ratio of androgen to estrogen is altered, gynecomastia occurs. In an extensive study of patients with a wide variety of conditions that produced gynecomastia, SIITERI and MACDONALD (14) found that the one common hormonal denominator was a decreased ratio of testosterone to estrogen production. Consequently, gynecomastia may occur in men with either deficient androgen production or excessive estrogen secretion. In men with malignant testicular neoplasms, either one of these two mechanisms may be operative.

Excessive estrogen production occurs in patients with gonadotropin-producing neoplasms, most commonly choriocarcinoma and also less commonly in patients with embryonal carcinoma, teratocarcinoma, and seminoma. The cause of increased estrogen production in these patients may be twofold. When the testis is stimulated by excessive amounts of chorionic gonadotropin (HCG), more estrogen than androgen is produced (17). Consequently, endogenous HCG production by malignant testicular tumors stimulates the contralateral testis to produce increased amounts of estrogen. Paradoxically, for reasons that are not entirely clear, androgen production is not increased to a similar degree (8). Because several studies have demonstrated synergism between FSH and LH, suppressed FSH levels in patients with circulating HCG-$\beta$ may be one explanation for the relative insensitivity of the Leydig cell to chorionic gonadotropin. The summation of these events leads to a decrease in the androgen/estrogen ratio, producing gynecomastia.

In addition, KIRSCHNER _et al_. (9) have demonstrated that trophoblastic tumors may synthesize and secrete estradiol. They have demonstrated that choriocarcinomas of the testes have the ability to convert dehydroepiandrosterone sulfate to estradiol and they have suggested that estradiol synthesis by these tumors may be the cause of gynecomastia. Thus it is clear that patients with gonadotropin-secreting tumors have excessive estrogen production that leads to the development of gynecomastia. It is unclear whether the major source of this estrogen is from stimulation of the contralateral testis or direct secretion of estradiol by the tumor via altered androgen metabolism. Although certain malignant tumors produce chorionic somatomammotropin, it is not clear whether HCS causes gynecomastia. In the reported cases where gynecomastia has occurred in the presence of high circulating levels of HCS, elevated levels of HCG were also present (5, 11, 18).

In some patients with malignant testicular tumors, the cause of gynecomastia is decreased androgen secretion. Following unilateral orchiectomy, gynecomastia occasionally occurs. In these cases the gynecomastia may again be explained on a dual basis. With removal of one nomal testis, there is a fall in androgen secretion to which the hypothalamic-pituitary axis responds by increased LH secretion. The androgen deficiency produced by unilateral orchiectomy coupled with increased gonadotropin stimulation of the contralateral testis again alters the normal androgen/estrogen ratio and leads to gynecomastia.

On a practical level all patients with malignant testicular tumors who have gynecomastia should be evaluated for the presence of HCG-β. The measurement of this hormone in the serum is helpful not only in explaining the gynecomastia but also in providing a biochemical marker that may prove useful in detecting subclinical residual disease and directing adjunctive therapy. In the patient in whom gynecomastia develops following orchiectomy, if the serum level of HCG-β is undetectable, it is most likely that the gynecomastia is due to deficient androgen production and is not the result of estrogen secretion from trophoblastic tissue.

The endocrinology of testicular tumors is a fascinating subject and the recent development of sensitive specific radioimmunoassays for the measurement of tumor markers has opened a new area of investigation into the biology of the neoplasms.

## SUMMARY

The endocrine manifestations of testicular tumors can be produced by one of three mechanisms: (1) direct synthesis of androgens or estrogens by the tumors; (2) synthesis of gonadotropins that stimulate secondary secretion of androgens or estrogens; (3) alteration of the peripheral metabolism of androgens. In this manuscript we have discussed these mechanisms in relationship to steroid-secreting tumors and gonadotropin-secreting tumors. In postpubertal males, the most common manifestation of these tumors is the production of gynecomastia. Because the breast is a target organ for the action of both androgens and estrogens, gynecomastia occurs when there is an alteration in the normal androgen/ estrogen ratio. Consequently, gynecomastia may be produced by either deficient androgen production or excessive estrogen secretion. The endocrinology of testicular tumors is a fascinating subject and recent development of sensitive specific radioimmunoassays for the measurement of tumor markers has opened a new area of investigation into the biology of these neoplasms.

## REFERENCES

1. Braunstein, G.D. et al.: Ectopic production of human chorionic gonadotropin by neoplamss. Ann. intern. Med. 78, 39-45 (1973)
2. Braunstein, G.D. et al.: Discordance of human chorionic gonadotropin and alpha-fetoprotein in testicular teratocarcinomas. Cancer (Philad.) 31, 1065-1068 (1973)
3. Cochran, J. et al.: The endocrinology of human chorionic gonadotropin-secreting testicular tumors: New methods in diagnosis. J. Urol. (Baltimore) (In Press)
4. Dixon, F.J., Moore, R.A.: Tumors of the male sex organs. In: Atlas of Tumor Pathology; Dixon, F.J., Moore, R.A. (eds.). Washington, D.C.: Armed Forces Inst. Path., 1952, Sect. VIII, Fasc. 32

5. Frantz, A.G. et al.: Human placental lactogen in choriocarcinoma of the male. Measurement by radioimmunoassay. J. clin. Endocr. 25, 1136-1139 (1965)
6. Gabrilove, J.L. et al.: Feminizing interstitial cell tumor of the testis: Personal observations and a review of the literature. Cancer (Philad.) 35, 1184-1202 (1975)
7. Hobson, B.M.: The excretion of chorionic gonadotropin by men with testicular tumors. Acta endocr. (Kbh.) 49, 337-348 (1965)
8. Kirschner, M.A. et al.: Leydig cell function in men with gonadotropin-producing testicular tumors. J. clin. Endocr. 30, 504-511 (1970)
9. Kirschner, M.A. et al.: Estrogen production and its origin in men with gonadotropin-producing neoplasms. J. clin. Endocr. 39, 112-118 (1974)
10. Kliman, B. et al.: Estradiol secreting Leydig cell tumor. Proc. 55th Ann. Meet. Endocrine Soc. 1973
11. Payne, R.A., Ryan, R.J.: Human placental lactogen in the male subject. J. Urol. (Baltimore) 99-103 (1972)
12. Pierrepoint, C.G.: The metabolism in vitro of dehydroepiandrosterone and dehydroepiandrosterone sulfate by Sertoli cell tumors of the testis of two dogs with clinical signs of hyperestrogenism. J. Endocr. 42, 99-107 (1968)
13. Selvaggi, F.P. et al.: Interstitial cell tumor of the testis in adults - Two case reports. J. Urol. (Baltimore) 109, 436 (1973)
14. Siiteli, P.K., MacDonald, P.C.: Role of extraglandular estrogen in human endocrinology. In: Handbook of Physiology. 7. Endocrinology Vol. II. Greep, R.O., Astwood, E.B. (eds.). Washington, D.C.: Amer. physiol. Soc. 1973, pp. 615-629
15. Talerman, A.: Malignant Sertoli cell tumor of the testis. Cancer (Philad.) 28, 446-455 (1971)
16. Villee, D.B.: Development of endocrine function in the human placenta and fetus. Med. Progr. 281, 473-541 (1969)
17. Weinstein, R.L. et al.: Secretion of unconjugated androgens and estrogens by the normal and abnormal human testis before and after human chorionic gonadotropin. J. clin. Invest. 53, 1-6 (1974)
18. Weintraub, B.D., Rosen, S.W.: Ectopic production of human chorionic somatomammotropin by nontrophoblastic cancers. J. clin. Endocr. 32, 94-101 (1971)

# Testicular Cancer, Histologic Classification and Staging, Topography of Lymph Node Metastases

P. HERMANEK

From the clinical point of view, histologic classification and staging of tumors have two functions. They are intended to give suggestions for therapy and to provide the basis for an assessment of the end results. Every comparison of different methods of treatment is only meaningful so long as the prognostically different subgroups are known.

## HISTOLOGIC CLASSIFICATION AND PLANNING OF TREATMENT

In adults, the decisive question is: Does a tumor consist exclusively of seminoma structures or not? It is important to include among the non-seminomas all germinal tumors which do not consist of seminoma structures only. The question of dissection of retroperitoneal lymph nodes arises exclusively with non-seminomas, the dosage of abdominal radiotherapy differs for seminoma and non-seminoma, at least in the clinical stage I.

In the literature we see considerable differences in the frequency of seminomas among the germinal tumors of the testis. In the publications which have appeared since 1964 with more than 200 observations, we find values of 35-72% for seminomas. More seminomas are usually found in Europe. In our series of patients in Erlangen from 1969 to August 31, 1975, we observed 35% pure seminomas among 68 germinal tumors of the testicle.

In statistics such as these, only patients with a primary diagnosis may be included. If those patients who had been subjected to orchiectomy elsewhere and then transferred to a specialized clinic for further therapy are also included, the picture is blurred by selection.

The younger the patients the fewer seminomas are found in the series. But the different age distribution cannot of itself explain the difference in incidence of seminoma.

Geographical differences possibly play a role. In our opinion, the subtetly of the histologic examination is decisive. The more closely the pathologist investigates, the fewer seminomas he finds. It is important to embed as much of the tumor as possible. This is not only a theoretical consideration but it is also of considerable clinical significance. It has been claimed that patients with seminomas had similar survival rates in all series (2, 15). Figure 1 shows the end results in seminoma of all clinical stages published by various authors. At the same time, the reported frequency of seminoma can be seen in each case. The more seminomas an author has among his testicular tumors, the worse the results of seminoma therapy. The cause for this lies in

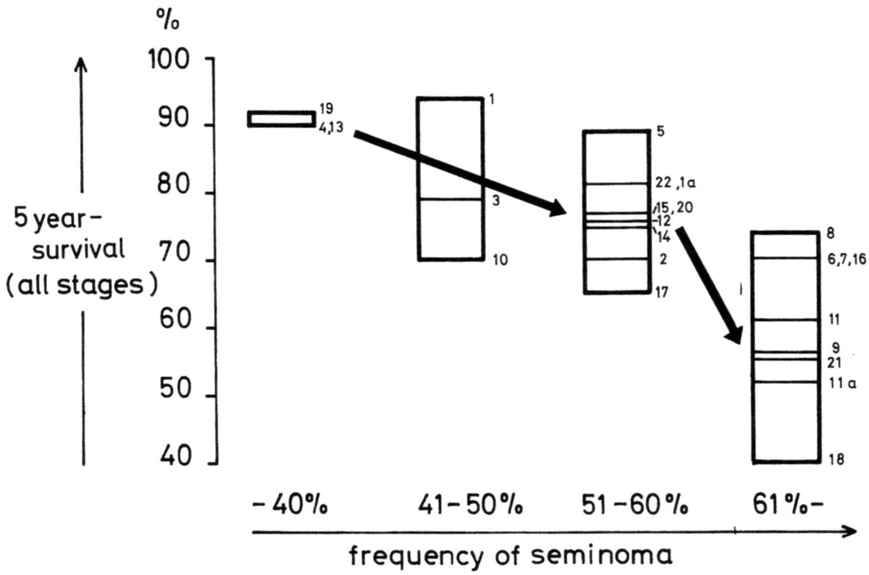


*Fig. 1. Seminoma. 5-year survival (all stages). Frequency of seminoma. 1, BATTERMANN (1); 1a, CADE (3); 2, CHAPMAN et al. (4); 3, COLLINS & PUGH (6); 4, DYKHUIZEN et al. (8); 5, EKMAN et al. (9); 6, FRANKE et al. (10); 7, HALAMA (12); 8, HINTZEN et al. (14); 9, KLAUA (16); 10, KUROHARA et al. (17); 11, KUTTIG & SURANIC (18); 11a, LUDVIK & JENTSCH (19); 12, MACKAY & SELLERS (20); 13, MAIER & SULAK (21); 14, MEIENBERG (23); 15, MILLER & SELJELID (24); 16, REINHARD (29); 17, ROBSON et al. (30); 18, RÖHL & HOCHBERG (31); 19, SAXENA (32); 20, SCHMIEDT & STAEHLER (33); 21, SHEPHERD (34); 22, SMITHERS (37)*

the fact that a proportion of non-seminomas is present among these so-called seminomas for which and "undertreatment" was proposed. The non-seminomas were falsely classified as seminomas, the irradiation was carried out with too small a dose, and abdominal dissection was not performed.

Other therapeutic decisions which depend on histologic classification are of less significance and principally involve the choice of chemotherapeutic agent. The files on this subject are by no means closed. SMITHERS (37) made the indication for mediastinal and supraclavicular irradiation in clinical stage I dependent on histology (only for embryonal carcinoma, not for teratocarcinoma).

For germinal tumors of the testicle in children, the decisive question is: Is this a pure teratoma? In this case - in contrast to adults - orchidectomy alone is sufficient therapy, and further treatment measures are unnecessary.

## CONTINUOUS SPREAD OF TUMORS

From the orchiectomy specimen, the pathologist must not only classify the tumor but also investigate the continuous progression of the tumor. In particular, he must establish:

1. Does the tumor invade the rete testis or epididymis?
2. Does the tumor invade the scrotal wall?

This is of practical significance. Because if the borders of the testis are exceeded, the tumor gains access to other areas of lymph drainage. Accordingly, the surgical or radiation therapy must be extended to the iliac and inguinal lymph regions.

## HISTOLOGIC CLASSIFICATION AND PROGNOSIS

The histologic classification of testicular cancer has a second task in giving information on the prognosis.

For seminoma, subdivision into typical, anaplastic, and spermatocytic seminoma is uncontested (22, 25). The anaplastic seminoma has a considerably worse prognosis; its tendency to metastasize is outstanding.

The non-seminoma raises problems. MOSTOFI's classification (25) is based on that of FRIEDMAN and MOORE (11). Besides this, the British classification by COLLINS and PUGH (6) is still very widespread in Europe. But nowadays the original version of 1964 is not usually used, but rather the modified version by PUGH (27) and MEIENBERG (23) (Table 1). The intermediate malignant teratoma type B and the anaplastic malignant teratoma are combined as malignant teratoma, undifferentiated. The tumors with teratomatous and seminomatous components are no longer listed as a separate group of combined tumors, but classified according to the appropriate teratoma. In our opinion, it is no longer of immediate interest to discuss the advantages and disadvantages of the American and British histologic classifications. The fact is that WHO has, in principle, adopted the American classification.

This WHO classification will therefore have to be used generally in the future so as to be internationally comprehensible, and in order to be able to make comparisons.

The principle of MOSTOFI's classification is to list all the components of tumors with different structures. Consequently we arrive at 14 subtypes of non-seminomas and 26 subtypes if infantile embryonal carcinomas are listed separately. This grouping is too complicated for clinical use. Therefore the old group classification of DIXON and MOORE (7) (Table 2) has a well-founded justification. It subdivides the many possible types of non-seminoma into four groups, each with a different

Table 1. British classification of non-seminomatous germ cell tumors

| Original classification[a] | Modified classification[b] |
|---|---|
| T., differentiated | Same |
| m.T., intermediate, type A | m.T., intermediate |
| m.T., intermediate, type B<br>m.T., anaplastic | m.T. undifferentiated |
| m.T., trophoblastic | Same |
| Cobined tumors | Classified according to teratomatous component |

[a] COLLINS and PUGH (6).
[b] PUGH (27); MEIENBERG (23).

Table 2. Prognostic classification of non-seminomatous germ cell tumors

| Prognostic groups[a] | 17-year survival[b] |
|---|---|
| III teratoma ± seminoma | 64% |
| IV teratocarcinoma (= teratoma + embryonal carcinoma) ± seminoma ± choriocarcinoma | 41% |
| II embryonal carcinoma ± seminoma | 28% |
| V choriocarcinoma ± embryonal carcinoma ± seminoma | 0% |

[a] According to DIXON and MOORE (7).
[b] NEFZGER and MOSTOFI (26).

prognosis. Consequently it is also of practical use for the statistical evaluation of therapy. Comparisons with older reports in the literature are also possible. The descriptive WHO classification can at any time be arranged in these DIXON and MOORE groups. Therefore our findings always include the MOSTOFI's classification and the group classification of DIXON and MOORE. For the time being, we still also use the modified British classification.

## STAGING OF THE GERMINAL TUMORS OF THE TESTIS

The UICC has not recommended any stages so far. The recently issued TNM and P classification (3) is valid for the trial period 1975-1979. It would be premature to discuss this today.

In the literature, there are various stage classifications of germinal tumors of the testicle. The simplest and most reliable clinical stage classification is shown in Figure 2. It is now decisive whether this clinical stage classification was undertaken on the basis of a lymphography or not. Table 3 shows how the number of cases of clinical stage I falls substantially after lymphography. Statements on clinical stages are therefore only informative when it is also stated whether a lymphography has been performed or not.

Table 3. Clinical staging without and with lymphography

| | VAHLENSIECK and WEISSBACH (39) | Erlangen 1969-Aug. 31, 1975 |
|---|---|---|
| No. of cases | 110 | 72 |
| Without lymphography | | |
| Stage I | 98 (89%) | 65 (90%) |
| Stage II | 2 ( 2%) | 5 ( 7%) |
| Stage III | 10 ( 9%) | 2 ( 3%) |
| With lymphography | | |
| Stage I | 53 (48%) | 45 (63%) |
| Stage II | 47 (43%) | 25 (35%) |
| Stage III | 10 ( 9%) | 2 ( 3%) |

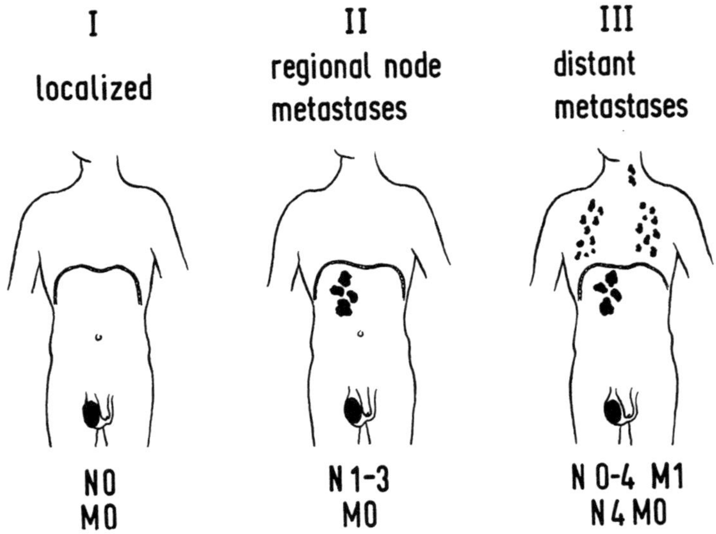


*Fig. 2. Clinical stages of testicular cancer (42). TNM classification (38)*

Even with lymphography, the determination of the clinical stage is not free from error (Table 4). Both false positive and false negative lymphographic findings occur.

Table 4. Lymphography. Frequency of false results

| | Literature | Erlangen 1969-Aug. 31, 1975 |
|---|---|---|
| False positive / All positive | 34/296 = 11.5% | 4/18 = 22% |
| False negative / All negative | 63/253 = 24.9% | 7/25 = 28% |

In addition to the clinical stage, a pathologic stage can also be established if a dissection is carried out. It may be seen from Table 5 how the histologic examination modifies the stage classification. It can be seen that for non-seminomas about 25-30% of patients with clinical and lymphographic stage I actually show regional lymph node metastases. In the clinical stage I without lymphography, this applies to about 50% of the patients.

## CRITERIA FOR THE COMPARISON OF TREATMENT RESULTS

One of the principal points of discussion in the treatment of non-seminomatous tumors of the testicle in stages I and II is: lymph node dissection or radiation? In the assessment of retrospective studies - and we have been mainly dependent on these up to the present time - four points must always be taken into consideration:

Table 5. Clinical and pathologic staging. Non-seminomas

| | Frequency of histologically demonstrable regional node metastases | |
|---|---|---|
| | WHITMORE (41) | Erlangen 1969-Aug. 31, 1975 |
| Clinical stage I | | |
| No lymphography | ∿50% | 45% |
| With lymphography | ∿25% | 33% |

1. A subdivision into clinical stages I and II is only logical if the determination of the clinical stage was carried out uniformly. In all the patients to be compared, the lymphography must either be taken into consideration or not; otherwise one can only group both stages together. A subdivision of the results according to the pathologic stages is actually interesting, but of no significance for a comparison between surgical therapy and radiation. It is not fair and not admissible to compare irradiated patients in clinical stage I with surgically treated patients of pathologic stage I.

2. In a comparison between lymph surgery and radiation therapy, the cases treated by surgery must include those patients in whom laparotomy indicated local inoperability. It is incorrect to compare all radiotherapeutically treated patients with the surgical patients in whom a dissection was carried out according to plan. Rather the surgical patients should include also those patients for whom a dissection was planned but not at all or not radically carried out after opening the peritoneal cavity because of the extent of the metastases.

3. In the course of time the techniques of lymphatic surgery and also, and especially, the methods of radiotherapy have considerably changed in all centers. Results with orthovoltage therapy cannot be identified with those of high voltage therapy. Consequently, collected statistics from large centers which include periods from about 1940 to 1970 have little information value with regard to the methods of treatment to be used today. In forming a judgment, only such statistics can be included in which high voltage therapy was applied exclusively and in which approximately equal lymphatic surgery procedures were used.

4. In the comparison of differently treated groups of patients a comparable histologic classification must finally be made.

## TOPOGRAPHY OF LYMPHATIC METASTASES OF TESTICULAR TUMORS

For years we have prospectively examined the dissection specimen topographically. An essential condition for this was the operative procedure of the Urological Clinic in Erlangen, which consists of an en bloc dissection from above caudally. Thus the pathologist receives a principal specimen (Fig. 3) which extends from the level of the origin of the superior mesenteric artery to the bifurcation of the aorta and on the side of the tumor still further caudally and including the testicular vein from the side of the tumor as far as the internal inguinal ring. Topographic orientation markings are provided by the

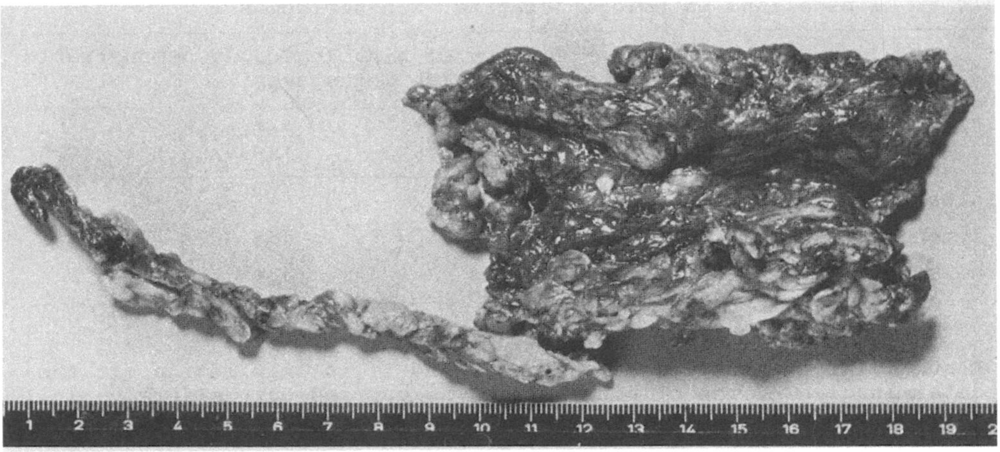


*Fig. 3. En bloc dissection of retroperitoneal lymph nodes. Surgical specimen*

surgeon. In addition, there are various marginal samples and random samples from other accurately defined areas. After cutting narrow laminae from the specimen, every lymph node and every suspicious formation is embedded and histologically examined in stepwise sections. Since 1973, our dissection preparations contain an average of 34 lymph nodes and 67 as a maximum.

From our results, a few points of clinical importance can be raised. (With reference to cases where the tumors have invaded the epididymis or the scrotum and after scrotal or inguinal preoperation, see (35)).

1. The normal primary site for lymphatic metastases of testicular cancer is the testicular lymph center, as CHIAPPA et al. (5) have described.

2. Metastases may occasionally occur in the lymph nodes along the testicular vein (Fig. 4). We saw this is 4 of 53 dissections (8%). It is important to note that, owing to metastases along the testicular vein, lymph drainage to the testicular lymph center may become blocked, and then spreading to the more deeply situated lumbar lymph nodes is possible if the testicular lymph center is negative for metastases.

3. The great majority of testicular tumors metastasize regularly, i.e., primarily into the testicular lymph center and/or along the testicular vein, and only secondarily in other lymph nodes. We saw this in 32 of 34 patients with retroperitoneal metastatic spread.

4. In one of our patients with a right-sided tumor, there was a variation in the position of the testicular lymph center. On the right side, paracaval and precaval, only two very small lymph nodes were found at the level of the bifurcation of the aorta. The right-sided testicular lymph center lay between the aorta and the vena cava at the level of the junction of the testicular vein.

5. In one patient there was an irregular, atypical metastazation in contralateral lymph nodes with a testicular lymph center negative for metastases, without there being a satisfactory explanation for it.

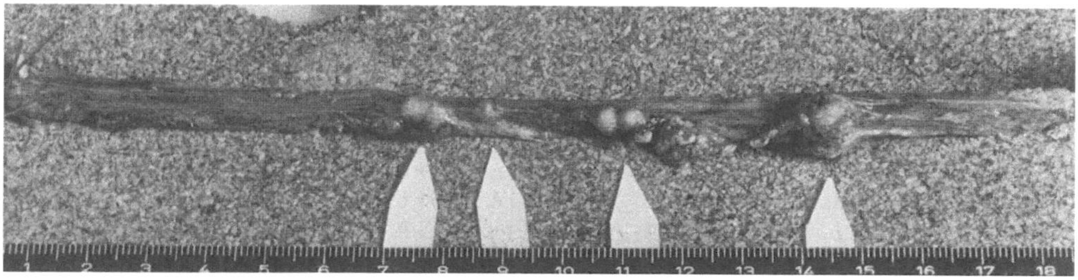

*Fig. 4. Lymph node metastases along the v. testicularis*

Accurate information on the topography of lymphatic spread is particularly important for the detailed procedure of abdominal node dissection. Our topographic investigations still suffer from the relatively small numbers (60 laparotomies, 53 dissections, and 7 exploratory laparotomies). But it may still be stated that where the testicular lymph center is negative for metastases and there are no metastases along the testicular vein, retroperitoneal node metastases occur exceptionally, provided that the tumor has not exceeded the border of the organ and no previous scrotal or inguinal operation has been performed. In retrospective investigations and with a somewhat different nomenclature, RAY et al. (28) at the Memorial Cancer Hospital came to essentially similar conclusions. This provides a foundation for the increasing tendency to modified bilateral dissection (13, 28, 36, 40, 41).

## SUMMARY

From the clinical point of view, histologic classification is intended to give suggestions for therapy (therapeutic classification) and to provide the basis for an assessment of end results (prognostic classification). In adults, the essential therapeutic question is: seminoma (only seminoma) or non-seminoma? The frequency of seminoma among the germinal testicular tumors is influenced by the subtlety of the histologic examination. The histologic report should include the MOSTOFI (25) classification and the prognostic group classification of DIXON and MOORE (7). Staging of testicular cancer and criteria for the comparison of treatment results are discussed. The topography of lymphatic metastases of testicular cancer was investigated. The great majority of testicular cancers metastasize regularly, i.e., primarily into the testicular lymph center and/or along the testicular vein, and only secondarily in other lymph nodes. This provides a foundation for the increasing tendency to modified bilateral retroperitoneal node dissection.

## REFERENCES

1. Battermann, J.J.: Supervoltage radiotherapy for patients with testicular tumors. Presented at International College of Surgeons. IXth European Federation Congress, Amsterdam 1975
2. Blandy, J.P., Hope-Stone, H.F., Dayan, A.D.: Tumors of the Testicle. London: William Heinemann Med. Books, 1970

3. Cade, I.: The clinical picture and management of testicular tumors. Clin. Radiol. 24, 385-391 (1973)
4. Chapman, R.H., Blandy, J.P., Hope-Stone, H.F., Pollock, D., Dayan, A.D.: Identification of favorable group of teratomas. Proc. roy. Soc. Med. 66, 1045-1047 (1973)
5. Chiappa, S., Uslenghi, C., Bonadonna, G., Marano, P., Ravasi, G.: Combined testicular and foot lymphangiography in testicular carcinomas. Surg. Gynec. Obstet. 123, 10-14 (1966)
6. Collins, D.H., Pugh, R.C.B., (Ed.): The pathology of testicular tumours. Brit. J. Urol. 36, Suppl. (1964)
7. Dixon, F.J., Moore, R.A.: Tumors of the male sex organs. In: Atlas of Tumor Pathology. Washington, D.C.: Armed Forces Inst. of Path. 1952, Fasc. 31b and 32
8. Dykhuizen, R.F., George, F.W., Kurohara, S., Rotner, M., Sargent, Ch. R., Varney, I.K.: The use of cobalt-60 telecurietherapy or X-ray therapy with and without lymphadenectomy in the treatment of testis germinal tumors; a 20-year comparative study. J. Urol. (Baltimore) 100, 321-328 (1968)
9. Ekman, H., Fritjofsson, A., Johansson, J.: Treatment of testicular tumours. Urol. int. (Basel) 20, 129-142 (1965)
10. Franke, H.D., Hilweg, D., Kürschner, H.D., Prévôt, H., Jr., Scherer, K.: Strahlentherapie maligner germinaler Hodentumoren. Urologe 10, 281-288 (1970)
11. Friedman, N.B., Moore, R.A.: Tumors of the testis. A report on 922 cases. Milit. Surg. 99, 573-593 (1946)
12. Halama, J.: Die Behandlung der Hodentumoren unter besonderer Berücksichtigung der generalisierten Stadien. Dtsch. med. Wschr. 95, 1002-1006 (1970)
13. Hermanek, P., Schmidt, Th.: The importance of intraoperative histological examinations in the surgical treatment of testicular cancer. In: Abstracts Intern. Acad. Path., 9th Internat. Congr., Helsinki, 1972, p. 47
14. Hintzen, C., Ewald, H.J., Engelking, R., Hoeffken, W.: Die Bedeutung der Lymphographie für die Behandlung der Hodentumoren. Chirurg 42, 321-326 (1971)
15. Hope-Stone, H.F., Blandy, J.P., Dayan, A.D.: Treatment of tumours of the testis. Brit. med. J. 1, 984-989 (1963)
16. Klaua, M.: Beitrag zur Klinik, Therapie und Prognose germinaler Hodentumoren. Dtsch. Gesundheitswesen 27, 1051-1055 (1972)
17. Kurohara, S.S., Webster, J.H., Badib, A., Boctor, Z., Woodruff, M. W.: The clinical features of the common testicular tumors. J. Urol. (Baltimore) 101, 587-592 (1969)
18. Kuttig, H., Sunaric, D.: Klinische Erfahrungen und Ergebnisse nach Telekobalttherapie maligner Hodentumoren. Strahlentherapie 127, 323-335 (1965)
19. Ludvik, W., Jentzsch, K.: Maligne Hodentumoren. In: Krebsbehandlung als interdisziplinäre Aufgabe. Kärcher, K.H. (ed.). Berlin-Heidelberg-New York: Springer-Verlag, 1975
20. MacKay, E.N., Sellers, A.H.: A statistical review of malignant testicular tumours based on the experience of the Ontario cancer foundation clinics, 1938-1961. Canad. med. Ass. J. 94, 889-899 (1966)
21. Maier, J.G., Sulak, M.H.: Radiation therapy in malignant testis tumors. Cancer (Philad.) 32, 1212-1226 (1973)
22. Maier, J.G., Sulak, M.H., Mittemeyer, B.T.: Seminoma of the testis: Analysis of treatment success and failure. Amer. J. Roentgenol. 102, 596-602 (1968)
23. Meienberg, O.: Zur Frage der Klassifizierung von Hodentumoren. Virchows Arch. path. Anat. 353, 10-26 (1971)
24. Miller, A., Seljelid, R.: Histopathologic classification and natural history of malignant testis tumors in Norway, 1959-63. Cancer (Philad.) 28, 1054-1062 (1971)

25. Mostofi, F.K.: Tumors of the testis, In: Mostofi, F.K., Price, E. B., Jr.: Tumors of the male genital system. In: Atlas of Tumor Pathology. Washington, D.C.: Armed Forces Inst. Path., 1973, 2nd. Series, Fasc. 8
26. Nefzger, M.D., Mostofi, F.K.: Survival after surgery for germinal malignancies of the testis. I. Rates of survival in tumor groups. Cancer (Philad.) 30, 1225-1232 (1972)
27. Pugh, R.C.B.: Personal communication cited by Meienberg (1971)
28. Ray, B., Hajdu, St.I., Whitmore, W.F., Jr.: Distribution of retroperitoneal lymph node metastases in testicular germinal tumors. Cancer (Philad.) 33, 340-348 (1974)
29. Reinhard, B.: Strahlentherapie bösartiger Hodentumoren: 5 Jahres-Ergebnisse. Strahlentherapie 144, 533-540 (1972)
30. Robson, Ch.C., Bruce, A.W., Charbonneau, J.: Testicular tumors: a collective review from the Canadian Academy of Urological Surgeons. J. Urol. (Baltimore) 94, 440-444 (1965)
31. Röhl, L., Hochberg, K.: Beitrag zur Klinik und Therapie der Hodentumoren. Urologe 7, 311-315 (1968)
32. Saxena, V.S.: Seminoma of the testis. Amer. J. Roentgenol. 117, 643-652 (1973)
33. Schmiedt, E., Staehler, G.: Die operative Behandlung der Hodentumoren. Röntgenbericht 2, 146-155 (1973)
34. Sheperd, R.T.H.: Germ cell tumours of the testis. Clin. Radiol. 17, 280-288 (1966)
35. Sigel, A.: Scrotal surgery of testis tumors - A fatal error? Chapter 21, this volume
36. Sigel, A., Hermanek, P., Chlepas, S.: Lymphchirurgie des Hodentumors. Chirurg 44, 494-501 (1973)
37. Smithers, D.: The treatment of patients with seminomas and teratomas of the testis. J. roy. Coll. Surg. Edinb. 17, 133-147 (1972)
38. UICC: TNM classification of malignant tumours, 2nd ed. Geneva: UICC 1974
39. Vahlensieck, W., Weissbach, L.: Hodentumoren. Wissenschaftl. Informationen Fresenius-Stiftung 7, 97-147 (1974)
40. Walsh, P.C., Kaufman, J.J., Coulson, W.F., Goodwin, W.E.: Retroperitoneal lymphadectomy for testicular tumors. J. Amer. med. Ass. 217, 309-312 (1971)
41. Whitmore, W.E., Jr.: Germinal tumors of the testis. In: Proc. 6th Nat. Cancer Conf. Philadelphia: J.B. Lippincott, 1968
42. Whittle, R.J.M.: Tumours of the testicle. Brit. J. Radiol. 30, 7-12 (1957)

# Scrotal Operation or Biopsy of Testicular Tumors – A Fatal Mistake?

A. SIGEL and F. KRIEGER

The operative treatment of testicular tumors fails for two reasons. The chief reason is that for many physicians the existence and the deadly significance of this disease is too little known. For this reason, the interval between the first medical consultation and surgery is 4-5 months on the average. Ten years ago, it was 6-8 months. The second reason - our topic - is the improper surgical approach. The scrotal operation always appears easier and more direct. However, it carries the risk of a deadly complication that the proper approach, the inguinal one, completely avoids. It is estimated that one-quarter to one-third of all testicular tumors are not properly excised.

1. What Happens Locally After Scrotal Resection? The testicular lymphatics anastomose exclusively with each other until they reach the retroperitoneal lymph nodes. Anastomoses of testicular lymphatics with those of overlying skin, of the groin, or of the scrotum do not exist in the normal case. Nor do the iliac nodes usually belong to the drainage of the testis (2-4, 6, 8, 10). Incision of the scrotum, like any other incision, cuts across lymphatics. They reanastomose either by direct proliferation of endothelium, or else they bypass the scar tissue by means of new collaterals with the skin and neighboring lymph channels (12, 14).

Thus, if a testicular tumor is removed by the scrotal approach, there is, by virtue of trauma to lymphatics, the risk of iatrogenic inguinal and iliac infiltration. For this reason the scrotal approach to testicular tumors has been discredited. Furthermore, the scrotal approach should be rejected because it does not prevent lymph-borne tumor embolism via the exposed spermatic cord (5, 9, 11).

How often this metastatic risk occurs one can only estimate 10-20%. In the case of pure seminomas this is totally unknown since the appropriate - and usually successful - radiation therapy does not allow for evaluation of iatrogenic metastasis. However, scrotal and inguinal irradiation are an absolute necessity, which is not the case with the inguinal surgical approach.

In the case of the non-seminoma, partial scrotectomy and inguinal dissection are the inevitable consequences of the wrong approach; in fact, bilaterally so, when the tumor-bearing side really contains tumor tissue.

2. What Happens Following the Scrotal Approach to Testicular Tumor (Mistakenly Operated on as Benign and not Excised)? A catastrophic situation occurs with bilateral carcinomatous infiltration of the scrotum (Fig. 1). Next, follow bilateral inguinal, perineal, and intrapelvic metastasis. The therapeutic consequences are hopeless: radiation and/or an attempt at radical excision. Cures are unheard of.

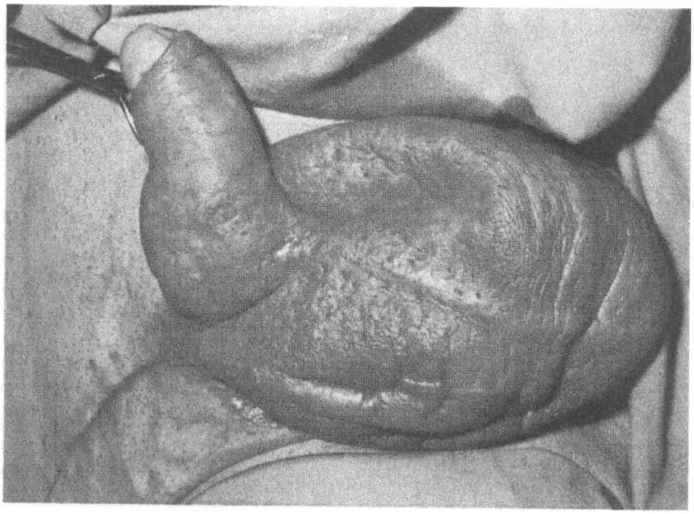

*Fig. 1. Sixty-two-year-old man: Teratoma of the right testis, mistakenly operated on by the scrotal approach as a hydrocele. Six months later, inguinal semicastration. Three months thereafter, total carcinomatous infiltration of the scrotum and penis. Radical excision was attempted; nevertheless, generalized metastasis followed and the patient died*

3. What Happens with Scrotally Biopsied Testicular Tumors? In the case where frozen section diagnosis is made and the tumor removed within a few minutes, the situation is a depicted under 1. If, however the diagnosis is incorrect, or it is not recognized until later, then the situation is as depicted under 2. This is then similar to the situation where a testicular tumor is not operated on until the tunica albuginea has been invaded and the scrotum infiltrated.

4. A related problem, not identical but rather smaller, arises in the case of the inguinal approach, the correct one, if an orchidopexy, hydrocelectomy, or other scrotal procedure was performed in the past (1, 7, 13, 15). Partial scrotectomy and inguinal dissection are necessary, although often negative. When positive, subsequent contralateral inguinal dissection also becomes necessary.

## CONCLUSION

a. The scrotal approach to testicular surgery or biopsy is justified only in cases where no suspicion of tumor exists, e.g., for andrologic indications.
b. Histologic diagnosis is to be made intraoperatively.
c. Out-patient punch biopsy is to be condemned.

(1) Scrotal Removal of the Testicular Tumor

= risk of lymphotraumatic infiltration of the scrotum and inguen
= risk operative tumor embolism via funiculus

(2) Scrotal Operation Without Removal of the Testicular Tumor

= diffuse bilateral infiltration of the scrotum

(3) Scrotal Biopsy of the Testicular Tumor

a) immediate histologic diagnosis and therapy → (1)
b) delayed therapy → (2)

## REFERENCES


1. Bowles, W.T.: Inguinal node metastases from testicular tumor developing after varicocelectomy. J. Urol. (Baltimore) 88, 266-267 (1972)
2. Busch, F.M., Sayegh, E.S.: Roentgenographic visualization of human testicular lymphatics: A preliminary report. J. Urol. (Baltimore) 89, 106-110 (1963)
3. Busch, F.M., Sayegh, E.S., Chenault, O.W., Jr.: Some uses of lymphagiograph in the management of testicular tumors. J. Urol. (Baltimore) 93, 490-495 (1965)
4. Chiappa, S., Uslenghi, C., Bonadonna, G., Marano, P., Rarasi, G.: Combined testicular and foot lymphagiography in testicular carcinomas. Surg. Gynec. Obstet. 123, 10-14 (1966)
5. Cooper, J.F., Leadbetter, W.F., Chute, R.: The thoracoabdominal approach for retroperitoneal gland dissection: Its application to testis tumors. Surg. Gynec. Obstet. 90, 486-496 (1950)
6. Gibert, P.: Intra-organ Lymphagiogram. J. Urol. (Baltimore) 96, 394-396 (1966)
7. GRAY's Anatomy, 25th ed. Philadelphia: Lea & Febiger, 1948
8. Jamieson, J.K., Dobson, J.F.: The lymphatics of the testicle. Lancet (1910), 493-495
9. Lewis, L.G.: Radioresistant testis tumors: Results in 133 cases; Five year follow-up. J. Urol. (Baltimore) 69, 841-848 (1953)
10. MOST: Über maligne Hodengeschwülste und ihre Metastasen. Wirchow's Archiv path. Anat. 154, 138-177 (1898)
11. Sayegh, E.S., Brooks, T., Sacher, E., Busch, F.M.: Lymphagiography of the retroperitoneal lymph nodes through the inguinal route. J. Urol. (Baltimore) 95, 102-107 (1966)
12. Sterns, E.E.: Current concepts of lymphatic transport. Surg. Gynec. Obstet. 138, 779 (1974)
13. Taylor, G.W., Nathanson, I.T.: Lymph node metastases. London: Oxford University Press, 1942
14. Wallace, S., Jackson, L., Dodd, G.D., Greening, R.R.: Lymphatic dynamics in certain abnormal states. Amer. J. Roentgenol. 91, 1187-1206 (1964)
15. Witus, W.S., Sloss, J.H., Valk, W.L.: Inguinal node metastases from testicular tumors developing after orchiopexy. J. Urol. (Baltimore) 81, 669-671 (1959)

# Surgical Treatment of Non-Seminomatous Germinal Testes Tumors

W. J. STAUBITZ

This presentation will be limited to the surgical management of non-seminomatous testes tumors.

Surgical management of non-seminomatous testes tumors can be considered to represent several phases of clinical management. Phase I is the removal of the primary tumor. Phase II is the ablation of actual or possible metastatic disease in the retroperitoneum. Phase III is the removal of metastatic lesions beyond the retroperitoneum.

In phase I, high inguinal orchiectomy is the well-established surgical procedure for the removal of the primary lesion. Any operation less than this is wholly inadequate. When a patient is seen with a scrotal mass, and clinical findings suggest a tumor, phase I should be performed without delay. Any form of biopsy is contraindicated. The tunica albuginea should not be incised until after the testis and cord are given to the pathologist. Incisional biopsy of the testis without complete removal opens new avenues for metastatic spread, as well as local seeding.

Phase I and phase II are not usually performed at the same time. With the entire primary tumor, the pathologist is able to perform serial sections to determine the exact histologic features of the tumor. Testis tumor often contains a variety of cellular elements that determine future therapy and prognosis. Therefore, before definite treatment can be planned, the pathologic findings must be thoroughly studied. If the tumor is predominantly seminoma, but contains other elements such as embryonal or choriocarcinoma, treatment must be directed in favor of the most malignant elements present.

In 1958, in an effort to evaluate the efficacy of lymphadenectomy and also to improve survivals, a prospective study was established (6). All patients with non-seminomatous testis tumors confined to stage I and stage II were to be treated, following radical orchiectomy, by transbadominal bilateral retroperitoneal lymphadenectomy. None were to receive pre- or postoperative irradiation. The guidelines established for this study have not varied in the 12 years, or to 1970, when the study was completed. Preoperative evaluation included history and physical examination, chest tomography, intravenous pyelograms, venacavagrams, and bilateral pedal lymphangiography. If clinical or radiographic evidence of disease outside the retroperitoneum existed (stage III), lymphadenectomy was not attempted.

## MATERIALS AND METHODS

### Surgical Technique

Our surgical approach is based on the fundamental knowledge of testicular lymphatic drainage investigated by JAMIESEN and DOBSON (2). Their work, recently confirmed by SAYEGH (4) and by CHIAPPA (1), shows the primary node receptacles are near L-2 on the left and are usually located between L-1 and L-3 on the right. They have further shown that crossover drainage does occur. It is more frequently from right to left. Furthermore, the phenomenon of retrogarde filling of para-aortic nodes has been documented. Respecting this complex and sometimes unpredictable lymphatic network, our intent is to remove all accessible lymph node-bearing tissue en bloc in the retroperitoneum.

A vertical xyphoid-to-pubis midline incision is made. Upon entering the abdominal cavity, a thorough search for metastatic disease is undertaken. If distant organs are involved, no dissection is attempted. If suspicious lymph nodes above the renal hilum are shown to contain metastatic tumor by frozen section, the case is considered unresectable.

If no metastatic disease is evident cephalad to the renal pedicles, mobilization of the right colon and small bowel is begun. The right lateral peritoneal reflection is incised, the ascending colon and cecum are mobilized. Subsequently, the parietal peritoneum of the small bowel mesentery is incised to the ligament of Trietz. The entire small intestine and right colon then can be eviscerated, exposing the retroperitoneum and major vessels. Dissection is begun at the level of the renal pedicles. Care is taken to remove all lymphatic and areolar tissue in the lateral pockets which are bounded by the vena cava or aorta, the renal pelvis, and the posterior abdominal wall.

The major vessels are circumferentially dissected clean. The spermatic arteries and veins are bilaterally included in the dissection. Both ureters are identified, tagged, and closely observed throughout the procedure. They mark the most lateral boundaries of dissection. The en bloc removal is then continued inferiorly, removing all nodal tissue behind and between the great vessels, allowing the aorta and vena cava to be lifted from their beds anchored only by the major lumbar tributaries. The inferior mesenteric artery is routinely sacrificed. No adverse effects have been noted to date. Dissection is carried distally to the bifurcation of the iliac vessels on the uninvolved side and to the internal ring on the ipsilateral side. If any segment of spermatic cord was left behind during the previous orchiectomy, it is removed.

At the completion of the procedure, all lymphatic and areolar tissue has been removed from the area bordered proximally by and including the renal pedicles, laterally by the course of the ureters and distally by the bifurcation of the iliac vessels and/or the internal ring on the involved side. An X-ray of the operative field is then taken. If, according to the previously obtained lymphangiogram, opacified nodes remain at the site of dissection, they are searched for and removed.

After the completed dissection, the mobilized duodenum, small bowel, and colon are replaced in their original positions and sutured to the parietal peritoneum, and a routine appendectomy is performed. The wound is closed in layers and retention sutures are employed.

## Complications

In the 65 patients treated, complications occurred in 8, or 12%. One postoperative death occurred. This resulted from massive intestinal bleeding with exsanguination secondary to multiple gastrointestinal ulcerations (Table 1).

Table 1. Major complications

| Description | No. of occurrence |
|---|---|
| Severe wound sinus | 1 |
| Postoperative hemorrhage reexplored controlled | 1 |
| Ureteropelvic junction obstruction due to periureteral fibrosis; relieved by lysis 1 year postoperative | 1 |
| Wound dehiscence | 1 |
| Ventral hernia repaired successfully 1 year after lymphadenectomy | 1 |
| Renal pedicle accident requiring intraoperative nephrectomy | 1 |
| Massive gastrointestinal bleeding 5th post-operative day. Patient expired. Autopsy revealed multiple gastrointestinal ulcerations | 1 |

Absence of ejaculation occurred in the majority of patients, although not uniformly so. Incomplete recording of preoperative and postoperative sexual histories precluded accurate documentation of the precise incidence. In those patients with failure of ejaculation, no adverse social or psychological reactions have become manifest to date.

## RESULTS

In an effort to obtain at least a 3-year follow-up, the results of 72 patients explored during the period of 1958 to 1970 are presented. Seven of these were found to be unresectable with extensive disease above the renal pedicle. Each received chemotherapy, either actinomycin D alone or in combination with cytoxin and methotrexate. Three had irradiation in addition to chemotherapy. Six died within 1 year and the other expired of disease in 5 years.

The results obtained in the 65 patients who were resectable are shown in Tables 2 and 3. These tables show the survival figures for 3 and 5 years in both stage I and II. They also reflect the survivals according to the histology of the primary tumor. Of these 65 patients, 20, or 30%, had metastatic tumor in the retroperitoneal nodes and are stage II. Fifteen of 20, or 75%, have survived 3 years, while 12 of 17, or 70%, have survived 5 years or more. In stage I patients, 42 of 45, or 93%, have lived 3 years and 31 of 36, or 86%, have lived 5 or more years.

Table 2. Stage I

| Histology of tumor | No. of patients | 3-year survival No. | (%) | 5-year survival No. | (%) |
|---|---|---|---|---|---|
| Embryonal cell carcinoma | 28 | 26/28 | ( 93%) | 20/23 | ( 87%) |
| Teratocarcinoma | 11 | 11/11 | (100%) | 7/8 | ( 87%) |
| Teratocarcinoma + embryonal cell carcinoma | 4 | 4/4 | (100%) | 3/3 | (100%) |
| Embryonal cell carcinoma + choriocarcinoma | 2 | 1/2 | ( 50%) | 1/2 | ( 50%) |
| Total | 45 | 42/25 | ( 93%) | 31/36 | ( 86%) |

Table 3. Stage II

| Histology of tumor | No. of patients | 3-year survival No. | (%) | 5-year survival No. | (%) |
|---|---|---|---|---|---|
| Embryonal cell carcinoma | 14 | 12/14 | (85%) | 10/12 | (83%) |
| Teratocarcinoma + embryonal cell carcinoma | 1 | 0/1 | ( 0%) | 0/1 | ( 0%) |
| Teratocarcinoma + choriocarcinoma | 2 | 1/2 | (50%) | 1/2 | (50%) |
| Embryonal cell carcinoma + choriocarcinoma | 3 | 2/3 | (75%) | 1/2 | (50%) |
| Total | 20 | 15/20 | (75%) | 12/17 | (70%) |

## DISCUSSION

This series represents a study of a single surgical procedure for definitive treatment of non-seminomatous germinal testis tumors confined to stage I and II following radical orchiectomy. In 1958, guidelines were established for the implementation of this study, and they have not varied during this period of 12 years.

During these 12 years, several other series have been reported in which patients with similar histology and stages have been treated by combinations of therapy and various anatomical routes for the performance of lymphadenectomy. In each of these studies, there was no protocol or plan established that would study a single modality, be it surgery or irradiation. Those series then represent a retrospective rather than a prospective study. MAIER et al. (3) did state that a protocol at Walter Reed General Hospital has been established to study two groups of patients; one confined only to irradiation of retroperitoneal lymph nodes following orchiectomy, and the other to preoperative irradiation, bitaleral retroperitoneal lymphadenectomy, and postoperative irradiation.

To our knowledge, the results of this prospective study have not been published as yet. We have also not uncovered in the literature the published results of any other prospective study established to evaluate the effect of a single therapeutic method directed at stage II patients.

Another area of controversy besides combination of therapy is that concerning the best method of performing the retroperitoneal lymphadenectomy. Recent publications (3, 5, 7) favor a unilateral approach. Those advocating this approach state that bilateral metastatic node involvement is rare. Our experience would differ from this. In the present series of 65 patients undergoing a bilateral retroperitoneal lymphadenectomy, 9% had bilateral involvement, but more important, over 30% of the stage II patients had bilateral extension of metastatic disease. This supports the work of JAMIESEN and DOBSON (2) who demonstrated the crossover of the lymphatic system draining the testes. Therefore, with one-third of stage II having this degree of node involvement, unilateral dissection in our opinion seems very inadequate, regardless of what route is used. Those favoring the unilateral route state that is lowers or eliminates the complication of retrogarde ejaculation. They are quite right about this. Unilateral dissection does have a much lower incidence of failure to ejaculate, whereas in bilateral dissection where the surgery is much more thorough and extensive, absence of ejaculation is common. With the bilateral dissection, using a midline incision, a wider dissection is possible and hence, disturbance of the sympathetic nerve chain occurs more frequently.

When dealing with a highly malignant disease in a young individual, it is our philosophy that all efforts must be directed toward achieving a curative result and that disturbances of nonfatal physiologic functions may result in order to attain the best survival figure. Therefore, with a more thorough dissection, the chance of removing all tumor is greater, and our survival figures attest to this.

## SUMMARY

Surgical management of germinal testis tumors other than seminoma is presented. Phase I consists of removal of the primary tumor; phase II, the surgical removal of retroperitoneal metastatic disease, and phase III, surgical management of chest metastasis. Seventy-two patients were explored with the intent of performing a simultaneous bilateral retroperitoneal lymphadenectomy. Each had a radical orchiectomy prior to exploration. Seven patients were found unresectable because of extensive disease above the renal pedicle and lymphadenectomy was not performed. The remaining 65 were found resectable and a transabdominal bilateral retroperitoneal lymphadenectomy was done. Of this number, 20, or 30%, had metastatic nodes. No other treatment was used. All had a 3-year follow-up and 53 were followed for 5 years or more. The 3-year survivals for stage I is 93%, and for stage II, 75%. Survivals of 5 or more years in stage I are 86% and in stage II, 70%.

Thus, this experience with pathologic stage II cases clearly demonstrates the capability of surgery as a primary treatment to control 70% of patients with retroperitoneal lymph node metastases. This surgical technique is therefore recommended as primary therapy in stage I and II non-seminomatous germinal testis tumors.

REFERENCES


1. Chiappa, S., Uslengmi, C., Bonadonna, G., Marano, P., Ravasi, G.: Combined testicular and foot lymphangiography in testicular carcinomas. Surg. Gynec. Obstet. 123, 10 (1966)
2. Jamiesen, J.K., Dobson, J.F.: Lymphatics of the testicle. Lancet (1910) 1, 493
3. Maier, J.G., Buskirk, K.E., Van Sulak, M.H., Perry, R.H., Schomber, D.T.: An evaluation of lymphadenectomy in the treatment of malignant testicular germ cell neoplasms. J. Urol. (Baltimore) 101, 356-359 (1969)
4. Sayegh, E., Brooks, T., Sacher, E., Busch, F.: Lymphangiography of retroperitoneal lymph nodes. J. Urol. (Baltimore) 95, 102 (1966)
5. Skinner, D.G., Leadbetter, W.F.: The surgical management of testis tumors. J. Urol. (Baltimore) 106, 84 (1971)
6. Staubitz, W.J., Magoss, J.V., Lent, M.H., Sigman, E.M., Grace, J. T.: Surgical management of testicular tumors. N.Y State J. Med. 59, 3459 (1959)
7. Walsh, P.C., Kaufman, J.J., Coulson, U.F., Goodwin, W.E.: Retroperitoneal lymphadenectomy for testicular tumors. J. Amer. med. Ass. 217, 309 (1971)

# Retroperitoneal Lymphadenectomy: Indications, Complications and Expectations

D. E. JOHNSON

The rapid development of multimodal therapy in the management of nonseminomatous testicular tumors demands a reappraisal of the role of lymphadenectomy in this disease. Radiotherapy has been used almost exclusively for the past 25 years in England and many European countries for treatment of all patients with testicular carcinoma, regardless of histologic type (1, 9, 10, 19, 26, 27); whereas, in the USA, lymphadenectomy either alone (29) or combined with irradiation (3, 7, 15, 24) has remained the popular choice. The purpose of this presentation is to report our experience gained from performing 152 retroperitoneal lymphadenectomies over the past 18 years and is an attempt at the present time to answer CALDWELL's (2) challenge: "Why retroperitoneal lymphadenectomy?"

## INDICATIONS

There are three major reasons for performing a retroperitoneal lymphadenectomy: (1) It is the only means for accurately assessing in the extent of the malignant disease (staging); (2) it reduces the amount of malignant disease present which should allow radiotherapy and/or chemotherapy a better opportunity to sterilize the area ("debulking"); and (3) it provides the oncologist with the necessary information regarding the efficacy of chemotherapy to determine rationally whether to continue or discontinue drug therapy.

Staging. After the diagnosis of a nonseminomatous germ cell tumor of the testis has been established, it is mandatory that an accurate assessment be made as to the extent of the disease (Table 1). In addition to performing the usual history and physical examination, serum determinations for chorionic gonadatropin and alpha-fetoprotein titers, routine laboratory studies for liver and bone disease, and excretory urography, a pedal lymphangiogram is required for evaluation of retroperitoneal nodal disease. Although the development and refinement of lymphangiography have done much to aid in the separation of patients with local versus regional disease, approximately one of six (14-16%) in whom the lymphangiogram is interpreted as normal will have microscopic disease when the lymph nodes are removed and carefully examined by the pathologist (22, 31). Consequently, to prevent the indiscriminate use of radiotherapy with its inherent risks, including retroperitoneal fibrosis (8), irradiation damage to bowel (21, 25, 30), radiation nephritis with associated renal hypertension (4, 11, 13, 17, 35), and permanent compromise of the bone marrow which may severely restrict adequate dosage of cytotoxic drugs should their use be required for subsequent visceral metastases (18), surgical removal of the retroperitoneal lymph nodes appears mandatory for adequate clinical staging.

Table 1. M.D. Anderson staging system for testicular neoplasms

| | |
|---|---|
| Stage I | Tumor limited to testicle with no evidence of spread through capsule or to spermatic cord |
| Stage II | Clinical or radiographic evidence of tumor extension beyond testicle but not beyond regional lymphatic drainage |
| Stage IIIA | Extension beyond diaphragm but still confined to lymphatic system as in mediastinal or supraclavicular lymphatics, or massive retroperitoneal disease |
| Stage IIIB | Disseminated disease as seen in generalized abdominal (visceral) or pulmonary metastases |

Our 5-year survival rates of 74, 93, and 100% for 72 patients with embryonal carcinoma, teratoma, and teratocarcinoma, respectively, who underwent only retroperitoneal lymphadenectomy and in whom the lymph nodes were subsequently negative on histologic examination support the premise that radiotherapy is unwarranted when the removed lymph nodes are free of disease (Fig. 1). The 5-year survival rate of 43.8% for 16 patients in whom the lymphangiogram was negative but in whom metastatic disease was present suggests that survival is not adversely affected by the procedure.

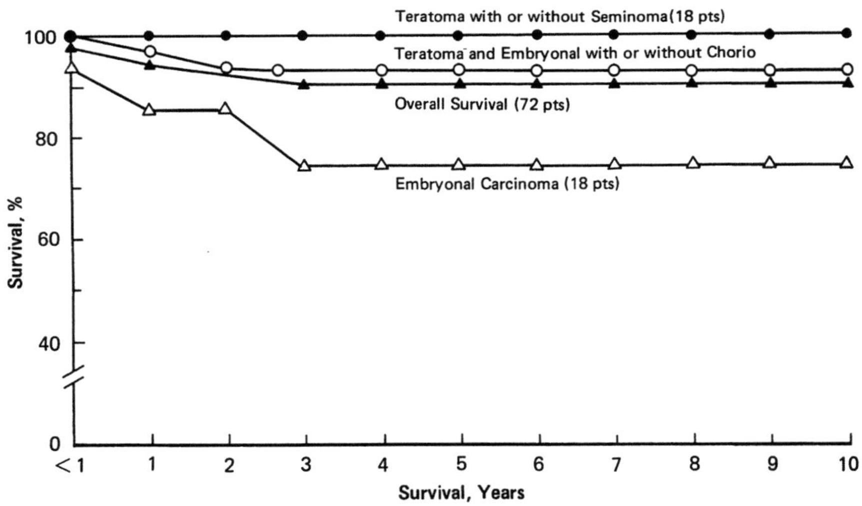


*Fig. 1. Survival rates according to histologic type*

Debulking. Considerable interest and discussion have heretofore focused on the value of using radiotherapy alone in treating patients with regional metastatic disease. Since 1968, the policy at Anderson Hospital in treatment for all clinically stage II nonseminomatous tumors has been to use combined therapy giving preoperative irradiation, 2500 rad tumor dose in 3 weeks, followed immediately upon completion with periaortic lymphadenectomy. During the postoperative convalescent period, usually beginning 3 weeks after surgery, an additional course of radiation, 2500 rad, is given in 3 weeks to the retroperitoneal area. The final 500-1000 rad is given through reduced portals to the area of known involvement marked with silver clips. The periaortic area is preferably treated with 25 meV megavoltage X-rays and the inguinal-iliac fields are treated with Cobalt-60.

The rationale for such an approach is based on the belief that preoperative irradiation should: (1) decrease the risk of spread of malignant cells at the time of surgery by rendering them less capable of reproduction and growth and making the retroperitoneal bed less suitable for the cells, (2) eradicate all microextensions of the tumor that were clinically unrecognized, and (3) make some tumors resectable under the influence of irradiation which otherwise would not have been. Postoperative irradiation has been utilized following lymphadenectomy as a further attempt to decrease the incidence of local recurrences. To date, there have been minimal complications associated with this combined therapy and no documented instances of local recurrences. In addition , during the 6 years that the "sandwich" technique has been utilized, there have been no cases in which extensive regional metastatic disease has precluded lymphadenectomy, which strongly supports the premise that preoperative irradiation has rendered some inoperable cases operable.

Monitoring Chemotherapy. The development of cancerocidal chemotherapeutic programs with the potential for cure in over 25% of patients with disseminated testicular carcinoma (23) has altered the indications for retroperitoneal lymphadenectomy in advanced disease. Once a complete remission has been obtained and maintained for a period of several months, exploratory laparotomy and bilateral retroperitoneal lymphadenectomy allows for a more accurate assessment of the disease status, and the findings serve as an accurate guide for determining the need for further chemotherapy.

Ten patients presenting initially at Anderson Hospital with advanced testicular malignant disease in whom either complete remissions or reduction in clinical stage were obtained with chemotherapy have been subjected to bilateral retroperitoneal lymphadenectomy 5-10 months following initiation of drug therapy (Table 2). Histologic examination of the removed lymph nodes revealed no residual tumor in four instances, adult teratomatous elements in three cases, and residual malignant disease in three patients. The absence of residual disease allowed the medical oncologist to tailor the need for subsequent courses on an individual basis rather than keeping patients on drugs for an empirical period of time. Benign transformations of the testicular carcinoma were at first puzzling, but increasing experience has shown that treatment with either radiotherapy or chemotherapy can result in the destruction of the poorly differentiated and less differentiated elements with only mature teratomatous elements remaining (Table 3). However, without surgical removal, these lesions cannot be differentiated from malignant disease requiring further aggressive therapy. In addition, we believe these areas of adult teratoma are best removed when their malignant potential has been ablated and before continued growth results in local problems. The finding of residual tumors in the removed nodes is a poor prognostic sign and demands continued aggressive therapy.

Table 2. Clinical summary

| Age at diagnosis | Primary tumor | Site of metastases | Treatment (MDAH) | Interval from beginning drugs to lymphadenectomy (months) | Pathologic finding | Further treatment | Status post-lymphadenectomy |
|---|---|---|---|---|---|---|---|
| 16 | Terato-carcinoma | Lung | Bleo-COMF[b] | 8 | Teratoma (neg. nodes) | None | 4 years-NED[c] |
| 24 | Embryonal carcinoma | Lung; supra-clavicular nodes | $VB_3$[b] | 5 | Extensive necrosis $\bar{c}$ teratoma & embryonal | Chemotherapy | 1 year - dead with disease |
| 19 | Embryonal carcinoma | Lung | Bleo-COMF | 7 | Embryonal | Radiation | 2 months - dead with disease |
| 20 | Embryonal carcinoma | Lung; supra-clavicular nodes | $VB_1$[b] | 10 | No tumor | Chemotherapy (1 course) | $2\frac{1}{2}$ years - NED |
| 23[a] | Embryonal carcinoma | Extensive retro-peritoneal Dx | $VB_3$ | 6 | No tumor | None | 6 months - NED |
| 33[a] | Embryonal carcinoma | Mediastinum | Bleo-COMF | 8 | No tumor | Chemotherapy (2 courses) | 3 years - NED |
| 20 | Embryonal carcinoma | Lung; supra-clavicular nodes | $VB_3$ | 5 | No tumor | Chemotherapy (4 courses) | 1 year - NED |
| 21 | Embryonal carcinoma | Lung | $VB_3$ | 6 | Foci teratoma | None | 6 months - NED |
| 22 | Terato-carcinoma | Supraclavicular nodes | $VB_3$ | 6 | Teratoma $\bar{c}$ embryonal | Chemotherapy | 6 months - alive with disease |
| 19[a] | Embryonal carcinoma | Lung; supra-clavicular nodes | $VB_3$ | 9 | Teratoma | Chemotherapy | 2 months - NED |

[a] There were previous attempts at node dissections by referring physician, but the patients were considered inoperable.

[b] See text.

[c] No evidence of disease.

Table 3. Benign transformation of retroperitoneal metastases from testicular carcinoma

| Author | Primary tumor | Treatment of retroperitoneal metastases |
|---|---|---|
| DUARI (6) | Teratoma with seminoma | Radiotherapy |
| SMITHERS (26) | Teratoma with seminoma | Chemotherapy |
| WILLIS and HAJDU (34) | Embryonal carcinoma | Chemotherapy |
| | Embryonal carcinoma | Radiotherapy |
| | Embryonal carcinoma | Radiotherapy |
| DEES (5) | Embryonal carcinoma | Chemotherapy |
| MERRIN et al. (16) | Embryonal carcinoma (7 patients - details absent) | Chemotherapy |

## COMPLICATIONS

Complications following retroperitoneal lymphadenectomy in our 152 patients have been minimal (6.5%), and have consisted of wound infection in 5 instances, lymphocyst formation in 2 cases, postoperative pancreatitis in 2 cases, and chylous ascites in 1 case. There have been no operative deaths. The mean and median hospital stay has been 10 days.

The formation of a lymphocyst following pelvic lymphadenectomy is a frequent occurrence but usually does not require surgical intervention. Similar situations may be encountered following retroperitoneal lymphadenectomy, and the diagnosis should be suspected in any patient who develops renal obstructive symptoms (flank pain, fever, mass) during the early postoperative convalescent period. A presumptive diagnosis can usually be made upon palpating an abdominal mass, usually located lateral to the midline and developing within 2-6 weeks following surgery. Its rapid formation following lymphadenectomy aids in differentiating it from recurrent disease. The diagnosis is confirmed by lymphangiography (Fig. 2). In one of our cases, surgical intervention became necessary due to progressive hydroureteronephrosis associated with flank pain. The preoperative roentgenogram demonstrated a large mass displacing the left ureter anteriorly and laterally with moderate hydroureteronephrosis. Lymphangiograms confirmed the diagnosis of a large retroperitoneal lymphocyst (Fig. 3). A large, thick-walled cyst adherent to the surrounding structure was found at surgery. The roof of the cyst was excised and an omental flap was used to fill the evacuated space. The patient's postoperative course was uneventful with gradual relief of the obstruction.

The occurrence of acute pancreatitis in two of our patients may have been coincidental findings, but we believe that it may well reflect excessive superior retraction in an attempt to gain wider exposure at the level of the renal vessels. In retracting the abdominal viscera upward, care should be exercised in packing the organs so as to prevent unnecessary injury, especially to the pancreas. Chylous ascites was demonstrated in one of our patients, and although his postoperative recovery was prolonged, this complication regressed on conservative therapy and did not require either drainage or surgical intervention.

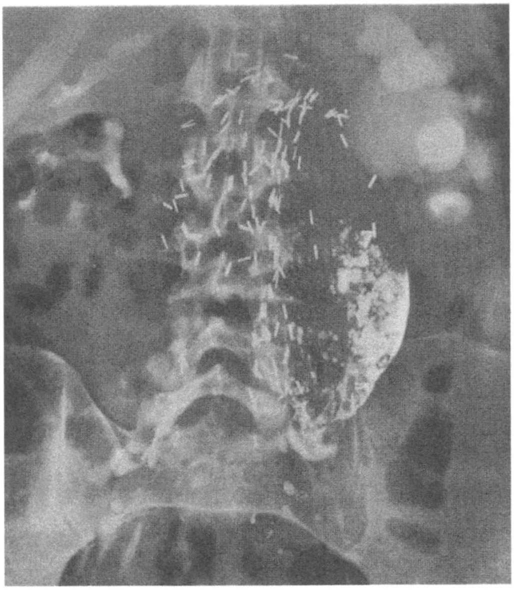

*Fig. 2. Postoperative lymphocyst obstructing left kidney*

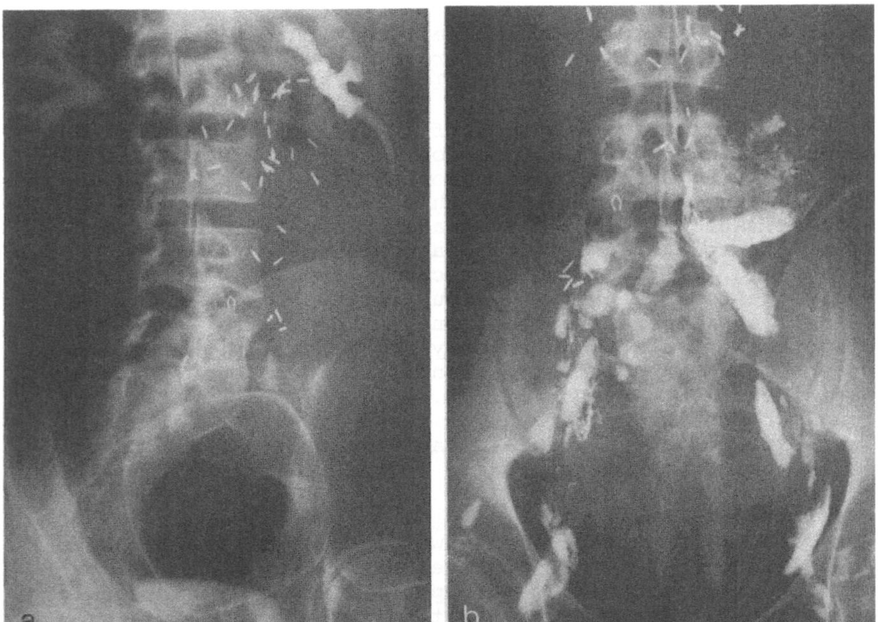


*Fig. 3a and b. Postoperative lymphocyst. (a) Displacement of the left ureter is noted shortly after retroperitoneal node dissection for embryonal carcinoma of the testicle; (b) Lymphangiogram demonstrates distortion of the ureter due to lymphocyst*

The major drawback of retroperitoneal lymphadenectomy and the complication which has received far too excessive emphasis by the proponents for "radiation therapy alone" is that of ejaculatory impotence or sterility following the procedure. Erectile impotence has not occurred in any of the 152 patients undergoing retroperitoneal lymphadenectomy in our series.

Questionnaires returned from 50 patients undergoing lymphadenectomy revealed that 42 had a decrease of 50% or greater in semen volume and 20 (40%) had a dry ejaculate. All patients returning the questionnaires who had undergone a unilateral dissection had a significant decrease in ejaculatory volume and consequently we could not confirm any trend toward preservation of ejaculation for the modified procedure. More importantly, however, only 12 of the 37 married patients stated that they wanted to have children following lymphadenectomy; in seven of these married units, uncomplicated pregnancy and delivery have successfully resulted. Although retroperitoneal lymphadenectomy obviously compromises semen volume, the findings that most patients are not anxious to have further children after surgery and that the majority of those who desire children have been successful, enhances our belief that this complication has been overemphasized.

## EXPECTATIONS

Our 5-year survival rate for 72 patients with nonseminomatous germ cell tumors of the testis who received no form of therapy other than retroperitoneal lymphadenectomy and in whom the removed lymph nodes showed no evidence of malignant disease was 90.8%. Five-year survival rates according to the histologic characteristics of the primary tumor for this group of patients were as follows: 74.4% for 18 patients with embryonal carcinoma, 93.0% for 36 patients with teratocarcinoma, and 100% for 18 patients with teratoma. Five-year survival rates analyzed according to the type of lymphadenectomy failed to show any statistical difference between those patients undergoing bilateral as opposed to unilateral lymphadenectomy; 5-year survival rates were 87.5% as opposed to 92.6%, respectively. These results are in agreement with others (14, 32) in that bilateral lymphadenectomy has no advantage over carefully performed unilateral lymphadenectomy in stage I disease. Based on this recent cumulative experience, we have changed our policy of performing only modified bilateral dissections (20) for left-sided tumor. However, since contralateral spread of tumor occurs occasionally in the absence of ipsilateral involvement (especially for a right-sided tumor) (12) and because of RAY's findings (20) of a higher proportion of positive nodes in patients with right-sided tumors undergoing bilateral as opposed to unilateral dissections, we believe that a bilateral dissection is required for all clinically stage I patients with right-sided tumors.

The 5-year survival rates for the 16 patients who were initially clinically assessed as stage I but in whom metastatic disease was confirmed histologically and subsequently treated with postoperative irradiation was 48.3%. Whether surgery alone without additional radiation therapy, as suggested by STAUBITZ et al. (29), would give equal or better survival rates awaits a prospective randomized clinical study.

Combined ("sandwich") therapy was utilized in 19 patients with positive lymphangiograms (stage II). The 5-year survival rate was 73.9%. The addition of prophylactic chemotherapy in 6 of the 19 patients did not appear to improve survival.

The discrepancy between the 48.3% survival rate for patients with unsuspected microscopic disease discovered histologically after retroperitoneal lymphadenectomy and treated with postoperative irradiation and the 73.9% survival rate for patients with more extensive disease discovered preoperatively and treated with the sandwich technique is disturbing. Although the small numbers of patients in each group preclude any statistically significance, this difference may reflect differences in the histologic character of the retroperitoneal metastases. The retroperitoneal metastases consisted of embryonal carcinoma in 9 of 13 patients with clinical stage I disease as opposed to only 4 of 19 patients with clinical stage II disease.

## CONCLUSIONS

The use of retroperitoneal lymphadenectomy in the management of 152 patients with nonseminomatous germ cell tumors of the testis treated at Anderson Hospital has been reviewed. Complications consisting of wound infection (six cases), acute pancreatitis (two cases), lymphocyst formation (two cases), and chylous ascites (one case) developed in 6.4% of patients. Although ejaculatory impotence is common postoperatively, only 12 marriage units were desirous of having children and 7 of these have had uncomplicated and successful pregnancies. No instances of erectile impotence developed in this series.

The indications for the procedure have been defined with regard to accurate staging, combined therapy, and, in selected instances of advanced disease, as a means of monitoring the effects of chemotherapy. The importance of this operative procedure in the multimodal management of patients with nonseminomatous germ cell tumors of the testis cannot be overemphasized.

## REFERENCES


1. Boden, G., Gibb, R.: Radiotherapy and testicular neoplasms. Lancet (1951) II, 1195-1197
2. Caldwell, W.L.: Why retroperitoneal lymphadenectomy for testicular tumors? Sth. med. J. 62, 1232-1236 (1969)
3. Castro, J.R.: Lymphadenectomy and radiation therapy in malignant tumors of the testicle other than pure seminoma. Cancer (Philad.) 24, 87-91 (1969)
4. Dean, A.L.: Treatment of testis tumors. J. Urol. (Baltimore) 76, 439-446 (1946)
5. Dees, J.E.: Metastatic embryonal cell carcinoma of testis: an apparent 8-year cure. J. Urol. (Baltimore) 110, 90-92 (1973)
6. Duari, M.: A primary malignant testicular tumour with unusual metastases. Brit. J. clin. Pract. 21, 195-200 (1967)
7. Dykhuizer, R.F., George, F.W., III, Kirohara, S., Ratner, M., Sargent, C.R., Varney, J.K.: The use of cobalt 60 telecurietherapy or X-ray therapy with and without lymphadenectomy in the treatment of testis germinal tumors; a 20-year comparison study. J. Urol. (Baltimore) 100, 321-328 (1968)
8. Earle, J.D., Bagshaw, M.A., Kaplan, H.S.: Supervoltage radiation therapy of the testicular tumors. Amer. J. Roentgenol. 117, 653-661 (1973)
9. Gordon-Taylor, G., Wyndham, N.R.: On malignant tumors of the testicle. Brit. J. Surg. 35, 6-7 (1947)

10. Hope-Stone, H.F., Blandy, J.P.: Treatment of tumors of the testis. Brit. med. J. 984-989 (1963)
11. Host, H., Stokke, T.: The treatment of malignant testicular tumors at the Norwegian Radium Hospital. Cancer (Philad.) 12, 323-329 (1959)
12. Jamieson, J.K., Dobson, J.F.: The lymphatics of the testicle. Lancet (1910) I, 493-495
13. Lee, F., Perez, C.A.: Radiation therapy in the management of testicular tumors. J. Urol. (Baltimore) 111, 201-204 (1974)
14. Maier, J.G., Buskirk, K.E., Van Sulak, M.H., Perry, R.H., Schomber, D.T.: An evaluation of lymphadenectomy in the treatment of malignant testicular germ cell neoplasms. J. Urol. (Baltimore) 101, 356-359 (1969)
15. Maier, J.G., Sulak, M.H.: Radiation therapy in malignant testis tumors. Part II. Carcinoma. Cancer 32, 1217-1226 (1973)
16. Merrin, C., Baumgartner, G., Wajsman, Z.: Benign transformation of testicular carcinoma by chemotherapy. Lancet (1975) I, 43-44
17. Notter, G., Ranudd, N.E.: Treatment of malignant testicular tumors. Acta radiol. Ther. (Stockh.) 2, 272-300 (1964)
18. Nicholson, T.C., Wash, P.C., Ratner, M.B.: Lymphadenectomy combined with preoperative and postoperative cobalt 60 teletherapy in the management of embryonal carcinoma and teratocarcinoma of the testis. J. Urol. (Baltimore) 112, 109-110 (1974)
19. Peckham, M.J., McElevain, T.J.: Radiotherapy of testicular tumors. Proc. roy. Soc. Med. 67, 300-303 (1974)
20. Ray, B., Hajdu, S.I., Whitmore, W.F.: Distribution of retroperitoneal lymph node metastases in testicular germinal tumors. Cancer (Philad.) 33, 340-348 (1974)
21. Roswit, B., Malsky, S.J., Reid, C.B.: Severe radiation injuries of the stomach, small intestine, colon, and rectum. Amer. J. Roentgenol. 114, 460-474 (1972)
22. Safer, M.L., Green, J.P., Crews, Q.E., Jr., Hill, D.R.: Lymphangiographic accuracy in the staging of testicular tumors. Cancer (Philad.) 35, 1603-1605 (1975)
23. Samuels, M.L., Johnson, D.E., Holoye, P.Y.: Bleomycin combination chemotherapy program in stage 3 testicular neoplasia: results in 101 patients. Cancer Chemother. Rep. 59, 563-570 (1975)
24. Schroeder, A.F., Crews, Q.E., Jr., Rotner, M.B.: Combined treatment of nonseminomatous testicular cancer. In: Frontiers of Radiation Therapy and Oncology. Basel: S. Karger, 1970, Vol. 5, pp. 240-250
25. Sell, A., Skov, J.T.: Acute gastric ulcers induced by radiation. Acta radiol. (Stockh.) 4, 289-297 (1966)
26. Smithers, D.W.: Maturation in human tumors. Lancet (1969) II, 949-952
27. Smithers, D.W., Wallace, E.N.K.: Radiotherapy in the treatment of patients with seminomas and teratomas of the testicle. Brit. J. Urol. 34, 422-435 (1962)
28. Smithers, D.W., Wallace, E.N.K., Wallace, D.M.: Radiotherapy for patients with tumors of the testicle. Brit. J. Urol. 43, 83-92 (1971)
29. Staubitz, W.J., Early, K., Magoss, I.V., Murphy, G.P.: Surgical treatment of nonseminomatous germinal testis tumors. Cancer (Philad.) 32, 1206-1212 (1973)
30. Sylveni, B., Vikterlof, K.J., Schnurer, L.B.: Gastric ulceration following cobalt teletherapy. Acta radiol. Ther. (Stockh.) 8, 183-188 (1969)
31. Wallace, S., Jing, B.S.: Lymphangiography: diagnosis of nodal metastases from testicular malignancies. J. Amer. med. Ass. 213, 94-96 (1970)

32. Walsh, P.C., Kaufman, J.J., Coulson, W.F., Goodwin, W.E.: Retroperitoneal lymphadenectomy for testicular tumors. J. Amer. med. Ass. 217, 309-312 (1971)
34. Willis, G.W., Hajdu, S.T.: Histologically benign teratoid metastasis of testicular embryonal carcinoma: report of five cases. Amer. J. clin. Path. 59, 338-343 (1973)
35. Wilson, C., Ledingham, J.M., Cohen, M.: Hypertension following X-irradiation of the kidneys. Lancet (1958) I, 9-16

# The Combined Surgical and Chemotherapeutic Approach to Non-Seminomatous Cancer of the Testicle

W. VAHLENSIECK, and L. WEISSBACH

A total of 250 patients with testicular tumors were treated in our institution from 1926 until May 1975. Of these 233 (93.2%) were germ cell and 17 (6.8%) non-germ cell tumors. Between January 1966 and July 1975 we treated 143 patients with germinal tumors of the testicle. We were able to reexamine the histology in 123 out of 143 patients. This was done in cooperation with our pathologist Prof. Gedigk and Priv.-Doz. Dr. Mueller and Dr. Tschubel who confirmed the correct classification of the tumors. In 20 patients, however, who had their orchiectomy done outside our hospital, we were unable to reexamine the histology; we exclude those patients (14%) from our study.

Using the classification of DIXON and MOORE we were able to divide our 123 patients into 36 (29.3%) with seminoma and 87 (70.7%) with non-seminomatous tumors (Fig. 1). Using the nomenclature of COLLINS and PUGH we registered 36 (29.3%) pure seminomas, 12 (9.7%) combined tumors, and 70 (61.0%) teratomas (Fig. 2).

All 123 patients were treated using the same regimen as outlined in Figure 3. With regard to non-seminomatous tumors of the testicle, to which we will limit our discussion, they follow exactly the combined surgical and chemotherapeutic treatment as demonstrated in the right upper quadrant of the figure (8-10, 12, 13).

| Classification | 123 Germcell tumors (I/66 – VII/75) | | | |
|---|---|---|---|---|
| Dixon and moore | Stage | No. | Total | (%) |
| Seminoma | $T_{1-4}$ $N_{0,x}$ $M_0$ | 22 | | |
| | $T_{1-4}$ $N_1$ $M_0$ | 10 | 36 | 29.3 |
| | $T_{1-4}$ $N_{x,1,2}$ $M_1$ | 4 | | |
| Non-Seminomatous tumors | $T_{1-4}$ $N_0$ $M_0$ | 36 | | |
| | $T_{1-4}$ $N_{1,2}$ $M_0$ | 28 | 87 | 70.7 |
| | $T_{0\ 4}$ $N_{x,0-2}$ $M_1$ | 23 | | |

*Fig. 1*

| Classification<br>Collins / PUGH | 123 Germcell tumors (I/66 – VII/75)<br>Stage | No. | Total | % |
|---|---|---|---|---|
| Seminoma | $T_{1-4}$ $N_{0,x}$ $M_0$ | 22 | 36 | 29.3 |
| | $T_{1-4}$ $N_1$ $M_0$ | 10 | | |
| | $T_{0-4}$ $N_{x,1,2}$ $M_1$ | 4 | | |
| Combined tumors | $T_{1-4}$ $N_0$ $M_0$ | 4 | 12 | 9.7 |
| | $T_{1-4}$ $N_1$ $M_0$ | 7 | | |
| | $T_{1-4}$ $N_{1-2}$ $M_1$ | 1 | | |
| Teratoma | $T_{1-4}$ $N_0$ $M_0$ | 35 | 75 | 61.0 |
| | $T_{1-4}$ $N_{1-2}$ $M_0$ | 21 | | |
| | $T_{0-4}$ $N_{x,0-2}$ $M_1$ | 22 | | |

*Fig. 2*

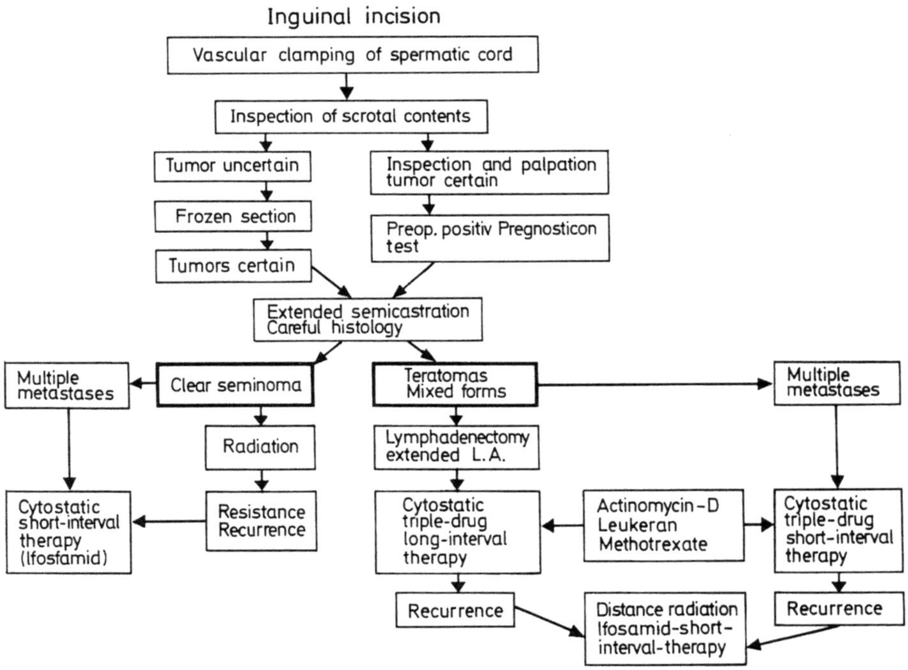


*Fig. 3. Operative and cytostatic treatment of germinal tumors of the testis*

Three different situations have to be considered.

1. The first is the case where we are unable clinically or by histologic examination of the retroperitoneal lymph nodes to demonstrate any metastasis. In this case the patient was started on the operative day on a cytostatic triple-drug long-interval therapy. When LI et al. introduced this regimen, they used massive doses in the 1st month after surgery 3 consecutive times (3). Contrary to this, we used triple-drug long-interval therapy every 3 months up to a total of 2 years. During surgery and on the following days the patients received 0.5 g of actinomycin D i.v. and starting on the 3rd postoperative day 15 mg chlorambucil and 10 mg methotrexate p.o. To prevent ulcerative stomatitis we stopped treatment at any sign of soreness of the mouth. We also stopped the treatment if the lymphocytes dropped below 2000. The drug was not given longer than 14 days. Every 3 months we repeated the treatment with the same drugs and doses for 5 consecutive days. This treatment was done on an in-patient basis in order to monitor and examine the patient closely.

2. Our approach was quite different when the clinical examination or the histologic examination of the retroperitoneal lymph nodes demonstrated metastasis, which we saw in 37.5% of our patients. In this case we start chemotherapy on the day of the operation using the same drugs in the same doses as outlined above. We then added a so-called short-interval therapy which means we repeated the treatment every month. As there was no evidence of recurrence after the third session, we switched over to the long-interval therapy. However, if we did find any progression of the disease (elevation of LDH, Pregnosticon test positive, metastases demonstrated by X-ray) a switch to a different drug was made. Years ago we used mitramycin, vincristine, or a similar drug. In the last few years, however, we prefer treatment with Ifosfamid in combination with low-dose radiation therapy.

3. In the patients presenting with solitary metastasis, which was found in 16.7% of our patients, we prefer a similar approach. Again we perform retroperitoneal lymphadenectomy and starting the day of operation, triple-drug short-interval chemotherapy. If this is followed by a complete remission, we switch after one or two short-interval treatments over to a long-interval therapy. When there is no progression of the disease, we plan surgical excision of the solitary metastasis. At this time the patient is on short-interval treatment and when stabilized, we switch over to the long-interval therapy. If, however, there is progression of the disease or further metastases show despite lymphadenectomy and triple-drug therapy, we switch to a different chemotherapy. Ifosfamid in combination with low-dose radiation therapy has been the treatment of choice in these cases in recent years.

Although we were not used to radiotherapy of non-seminomatous testicular tumors, we were impressed by the results obtained using the combination of low-dose radiation therapy and chemotherapy with Ifosfamid. This was especially true in the patient with generalized metastasis. HOEFER-JANKER and SCHEEF developed this mode of treatment (2). This so-called distant radiotherapy started out with 500 rad over a time period of 5-10 days. The fields radiated included all areas with metastases. For example, if only the abdominal cavity is involved we give 100 rad daily to this area. In a case of generalized metastasis to the thoracic and abdominal area, we employ 50 rad daily to each area. We think that the main effect of this distant radiotherapy is to produce and increase the permebility of the cell membrane and the nucleus for water-soluble substances to which the hydrophilic, cytostatic-active metabolites of Ifosfamid belong. In addition, we think that the repeated low dosage of radiation therapy leads to a prolongation of the G-2 phase which then can be attacked by the chemotherapeutic agent quite easily.

As soon as the treated patient has finished his course of radiotherapy, that is, between the 5th and 10th day, we give him 60 mg/kg Ifosfamid body weight in 5% solution i.v. up to a total dosage of 300 mg/kg body weight. Ifosfamid is, like cyclophosphamide, a oxazophosphorin derivative which has lost its typical Lost-configuration. The water solubility of Ifosfamid and its metabolites is much greater than in any other cytostatic-active N-phosphamide ester. We think that this explains the broad application, the only slight myelotoxicity, and the high nephrotoxicity.

Table 1 shows the effectiveness of our distant-radiation therapy in combination with Ifosfamid therapy. In the upper half of the figure are the patients with generalized metastases who underwent triple-drug therapy only. Despite the fact that we saw some remissions in this group, most of the patients (10) died within the 1st year and 2 patients died in the second year. In contrast to this, the 2 patients who lived longer underwent lymphadenectomy followed by triple-drug interval therapy over a period of 2 years. The group of patients in the lower half of the figure who were treated with distant radiation therapy and Ifosfamid seem to show a trend toward a better prognosis. HOEFER-JANKER and SCHEEF (2) recently reported that they achieved the best effects with this kind of treatment provided there is no other chemotherapy or radiation therapy before the regimen is started. This means that in the future we should abandon primary triple-drug therapy completely. In stage I, according to the good results of STAUBITZ et al. (6), we would recommend no further treatment after lymphadenectomy. In stage II, however, and in isolated metastases we would recommend that following lymphadenectomy two to three courses of distant radiation therapy could be combined with short-interval Ifosfamid every 4 weeks. In a patient with generalized metastases we pursue a similar regimen following orchiectomy. If, however, there is a progression of the tumor we try a triple-drug therapy or combined chemotherapy with actinomycin, bleomycin, and vincristine.

Table 1. Results of chemotherapy on metastatic non-seminomatous testicular tumors

| Therapy | | Year 1. | 2. | 3. | 4. | 5. |
|---|---|---|---|---|---|---|
| Triple-drug therapy | living | | | 1 | | 1 |
| Total | dead | 10 | 2 | | | |
| Distant-irradiation and Ifosfamid | living | 4 | 1 | 2 | 1 | |
| Total | dead | 12 | 6 | | | |

The technique of retroperitoneal lymphadenectomy should be discussed. Before 1966 we treated 20 patients with testicular tumors using extraperitoneal unilateral lymphadenectomy, but did not achieve any improvement of the prognosis. Since then we have only used transperitoneal bilateral lymphadenectomy. We, as well as other authors, reported a high incidence of impotence (90%) after radical lymphadenectomy. This impotence consisted of an inability to ejaculate with preservation of the ability for erection and orgasm. We tried to find a way to preserve the sympaticus going to the seminal vesicles and the ductus deferens. Looking at the distribution of metastases we found that out of 41 patients with left-sided testicular tumor, three patients had para-aortal bilateral metastases. This demonstrated that a crossover is possible. That means also, that one should always do a bilateral complete lymphadenectomy. Because we did not find any lymph nodes positive on the right side along the iliac vessels, we concluded that you may not have to do the lymphadenectomy in the right parailiac area in the case of left-sided testicular tumors. We still have to prove, however, whether the ability to ejaculate can be preserved using this technique.

In a group of 35 patients with right-sided testicular cancer we found in 11 cases metastases on both sides of the aorta and in 2 cases along the iliac vessels on the contralateral side. From this we draw the conclusion that in the future we will have to consider bilateral para-iliac and para-aortic lymphadenectomy for right-sided testicular tumors. SIGEL et al. (5) recently asked whether a lymphadenectomy is still indicated in the case of metastases above the renal vessels. The same question applies in the case of generalized massive retroperitoneal metastases. Looking at our patient material, we found that most of the deaths were in this group of patients. However, we were able in this type of situation, at least macroscopically, to remove all the tumor tissue. In 3 cases we had to remove a kidney which we call an "extended lymphadenectomy". Two patients out of this group who were also treated with drugs following lymphadenectomy lived longer than 4 years. We think that one should always try a radical lymphadenectomy unless invasion of the major vessels makes this procedure technically impossible. The postulate will be reinforced by the concept that modern chemotherapy works much better after the bulk of the tumor has been removed.

The complication rate of transperitoneal bilateral lymphadenectomy is minimal if you exclude the loss of ejaculation. As to see in Table 2 we had only a very few complications in 97 transperitoneal bilateral lymphadenectomies. We developed a better technique and no longer observe any retroperitoneal hemorrhage, lymphocele, or injury to the vessels or ureters. The death of one of our oldest patients (57 years) was due to wound infection and dehiscence.

Table 2. Complication rate of 97 transperitoneal, bilateral lymphadenectomies (87 Non-seminomatous testicular tumors - 9 Seminomas $\{N_2\}$ - 1 Ovarian carcinoma)

| | |
|---|---|
| Wound dehiscence | 3 x |
| Retroperitoneal hemorrhage | 2 x |
| Lymphocele (one with chylascites) | 2 x |
| Ileus | 2 x |
| Injury to renal artery | 1 x |
| Injury to ureter | 3 x |
| Exitus letalis | 1 x |

Our results in 96 transperitoneal bilateral lymphadenectomies for initially diagnosed teratomas (including the group that was not double-checked histologically) demonstrate that with stage I we should expect an excellent prognosis. But even in stage II, and in patients with isolated distant metastases, we achieved results which would not have been possible without lymphadenectomy. We are convinced that in the future , with improvements in cytostatic treatment, even better results will be achieved (Table 3).

Table 3. Survival rate after transperitoneal, bilateral lymphadenectomy

| Years | Stage | Total | Dead | Living |
|---|---|---|---|---|
| | I | 5 | | 5 |
| 1966-1969 | II | 3 | 2 | 1 |
| | III | 2 | 1 | 1 |
| | I | 25 | 4 | 21 |
| 1970-1973 | II | 24 | 7 | 17 |
| | III | 10 | 6 | 4 |
| | I | 14 | | 14 |
| 1974-VII/75 | II | 9 | 3 | 6 |
| | III | 4 | | 4 |
| | | 96 | 23 | 73 |


SUMMARY

Of 250 testicular tumors treated up to May 1975 233 (93.2%) were germ cell and 17 (6.8%) non-germ cell tumors. Reexamining the histology of the last 123 patients only 29.3% had pure seminomas and 70.7% had non-seminomatous tumors. The results of regimens of combined surgical (extended semicastration and lymphadenectomy) and chemotherapeutic (triple-drug as well as Ifosfamid in combination with low-dose radiation) treatment are presented, as well as modifications of treatment for stage II (37.5%) and stage II (16.7%).

There were good results after 96 transperitoneal bilateral lymphadenectomies. But even in stages II and III results were achieved which would not have been possible without lymphadenectomy. It is pointed out that in the future, with improvements in cytostatic therapy, even better results including treatment of stage IV tumors can be expected.


REFERENCES


1. Hoefer-Janker, H., Scheef, W., Günther, U., Hüls, W.: Erfahrung mit der fraktionierten Ifosfamid-Stoßtherapie bei generalisierten malignen Tumoren. Med. Welt 26, 972 (1975)
2. Hoefer-Janker, H., Scheef, W.: Kombinierte radiologisch-zytostatische Behandlung mit Ifosfamid bei generalisierten malignen Hodentumoren. Röntgen-Ber. 2, 186 (1973)
3. Li, M.C., Whitmore, W.F., Jr., Golbey, R., Grabstald, H.: Effects of combined drug therapy on metastatic cancer of the testis. J. Amer. med. Ass. 74, 1291 (1960)
4. Scheef, W.: Problems, experience and results of clinical investigations with Ifosfamid. In: Proc. VIIth Internat. Congr. Chemother., Prague, 1971. Munich: Urban & Schwarzenberg, 1972
5. Sigel, A., Hermanek, P., Schlepas, S.: Lymphchirurgie des Hodentumors. Chirurg 44, 494 (1973)

6. Staubitz, W.J., Early, K.S., Magoss, J.V., Murphy, G.F.: Surgical treatment of testis tumor. J. Urol. (Baltimore) 111, 205 (1974)
7. Staubitz, W.J., Magoss, J.V.: Surgical treatment of non-seminomatous germinal testes tumors. Presented at Internat. Coll. Surg., Amsterdam Juli 1975
8. Vahlensieck, W.:"Erweiterte Semikastration," Lymphadenektomie, Radiotherapie und zytostatische "Triple-Drug-Intervalltherapie" bei germinalen Hodentumoren. Z. Urol. 61, 538 (1968)
9. Vahlensieck, W.: Therapie und Prognose bei Hodentumoren. Med. Welt 21, 1761 (1970)
10. Vahlensieck, W.: Hodentumoren. Therapiewoche 23, 450 (1973)
11. Vahlensieck, W.: Lymphadenectomy combined with chemotherapy. Presented at Internat. Coll. Surg., Amsterdam, Juli 1975
12. Vahlensieck, W., Weißbach, L.: Operative and cytostatic treatment of germinal tumors of the testis. Int. Urol. Nephrol. 5, 85 (1973)
13. Vahlensieck, W., Weißbach, L.: Hodentumoren. Fortschr. Med. 91, 667 (1973)
14. Vahlensieck, W., Weißbach, L.: Hodentumoren. Wiss. Inform. (Dr. Fresenius) 7, 97 (1974)

# Chemotherapy in Testicular Tumors

F. KÖRNER

There is no doubt today about the value of cytostatic therapy of testicular tumors. Testicular tumors require intensive therapy. Previous chapters have dealt with operative and high-voltage therapy.

Cytostatic therapy can always be a supplementary - often a crucial - means of therapy only.

Clinical experience has demonstrated only a few cytostatic agents to be effective upon the cellular growth of testicular tumors. Hormone and isotope therapies have been ineffective.

Two German clinical centers which have engaged themselves especially with the therapeutic problems of testicular tumors employ two different ways of administering therapy.

In view of good results at American hospitals VAHLENSIECK of the Bonn University Hospital prefers the so-called triple-drug therapy wherein a combination of several cytostatic drugs are administered at certain intervals.

Table 1. Initial chemotherapy of metastasizing testicular teratoma

| | | | |
|---|---|---|---|
| Day 1: | Adriamycin (Adriblastin) | 75 mg/m$^2$ | |
| | Bleomycin | 2 x 15 mg | i.m. |
| | Vincristine | 1 mg | |
| Day 8: | Bleomycin | 2 x 15 mg | i.m. |
| | Vincristine | 1 mg | |
| Day 15: | As on day 8 | | |
| Day 22: | Start as on day 1 | | |
| Total dosage: | Adriamycin | 550-600 mg/m$^2$ | (~6 months) |
| | Bleomycin | ca. 300-400 mg | ( 3-4 months) |
| | Vincristine until neurotoxicity | | |

From SEEBER et al. (12).

The Essen Tumor Hospital uses a different therapeutic combination for the treatment of testicular tumors (Table 1). As a result of the author's experience at Freiburg University Hospital and influenced by the publications of Prof. DRUCKREY and co-workers, we first carry out long-term monotherapy with N-Lost (Endoxan) which will be described in detail below. In spite of this monotherapy and in spite of the different combined therapies mentioned above, many tumor patients succumb to retroperitoneal metastases, supraclavicular metastases, and ultimately to metastases of the entire organism.

Especially when a retroperitoneal lymphadenectomy meets with metastases, further metastases may develop about 10 months after the initial treatment was started.

These metastases of malignant testicular tumors - that is teratomas - have until recently resisted effective therapy.

New results in cell research, especially triggered by investigations on hemoblastoses, have led to a hopeful change. SCHUMANN of Hornheide, by means of his cell kinetic investigations, furnished us with the key to our own clinical procedure, while we in turn furnished him with a fresh human tumor specimen speeded to him by helicopter within one hour.

According to SCHUMANN seminoma cells remarkably seem to display a similar rhythm of division as the various kinds of teratoma. The duplication rate is between 24 to 30 h.

Thus the length of every cell cycle can be computed. Furthermore, experimental investigations have shown the phase of cell division at which a cytostatic agent develops its specific effect. The phases of a cell cycle are commonly abbreviated $G_1$ and $G_2$ - i.e., growth phases one and two; S - the synthetic phase, and M - the mitotic phase.

In other words, one cytostatic agent does not affect the total spectrum of cell division but only one specific phase. Knowing the duplication rate the timing of every phase of cell division can be accurately predicted.

These, at first sight, seemingly theoretical considerations on cell kinetics have, nevertheless, resulted in a fundamental change of our clinical and therapeutic approach to malignant tumors. Thus our aim of a tailor-made cytostatic therapy for every kind of malignant tumor is not as much of a distant prospect as it used to be. Although we still do not know why cytostatic drugs have a selective effect on tumor cells - while not on normal cells - in currently applied doses, we taken therapeutic advantage if this empirically experienced phenomenon.

Thus we have synchronized our treatment with the subsequent phases of cell division, although it must be kept in mind that the synchronization can only be partial.

Our therapeutic concept is as follows:

The cell growth of a tumor is brought to a halt within a certain phase of cell division by relatively small doses of cytostatics, while all other cells in various phases of cell division are not prevented from developing up to this point. This point of interference becomes the starting point for tumor cells to fall in step. The synchronization of cell growth by the initial cytostatic agent allows a consequent cytocidal attack via other therapeutic means, including both chemo- as well as high-voltage therapy.

Thus the very same chemotherapeutic agent may be used as a cytostatic agent in small doses, whereas in high doses it becomes a cytocidic therapeutic tool.

Therefore, both steps of the so-called synchronized therapy can be achieved by chemotherapy, depending only on the dose used. High-voltage therapy, however, is restricted to the second step, the <u>destruction</u> of cells.

Our cytostatic agent of choice proved to be Ifosfamid. In close cooperation with Dr. SCHUMANN we developed the following therapeutic procedure as to malignant metastatic testicular tumors, using in addition to Ifosfamid, (1) vincristine, (2) bleomycin, (3) adriamycin.

We used bleomycin and adriamycin in doses of 15 mg and 50 mg per square meter of body surface respectively. We administered both drugs twice within a 24 h interval and completed therapy with 3 g of Ifosfamid 15 h after the initial bleomycin or 24 h after adriamycin therapy (Table 2).

Table 2. Therapy of metastasizing testicular tumor. Synchronization

| | | | | |
|---|---|---|---|---|
| Vincristine | | | | Ifosfamid: 2 x/week |
| 1.5 mg i.v. | | 8 h | | 3 g in 500 ml levulose |
| Bleomycin | | Bleomycin | | Ifosfamid: 1 x/week |
| 15 mg i.v. | 24 h | 15 mg i.v. | 15 h | 3 g |
| Adriblastin | | Adriblastin | | Ifosfamid: 1 x/week |
| 50 mg/$m^2$ | 24 h | 50 mg/$m^2$ | 24 h | 3 g |

Our current therapeutic approach, based on a total of 150 cases, is as follows:

Depending on the result of the sensibility test with regard to the synchronization of tumor cells, we administer vincristine, bleomycin, or adriamycin in relatively small doses, the cytocidal agent of choice being Ifosfamid. Weight, general condition, and an exact and regular control of the red and white blood cell count determine the dose to be applied, normally 3 g with respect to an otherwise healthy individual of about 70 kg. Cell kinetic investigations define the length of the time interval from the administration of the synchronizing drug up to the application of Ifosfamid. The most favorable time interval between the application of vincristine and Ifosfamid is exactly 8 h, a single dose of vincristine already leading to a good synchronization. Bleomycin and adriamycin are likely to synchronize the cell growth more effectively when administered in two doses within a 24 h interval.

Patients with testicular tumors without detectable metastases and without preoperative therapy are treated in the following manner: Inguinal semitestectomy and instantaneous lymphadenectomy are performed. During the operation the patients are given 2 g Ifosfamid in an infusion and 1 g per day during the three postoperative days.

In the case of a complete operative elimination of metastases of the retroperitoneal lymph nodes, follow-up radiotherapy is nevertheless applied. As to radiotherapy, we make no difference between patients with or without metastases. They are both irradiated by high-voltage therapy, the tumor dose being 4000 rad. Trofosfamid (Ixoten) is then given in daily doses of 200 mg for a period of 3 months. At 3-month intervals reinduction therapy is enforced with vincristine or bleomycin or adriamycin under synchronizing conditions. If a patient after one year does not show any clinical or X-ray signs of metastases, we assume that he will develop none in the future and consider him safe and sound after 2 years.

In the case of extensive metastases which show up both clinically and on X-ray, the situation is completely different. If an undescended semicastration has not yet been executed, the testicle will be removed and the tumor tissue analyzed cell-kinetically. The result of the sensibility test will then determine a synchronized treatment with vincristine/Ifosfamid twice a week until paresthesia of hands and feet occur. Likewise, bleomycin and adriamycin can be administered in the above mentioned order. In most cases this treatment results in a quick regression of the metastases permitting a radical operation within 4-6 weeks. After healing of the wounds, a new synchronized treatment is started with the drugs just mentioned according to the result of the sensibility test. A comparison of the primary and metastatic tumor tissue is made possible by this procedure, not only histologically but also cell-kinetically. Further treatment is carried out in the above-mentioned manner.

Among the 22 patients with testicular tumors and metastases treated between the January 1, 1974 and September 15, 1975, 4 had a seminoma, 13 a teratoma, 4 a trophoblastic teratoma and 1 patient a myoleiosarcoma. Of the 4 patients with seminoma two have a complete remission after 8 and 14 months, 1 a partial remission, and 1 patient died. Of the 13 patients with teratoma 9 have a complete remission and 4 died. One of these 9 patients died intercurrently due to a pneumonia. At autopsy we did not find any macroscopic and histologic signs of metastases. Of the 4 patients with trophoblastic teratoma 3 are in complete remission, and 1 died. The 1 patient with a myoleiosarcoma is in partial remission. Thus 14 of the 22 patients are in complete remission, the longest time being 18 months; the average period is between 8 and 12 months. Of the rest 2 are in a partial remission and 6 patients died. Of the patients who died, all except 1 had a complete remission first. They suffered a relapse, 2-4 months on an average after complete remission. The recurrences could then no longer be mastered. During the same period we treated, in our department, 24 patients with testicular tumors without metastasis: 11 had so-called pure seminomas and 13 patients had teratomas of different types. All of these patients are still alive without visible signs of metastasis.

Two typical cases will help to elucidate the treatment of patients with malignant testicular tumors.

Case 1. This was a primary teratoma of the retroperitoneum larger than a child's head with a supraclavicular metastasis as big as a fist. The patient was first operated on externally and a sample excision was taken from the supraclavicular tumor. The operation was not completed, because the tumor was considered to be inoperable. After admission to our department, the patient was first subjected to synchronized treatment with vincristine and Ifosfamid. After this treatment was repeated 8 times (i.e., after 4 weeks), the tumors had decreased in size to such a degree that we were able to remove first the retroperitoneal tumor and to operate on the supraclavicular metastasis 2 weeks later.

The histology of the abdominal tumor showed extensive necrosis and granular tissue as compared to the histologic picture of the supraclavicular metastasis. In this instance only localized tumor tissue in small regions could be found peripherally. In the supraclavicular tumor only cicatricial and granular tissue were present without signs of the earlier tumor tissue.

After operation the patient was synchronized with bleomycin and Ifosfamid for a period of 3 weeks. Now, 12 months after operation, the patient is free of metastases both clinically and radiologically. He has taken up light work.

Case 2: This patient underwent a left semicastration outside our hospital due to a teratoma with extensive pulmonary metastases. He was transferred to our department for special treatment. At the time of admission we found subsequently developed and extended metastases in his lungs. We started synchronized treatment with vincristine and Ifosfamid. By repeating this synchronized treatment 5 times, the lung metastases disappeared completely. Then the retroperitoneal metastases were removed. Further reinduction therapy with bleomycin/Ifosfamid over a period of 6 weeks completed the treatment.

## SUMMARY

Surprisingly good clinical results are obtained by means of the so-called synchronized treatment with vincristine or bleomycin or adriamycin combined with Ifosfamid when cell-kinetic conditioning factors are taken into consideration. The results could neither be obtained with monotherapy nor by the aid of various combined therapies. Of 22 patients affected by metastasizing malignant testicular tumors a complete remission could be achieved in 14 continuing up to a period of 18 months. Six patients died. The answer to what extent these therapeutic results will be confirmed over a longer observation period, has, however, to be put off until a later date.

## REFERENCES

1. Drings, P., Fritsch, H.: Erste Erfahrungen mit Bleomycin bei metastasierenden Tumoren. Therapiewoche 22, 4569 (1972)
2. Hartwich, G., Fuchs, H.F., Neidhardt, B.: Zytostatische Behandlung teilsynchronisierter Tumoren. Fortschr. Med. 2, 46 (1972)
3. Hartwich, G., Tschätsch, W., Lutz, H.: Zytostatische Kombinations-Behandlung mit Vincristinsulfat und Ifosfamid. Dtsch. med. Wschr. 98, 1203 (1973)
4. Hoefer-Janker, H., Scheef, W.: Kombinierte radiologisch-zytostatische Behandlung mit Ifosfamid bei generalisierten malignen Hodentumoren. Röntgen-Ber. 2, 186 (1973)
5. Klein, H.O., Lennartz, K.J., Habicht, W., Eder, M., Gross, R.: Synchronisation von Ehrlich-Aszites-Tumorzellen und ihre Bedeutung bei der Anwendung eines alkylierenden Zytostatikums. Klin. Wschr. 48, 1001 (1970)
6. Klein, H.O., Gross, R., Lennartz, K.J.: Untersuchungen zur Proliferationskinetik und Synchronisation menschlicher Tumorzellen und ihre Bedeutung für die zytostatische Therapie. Verh. dtsch. Ges. inn. Med. 77, 738 (1971)
7. Körner, Fr., Lund, S.: Zytostatische Tumortherapie unter Teilsynchronisationsbedingungen mit besonderer Berücksichtigung der malignen Hodentumoren. MMW 117, 1345-1348 (1975)
8. Körner, Fr.: Controlled chemotherapy in testicular tumors. In: 2nd Int. Symposium on Pulse-Cytometry. European Press, Geneva/Belgium, 1976

9. Lund, S., Körner, Fr.: Die Therapie metastasierender Hodentumoren. Hamburger Ärzteblatt 7, 184-185 (1975)
10. Rathert, P., Terhorst, B., Lutzeyer, W.: Bleomycin bei malignen Genitaltumoren des Mannes. Urologe A 13, 67 (1974)
11. Schumann, J.: Personal communication
12. Seeber, S., Gallmeier, W.M., Höffken, K., Osieka, R., Bruntsch, U., Schmidt, C.G.: Neue Chemotherapiemöglichkeiten be der Behandlung metastasierender Hodencarcinome. Dtsch. med. Wschr. 100, 1319-1324 (1975)
13. Umezawa, H., Ishijuka, K., Kimura, J., Iwanaga, J., Tatzeucki, T.: Biological studies on individual bleomycins. J. Antibiot. 21, 592 (1968)
14. Vahlensieck, W.: Hodentumoren. Wissenschaftl. Informationen Fresenius-Stiftung, Aktuelle Nephrologie. Heft 1, 1974
15. Wüst, G.: Aktuelle Probleme der Therapie maligner Tumoren. Stuttgart: G. Thieme, 1973

# Chemotherapy of Seminoma

W. F. WHITMORE, A. SMITH, A. YAGODA, ST. CVITKOVIC, and R. GOLBEY

## INTRODUCTION

Germinal tumors of the adult testes have proved remarkably responsive to a wide range of chemotherapeutic agents (1, 4, 8). Although the control of patients with seminoma treated by orchiectomy and irradiation is good, treatment failures do occur after such therapy. MACKENZIE (5) reported Memorial Sloan Kettering Cancer Center (MSKCC) experience with the chemotherapy of seminoma and this is a further review of that subject.

## CASE SELECTION

In the period 1946-1971 a total of 42 patients who received chemotherapy with a histologic diagnosis of seminoma were identified in MSKCC files. From this group 23 patients were selected for analysis on the basis of the following criteria:

1. No histologic evidence of neoplasm other than seminoma either in the primary tumor, or in any biopsied metastasis, or at autopsy if performed.
2. At least one objective criterion for evaluation of chemotherapeutic effect present and not made unevaluable by concomitant radiotherapy.
3. Chemotherapy and patient survival judged sufficient to permit evaluation of potential response.

In spite of the restriction imposed by these criteria the composition of the patients was heterogenous relative to such variables as age, duration of disease, sites of metastases, and details of radiotherapy and/or chemotherapy.

## RESULTS

The 23 patients selected for analysis included one 27-year-old female with a primary mediastinal seminoma and 22 males, 18 with a primary tumor in the testis, and 4 with an apparently primary tumor in the mediastinum. The ages of the male patients ranged from 20 to 52 years with an average of 33 years and a median of 32 years. There were no age differences in patients with primary testicular or mediastinal tumors. The duration of the disease from the first symptom of tumor to the first chemotherapy varied from less than 1 month to 33 months with the average interval less than 8 months and a median interval of 4 months.

Of the 23 patients 21 had stage III neoplasm at the time of chemotherapy. This is defined as a tumor beyond the retroperitoneal lymph nodes in patients with a primary in the testis and beyond the supraclavicular lymph nodes in those with a primary in the mediastinum. Two patients had Stage II neoplasm: one (#60 15 98) with a primary testis tumor had only a huge retroperitoneal mass which failed to respond objectively to irradiation (3600 rad in 3+ weeks) or to successive trials of chlorambucil, actinomycin D, L-sarcolysin, and mithramycin; the other patient (#60 18 57) had only pelvic and retroperitoneal masses and responded to combined chemotherapy and irradiation.

Of the 23 patients only 3 never received any irradiation. All 3 had Stage III disease: 2 are free of evidence of neoplasm following chemotherapy and 1 died at 4 months of progressive disease while receiving 4-fluoro-orotic acid. Twenty patients received radiation therapy before, during, and/or after chemotherapy, often to multiple sites and sometimes with repeated courses to the same site.

The chemotherapeutic agents utilized and the responses achieved are shown in Table 1. Over the 35 years spanned by this experience there have been important changes: (1) in drugs and drug regimens, (2) in criteria for assessment of therapeutic response, (3) in chemotherapeutic expertise derived from cumulative clinical experience. These considerations and the other uncontrolled variables in this patient group make conclusions from these data necessarily tentative. There were 34 trials in 23 patients. Judgments regarding the adequacy, both in terms of dose and duration, of drug trials were liberal; many of the trials would be considered inadequate by modern standards. However, the fact, for example, that in one patient (##13 30 67) a single dose of 0.4 mg/kg $HN_2$ produced a rapid, complete, and sustained remission of pulmonary metastases or, that chlorambucil 0.15 mg/kg orally daily for 4 weeks on - 4 weeks off, serially, was responsible for complete and sustained remission in two patients (##70 44 87, ##61 62 87) without manifestations of drug toxicity helps to justify a liberal interpretation of the adequacy of the drug trials. All responses were judged on the basis of objective parameters (measurable tumor) but not all would meet current criteria for qualification as favorable responses. It is apparent (Table 1) that the greatest number of trials and all of the favorable responses occurred with alkylating agents or with drug combinations that included alkylating agents.

In recognition of deficiencies in the data base which make a more sophisticated analysis impossible, results have been categorized into four broad groups:

1. No response (N): Twelve patients had no evident benefit from chemotherapy. Survival from onset of disease until death averaged less than 2 years in this group.

2. Partial response (P): Incomplete and/or unsustained remissions in whole or in part as a consequence of chemotherapy occurred in six patients. Although survival from first evidence of neoplasm until death in these six patients was approximately 1 year greater than in the no-response group, inspection of the records suggests that this was a consequence of the longer natural history of the tumors in this group rather than of chemotherapy.

3. P/C response (P/C): Complete and sustained remissions clearly attributable in part to chemotherapy and in part to irradiation occurred in two patients. In one patient (##13 30 67) bilateral pulmonary metastases responded completely to a single dose of $HN_2$ (0.4 mg/kg i.v.) while adjunctive irradiation was utilized to treat bone metastases in the spine; this patient was apparently well when last seen more than

Table 1. Chemotherapy in patients with seminoma

| Drug(2) utilized | Response | | | | |
|---|---|---|---|---|---|
| | N | P | P/C | C | Total Trials |
| Clb | 5 | 2 | 0 | 2 | 9 |
| $HN_2$ | 1 | 1 | 1 | 0 | 3 |
| Ctx | 2 | 1 | 0 | 0 | 3 |
| L-sarcolysin | 2 | 0 | 0 | 0 | 2 |
| Thiotepa | 1 | 0 | 0 | 0 | 1 |
| Phosphonitrile | 1 | 0 | 0 | 0 | 1 |
| 5-fluoro-orotic acid | 1 | 0 | 0 | 0 | 1 |
| Mithramycin | 1 | 0 | 0 | 0 | 1 |
| Vinblastine | 2 | 0 | 0 | 0 | 2 |
| Ctx + Cib | 0 | 1 | 0 | 0 | 1 |
| Ctx + Vcr | 1 | 0 | 0 | 0 | 1 |
| Act. D + Clb | 2 | 0 | 1 | 1 | 4 |
| Act. D + Mtx + Clb | 2 | 1 | 0 | 0 | 3 |
| 5 FU + Ctx + Vcr + Mtx | 0 | 1 | 0 | 0 | 1 |
| 5 FU + Clb + Vcr + Mtx | 1 | 0 | 0 | 0 | 1 |
| | 22 | 7 | 2 | 3 | 34[a] |

N = No response; P = Partial regression; P/C = Complete regressions at least partially due to chemotherapy; C = Complete regression due solely to chemotherapy.
[a] Some patients had more than one trial
Clb. = Chlorambucil; $HN_2$ = Nitrogen mustard; Ctx = Cyclophosphamide; Vcr = Vincristine; Mtx = Methotrexate; Thiotepa = Triethylene-thiophoshoramide.

9 years after chemotherapy and irradiation. The other patient (# 60 18 57) with metastatic tumor in the retroperitoneal and pelvic lymph nodes demonstrated tumor regression with actinomycin D (1 mg i.v. x 4 days given once only) plus chlorambucil (10 mg daily p.o., 3 weeks on - 1 week off, serially) and was then given adjunct irradiation to the retroperitoneum and mediastinum; he was maintained on chlorambucil for 3 1/2 years and remains free of evidence of neoplasm more than 4 years after all therapy was discontinued.

Complete response (C): Three patients had complete remissions attributable solely to chemotherapy. One patient (#70 44 87) had lymphangiographic evidence of retroperitoneal lymph node involvement, a mediastinal mass, and a group of supraclavicular lymph nodes which biopsy proved to contain seminoma. He never received irradiation and the neoplasm regressed on chlorambucil 12 mg daily p.o., 30 days on - 30 days off (partial regression after one course, complete regression after the second course). This regimen was continued for 3 1/2 years and he remains free of neoplasm more than 2 years after all treatment was discontinued.

A second patient (#61 62 87) received retroperitoneal irradiation for stage I testicular seminoma and less than 1 year later developed a mediastinal mass which regressed completely (within 2 months) on chlorambucil 10 mg daily p.o., 30 days on - 30 days off for 2 years, and 30 days on - 60 days off for 3 additional years. He remains free of tumor less than 1 year off all treatment.

The third patient (#24 77 56) had a primary mediastinal seminoma with pulmonary, axillary lymph node, and cervical lymph node metastases. He was treated initially with actinomycin D and chlorambucil (actinomycin D 0.75 mg i.v. daily x 5 days followed 10 days later by 25 days of chlorambucil 10 mg orally daily in conjunction with three 5-day courses of 0.5 mg actinomycin D daily i.v.) Maintenance was with chlorambucil 10 mg p.o., daily, 21-28 days on - 2 months off, for approximately 5 years and with chlorambucil 10 mg p.o. daily, 1 month on - 3 months off, for 4 additional years. Regression was first recorded at 6 weeks and was considered complete 4 months following initiation of chemotherapy. He never received irradiation. He remains free of neoplasm 2 years off all treatment.

Perusal of the records relative to patient age, duration of neoplasm, and site of primary tumor revealed no features that distinguished those destined for successful treatment from those destined to be failures.

Not unexpectedly, patients who received chemotherapy after extensive prior irradiation sometimes demonstrated increased hematologic toxicity to chemotherapy and, more or less independently of the latter, fewer favorable responses to chemotherapy.

Although this experience included illustrations of tumor which responded to chemotherapy but not to irradiation, or to irradiation but not to chemotherapy, or to both, or to neither, quantitative data on these various events is not meaningful.

## DISCUSSION

The image of seminoma as a relatively slow-growing, remarkably radiosensitive and radiocurable tumor is tarnished by the aggressive and often rapid course, and the radioresistance and chemotherapeutic resistance in most of the patients here reviewed. On the other hand, this group of patients was adversely selected since, in general, they presented failures of conventional, usually successful treatment. Although patients with biopsy-proved tumor other than seminoma were excluded from this review, few of this group of patients known to have died were subjected to autopsy. DIXON and MOORE (3) found non-seminomatous metastases in 35% of their 23 patients with seminoma. MAIER et al. (6) concluded that the overall incidence of metastasis other than seminoma in patients with apparently pure testicular seminoma is 7%.

A multitude of uncontrolled variables makes hazardous too literal an interpretation of the data. However, the overall response rate of almost 50% (11/23) and the sustained complete remission rate of 13% (3/23) attained with chemotherapy, indicate a role for chemotherapy, at least in selected patients with seminoma. It should be pointed out that the three complete responses achieved with chemotherapy alone might have been achieved with radiotherapy alone. (One patient had received retroperitoneal irradiation only and subsequently developed mediastinal disease which responded to chemotherapy and the other two received no irradiation whatsoever.) It is of parenthetic interest that the response rates achieved with the chemotherapy of seminoma are not dissimilar to those achieved in germinal tumors other than seminoma with a variety of chemotherapeutic agents.

CHEBOTAREVA (2) reported 38 remissions among 42 patients with seminoma treated with L-sarcolysin, 19 of whom were "alive and fit for work 2 to 6 years after the treatment was instituted." Selection factors may have contributed to these good results. Although the precise duration of therapy is not specified for CHEBOTAREVA's patients it may be inferred that treatment intervals ranged from about 6 weeks to about 12 weeks with a total dose of 200-250 mg L-sarcolysin administered at a rate of 25-50 mg per week.

The present and published experiences (7) justify little in the way of categorical recommendations regarding drug(s) or drug(s) regimen. Alkylating agents have had the greatest number of trials and have produced the greatest number of responses but limitations in the data prevent definitive conclusions and certainly many other agents warrant trials.

The three complete responses attributable solely to chemotherapy were in favorably selected patients who may be more representative of the vast majority of seminomas on which our favorable image of this neoplasm is based than of the adversely selected group of patients who make up the majority of the cases here reviewed. In any event, these three cases clearly indicate the sometimes remarkable sensitivity of this neoplasm to alkylating agents and raise legitimate questions regarding the place of adjunct chemotherapy with alkylating agents in the "general population" of patients with seminoma.

Conventinal treatment by orchiectomy and irradiation produces 90% or better control in stage I seminoma, 50-80% control in stage II seminoma, and 20-50% control in stage III seminoma (7). This demonstrated failure of orchiectomy and irradiation invariable to control seminoma; the responsiveness of such tumors to chemotherapy, and the generally reversible and noncumulative (usually) effects of chemotherapeutic agents on bone marrow and other organs in contrast to the generally cumulative effects of irradiation provide a logical basis for systematic exploration of adjunct chemotherapy, at least in patients with stage II or stage III seminoma.

## SUMMARY AND CONCLUSION

1. Seminoma may occasionally be a rapidly growing, aggressive, radioresistant, and chemotherapy-resistant tumor.
2. Alkylating agents have had the greatest number of trials and have produced the best response rates in the management of seminoma, but a wide range of other agents warrants trials.
3. Adjunct chemotherapy is a logical consideration in patients with stage II and stage III seminoma.

## REFERENCES


1. Carter, S.K., Wasserman, T.H.: The chemotherapy of urologic cancer. Cancer (Philad.) 36, 729-747 (1975)
2. Chebotareva, L.I.: Late results of sarcolysin therapy in tumours of the testes. Acta Un. int. Cancr. 20, 380-381 (1964)
3. Dixon, F.J., Moore, R.A.: Testicular tumors: A clinicopathologic study. Cancer (Philad.) 6, 427-439 (1953)
4. Golbey, R.B.: The place of chemotherapy in the treatment of testicular tumors. J. Amer. med. Ass 213, 101-106 (1970)
5. Mackenzie, A.R.: The chemotherapy of metastatic seminoma. J. Urol. (Baltimore) 96, 790-793 (1966)
6. Maier, J.G., Mittemeyer, B.T., Sulak, M.: Treatment and prognosis in seminoma of the testis. J. Urol. (Baltimore) 90, 72-78 (1968)
7. Whitmore, W.F.: Germinal testis tumors in adults. In: 7th National Cancer Conf. Proc. (eds.) R.L. Clack, W.M. Stanley. Philadelphia: Lippincott, 1973, pp. 793-801
8. Whitmore, W.M.: 5ième Rapport: La chimiotherapie dans les tumeurs du testicle. Proc. 16th Congr. int. Soc. Urol. Brussels, Belgium, July 1973, pp. 485-499

# Radiotherapy in the Management of Testicular Tumors

H. F. HOPE-STONE

The old classification of seminoma and teratoma is too crude to allow either good retrospective or prospective survey, particularly in the teratomatous group. When the British Testicular Tumor Panel Registry (COLLINS and PUGH, 1964 (4)) was formed, its classification seemed more useful than that of DIXON and MOORE of America (5). The former classification divides histologically the groups into two - the seminomas, which are straightforward, and the teratomas (Table 1). It will be seen that the MTIA and MTA groups compare closely to the teratoma-carcinoma (group IV of DIXON and MOORE). More recently PUGH and COLLINS (10) modified the teratoma into MTI (the old MTIA) and MTU (the old MTIB and MTA).

Table 1. Comparison of British and United States classifications of commoner testicular tumors

| TTPR | | | DIXON and MOORE | |
|---|---|---|---|---|
| Seminoma | | | Seminoma pure | Group I |
| Teratoma | | | | |
| Teratoma differentiated | (TD) | | Teratoma pure or with seminoma | Group III |
| Malignant teratoma | | | | |
| Intermediate | | | | |
| - | MTIA | | Teratoma pure or mixed | Group IV |
| - | MTIB | MTU[a] | | |
| Malignant teratoma anaplastic | (MTA) | | Embryonal carcinoma | Group II |
| Malignant teratoma trophoblastic | (MTT) | | Chorion carcinoma | Group II |
| Combined tumor | | | | |
| Seminoma and teratoma | | | Teratoma with seminoma seminoma | Group III |

From BLANDY et al. (1).
[a]Malignant teratoma undifferentiated (8).

STAGING

A decision on how to treat the patient depends largely on the degree of spread when the tumor is first seen, and acceptance of the theory of occult metastases. Certain investigations are mandatory - a simple chest X-ray may show metastases, but if there is any doubt hilar and mediastinal tomography should be performed. If these are negative, one might have to consider whole lung tomography. Figure 1a shows a patient thought to have a solitary metastasis, but multiple metastases are seen on the whole lung tomograms (Fig. 1b). Lymphangiography is essential, but may be associated both with false positives and false negatives.

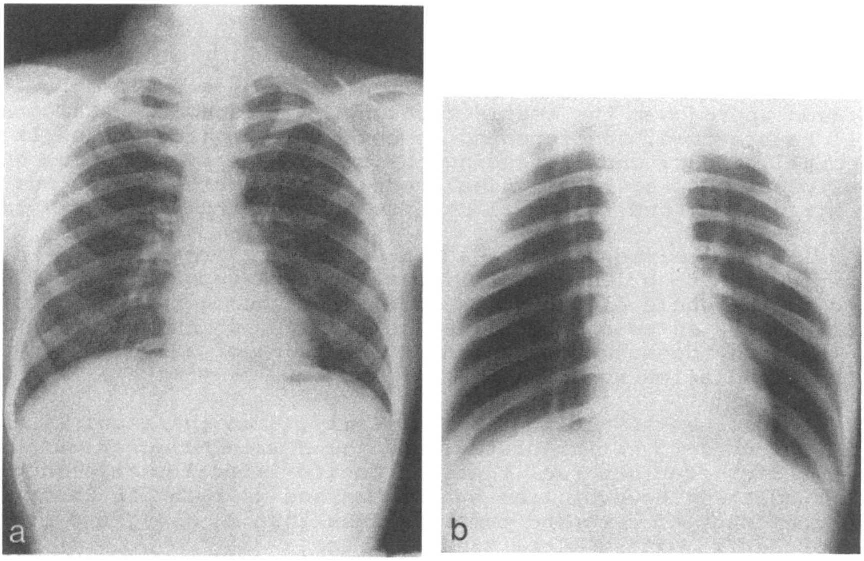

*Fig. 1. (a) Chest X-ray? solitary metastasis; (b) Tomograms showing multiple lesions*

In doubtful cases tomography of the lymphangiogram may be useful. If the lymphangiogram is negative, or there is failure to fill the nodes, then intra-venous pyelography (IVP) alone may be useful, as this may show quite marked deviation of the ureters. Sometimes both these investigations are negative, and if one is still suspicious then inferior cavography can be of value.

With the above information, combined with palpation of the abdomen under anesthesia, staging can be carried out. At the London Hospital we have used three main groups (1):

Stage I: No definite pelvic or para-aortic nodes can be demonstrated, but occult metastases are presumed to be present at these sites.

Stage II: Definite para-aortic or pelvic lymph nodes present; no known tumor is present above the diaphragm, but occult metastases are presumed to be present in the mediastinal or supra-clavicular nodes.

Stage IIIA: Supraclavicular and/or mediastinal nodes are present, and occult metastases are presumed to be present below the diaphragm.
B - Intra-pulmonary metastases are present, and occult metastases are presumed to be present in the nodes above and below the diaphragm.
C - Both supraclavicular nodes and intra-pulmonary metastases are present, and occult metastases are presumed to be present in the lymph nodes bolow the diaphragm.

The whole irradiation policy is therefore based on the presence of occult metastases. One should remember that prior to 1940, when irradiation was not generally used in the treatment of seminoma, the 5-year survival rate was less than 40%, whereas now it is over 90%, and this is surely due to eliminating these occult metastases by such treatment.

## TREATMENT POLICY

Orchiectomy through inguinal incision is first carried out. If the surgeon approaches the testis through the scrotum the tunica albuginea will be breached, thus opening up both the lymphatic channels to the inguinal glands, and increasing the chances of rapid venous spread. If the former occurs, the inguinal nodes and opposite testis must both be irradiated, and this will lead to unnecessary permanent sterility.

Stage I. The pelvic and para-aortic nodes are irradiated by one inverted T-shaped field, using a pair of parallel and opposed fields. We aim to give the whole of the lymph node area a homogeneous dose of irradiation. An IVP is used to outline the kidneys, which must be protected so that they do not receive a dose in excess of 2250 rad, in order to avoid irradiation nephritis (8).

If the scrotum was not incised initially, then the inguinal glands will not need to be irradiated, and the remaining gonad can be shielded. Some radiotherapists feel that the contra-lateral testis should always be irradiated. However, the author can see no point in this, since the incidence of a second tumor is less than 2% (11), and even if it does occur it can still be treated later.

At the London Hospital we have two patients who have developed tumors in the remaining testis 5 and 8 years after orchiectomy and irradiation: both are alive and well 12 and 20 years later, after a further full course of irradiation. It goes without saying that if the contra-lateral testis is not irradiated, fertility will be preserved. Megavoltage irradiation is to be preferred, since it is faster and easier for the patient, the skin reaction is reduced, accuracy of the set-up is guaranteed, and one large field can be used both anteriorly and posteriorly, thus avoiding the danger of over- or under-dosage at junction points. We give daily fractionations, treating 5 days a week for 4 weeks. The dose aimed at is 3000 rad for seminoma, 4000 rad for teratoma, and 4500 rad for the trophoblastic teratoma.

Stage II. Here the known involved para-aortic and pelvic nodes are treated first in the way already described. After a month's gap, to allow a rest and bone marrow regeneration, prophylactic irradiation is given to the mediastinum and supra-clavicular nodes, using a pair of parallel and opposed, standard T-shaped fields. The lungs are shielded, and care must be taken to prevent an overlap at the junction of the upper and lower fields, in order to eliminate the risk of overdosage to the spinal cord. The dose and fractionation is the same for both treatment areas.

Stage III A. Here the mediastinal and supraclavicular nodes are treated first, in the manner just described. Subsequently prophylactic irradiation is given to the pelvis and para-aortic nodes.

Stage III B and C. Here the problem is more difficult, as the whole of both lungs need to be irradiated, as well as the supraclavicular nodes. Since the tolerance level of the lung so treated is in the region of 2250-2500 rad, it is only in the relatively radiosensitive seminoma that this technique can be applied. Subsequently in this histological group prophylactic irradiation below the diaphragm should be given. Occasionally an MTIA teratoma may respond to this dose (Fig. 2a, b), but this is unusual, and other methods would need to be considered.

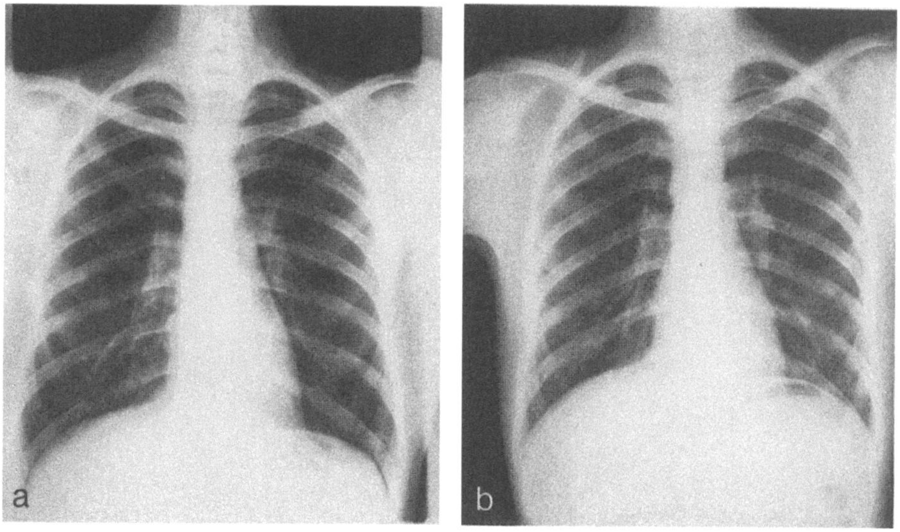


*Fig. 2. (a) Chest X-ray - MTIA tumor, with lung metastases; (b) Chest X-ray 3 years later, after 2250 rad, whole lung irradiation*

Radiation pneumonitis is the main problem with the above treatment, and can occur at even lower doses than we would wish to give. It presents with a dry cough, dyspnoea, and chest pain, but no fever. Radiologically there is a typical hilar flare (Fig. 3a), which may eventually settle down, or produce radiation fibrosis (Fig. 3b). This may also clear up in the next few months (Fig. 3c). Treatment may be with prednisone 10 mg t.d.s., combined with antibiotics (6) during the acute phase, but if fibrosis occurs then no treatment would be of any value.

## EFFECTS ON THE PATIENT

These should be relatively minimal. Nausea might occur, but this can be well controlled by Maxalon or Torecan, and a lot of reassurance - and it is as well to remember that a great deal of the nausea is probably psychologically induced; indeed, this was shown many years ago, in a controlloed trial, where patients treated for carcinoma of the

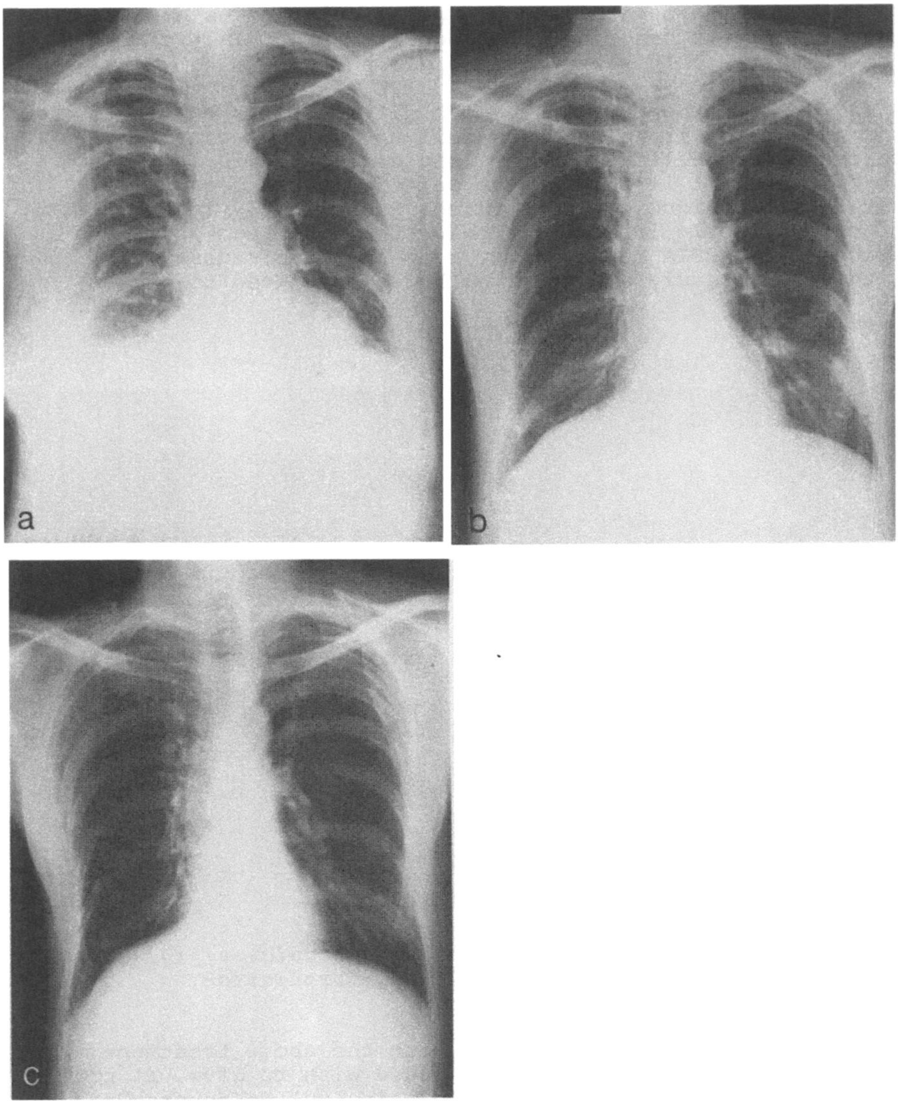

*Fig. 3. (a) Radiation pneumonitis - hilar flare; (b) Radiation fibrosis; (c) Clearing of lung fields 6 months later*

breast were given either a placebo, a standard anti-emetic drug, or the very latest drug - the very latest drug produced a 60% reduction in the nausea, the standard drug 50% and the placebo about 48%. Patients will certainly feel tired as treatment progresses, but indeed many of the author's patients continue to work during treatment. They are all treated as out-patients, as there is no real reason why they need to be in hospital. Diarrhoea may occur, but this can easily be controlled by mist, kaolin and morphine.

Bone marrow depression can be a problem. If the white cell count falls below 3000 then one might wish to stop treatment for a day or two; similarly, if the platelet count drops below 100,000. In some instances in the latter case an intra-muscular injection of 50 mg Decca Durabolin might improve the platelet count. Very rarely is it necessary to reduce the irradiated volume and treat only the para-aortic nodes, leaving the pelvic nodes to be irradiated at a later date.

Spinal cord damage should not occur if the known tolerance level of 4500 rad is not exceeded (2). The author has not seen any of the other major complications of irradiation such as small bowel fibrosis or stomach ulceration, both of which are reported in the American and Swedish literature. However, they were always associated with excessively high doses (greater than 5000 rad), and such a dose does not, in the opinion of the author, improve the cure rate, and yet it is associated with unnecessary morbidity.

## GONADS

The contra-lateral testis can be protected by both direct and indirect shielding. The measured gonad dose in the London Hospital series was between 50 and 150 rad. This of course will not cause long-term infertility, but it might do so in the short term. Thus the author warns patients not to attempt to start a family for about 12 months after treatment.

The genetic hazard is probably not of great importance, since the MRC report of 1956 (9) suggests that a dose of 50-200 rad to the remaining testis would add only 0.1% to the present level of 7-8% genetic mutation at the first generation.

## PALLIATION

Chemotherapy will play the major role, but the value of irradiation should not be forgotten. Thus, if local control of fungating tumor cannot be obtained, or if spinal cord, mediastinal or oesophageal compression occurs, irradiation can produce very rapid and useful relief of symptoms, and in the latter cases may even be life saving.

## CONCLUSION

Seminoma do well at all stages, and irradiation is accepted as the treatment of choice (Table 2).

The best treatment technique for teratoma, however, has for many years been controversial, particularly between the American and the British surgeons and radiotherapists. In 1963 the London Hospital series was carefully examined, and the cases classified pathologically, according to the DIXON and MOORE system. Two similar groups of teratoma were compared, one treated with radiotherapy alone and the other by radical node dissection. The results showed no statistical differences (7). Since surgery carried with it a much higher morbility rate (including impotence) and a possibly higher mortality rate, and since indeed

Table 2. Results in seminoma - The London Hospital, 1950-1972

| Clinical stage | No. of cases available | No. of survivors at years | 5-Year survivors (%) |
|---|---|---|---|
| 1 | 90 | 80 | 89 |
| 2 | 25 | 15 | 43 |
| 3 | 16 | 1 | 7 |

some of the so-called surgical cases were also given irradiation, the author and his colleagues could see no real evidence at all that radical surgery was of any real value.

Recently the London Hospital series has been brough up to date (3), and one very interesting point seems to emerge: Not only do the whole group of seminoma patients continue to do well but some of the teratoma (the MTIA) group are also doing very well. Thus the crude survival rate for stage I seminoma is 86%, and that of the MTIA group is 89%. More recently, we have compared all the teratoma groups, and the same trend continues (Table 3).

Thus the MTI teratomas, which correspond to DIXON and MOORE's group IV carcinoma, have a very high survival rate when treated by irradiation alone, and therefore there seems no place at all for radical node dissection. The latter does not improve the survival rate, and carries with it the risk of surgical morbility, and probability of impotence (so dreaded by patients of all ages).

It is only in the MTU group that one should consider other forms of treatment. It is highly unlikely that radical surgery would be of much value in the management of these patients, as the majority of the tumors have a tendency to hematogenous dissemination rather than lymphatic spread, and they show a high degree of anaplasticity. Removal of lymph nodes is unlikely to be of any value; indeed, one must look further to both the chemotherapists and immunologists in the management of this dangerous group of tumors.

Table 3. Results in malignant teratoma - Stage I (The London Hospital, 1950-1974)

| | No. of cases available | No. of survivors at 5 years | 5-Year survivors (%) |
|---|---|---|---|
| MTIA | 48 | 42 | 93[a] |
| MTU | 35 | 19 | 42 |

[a] 97% if two emigrants and one death from coronary thrombosis are excluded.

REFERENCES


1. Blandy, J.P., Hope-Stone, H.F., Dayan, A.D.: Tumours of the Testicles. London: Heinemann 1970
2. Boden, G.: Radiation myelitis of brain stem. J. Fac. Radiol. 2, 79-94 (1950)
3. Chapman, R.H., Blandy, J.P., Hope-Stone, H.F., Pollock, D., Dayan, A.D.: Identification of a favorable group of teratoma. Proc. Roy. Soc. Med. 66, 1045-1047 (1973)
4. Collins, D.H., Pugh, R.C.B.: Classification and frequency of testicular tumors. Brit. J. Urol. 36, Supplement 1-11 (1964)
5. Dixon, F.J., Moore, R.A.: Tumors of the Male Sex Organs. In: Atlas of Tumor Pathology. Washington, D.C.: Armed Forces Institute of Pathology 1962. VIII/31 B, 32
6. Hope-Stone, H.F.: Radiotherapy in the management of carcinoma of the lung. Brit. J. Dis. Chest 61, 57-69 (1967)
7. Hope-Stone, H.F., Blandy, J.P., Dayan, A.D.: Treatment of tumors of the testis. Brit. med. J. 1963/I, 984-989
8. Kunkler, P.B., Farr, R.F., Luxton, R.W.: The limit of renal tolerance to X-rays. Brit. med. J. Radiol. 25, 190-221 (1952)
9. Medical Research Council: Hazards to man of nuclear and allied radiations. M.R.C., H.M.S.O., 1956
10. Pugh, R.C.B.: The pathology of testicular tumors. Presented at Institute of Urology Seminar, London 1973
11. Whittle, R.J.M.: Tumors of the testicle. Brit. J. Radiol. 30, 7-12 (1957)

# VI. Subject Index

44 Special Topics in Carcinogenesis. Edited by E. GRUNDMANN (Symposium).
45 KOLDOVSKÝ, P.: Carcinoembryonic Antigens.
46 Diagnosis and Therapy of Malignant Lymphoma. Edited by K. MUSSHOFF (Symposium).
47 Investigation and Stimulation of Immunity in Cancer Patients. Edited by G. MATHÉ and R. WEINER (Symposium).
48 Platinum Coordination Complexes in Cancer Chemotherapy. Edited by T. A. CONNORS and J. J. ROBERTS (Symposium).
49 Complications of Cancer Chemotherapy. Edited by G. MATHÉ and R. K. OLDHAM (Symposium).
50 Cancer Registry. Edited by E. GRUNDMANN and E. PEDERSEN (Symposium).
51 Gliomas. Current Concepts in Biology, Diagnosis and Therapy. Edited by J. HEKMATPANAH (Symposium).
52 The Ambivalence of Cytostatic Therapy. Edited by E. GRUNDMANN and R. GROSS (Symposium).
53 A. CLARYSSE, Y. KENIS, and G. MATHÉ: Cancer Chemotherapy.
54 Malignant Bone Tumors. Edited by E. GRUNDMANN.
55 MATHÉ, G.: Cancer Active Immunotherapy, Immunoprophylaxis, and Immunorestoration.
56 Lymphocytes, Macrophages, and Cancer. Edited by G. MATHÉ, I. FLORENTIN, and M.-C. SIMMLER (Symposium).
57 Breast Cancer: A Multidisciplinary Approach. Edited by G. ST. ARNEAULT, P. BAND, and L. ISRAËL (Symposium).
58 B. S. SCHOENBERG: Multiple Primary Malignant Neoplasms.
59 Selective Heat Sensitivity of Cancer Cells. Edited by A. ROSSI-FANELLI, R. CAVALIERE, B. MONDOVI, and G. MORICCA.
60 Tumors of the Male Genital System. Edited by E. GRUNDMANN and W. VAHLENSIECK (Symposium).

Special Supplement: Biology of Amphibian Tumors. Edited by M. MIZELL.

MIX
Papier aus verantwortungsvollen Quellen
Paper from responsible sources
FSC® C105338

If you have any concerns about our products,
you can contact us on
**ProductSafety@springernature.com**

In case Publisher is established outside the EU,
the EU authorized representative is:
**Springer Nature Customer Service Center GmbH**
**Europaplatz 3, 69115 Heidelberg, Germany**

Printed by Libri Plureos GmbH
in Hamburg, Germany